MANAGEMENT OF PEDIATRIC OBESITY AND DIABETES

NUTRITION ◊ AND ◊ HEALTH

Adrianne Bendich, PhD, FACN, SERIES EDITOR

For other titles published in this series, go to
www.springer.com/series/7659

Management of Pediatric Obesity and Diabetes

Edited by

Robert J. Ferry, Jr., MD, FAAP

Le Bonheur Children's Hospital
The University of Tennessee Health Science Center
St. Jude Children's Research Hospital
Regional Medical Center of Memphis
Memphis, TN, USA

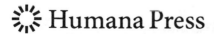 Humana Press

Editor
Robert J. Ferry, Jr., MD, FAAP
Le Bonheur Children's Hospital
UT Health Science Center at Memphis
Division of Pediatric Endocrinology and Metabolism
50 North Dunlap Street
Memphis, Tennessee 38103
USA
bob@uthsc.edu

ISBN: 978-1-60327-255-1   e-ISBN: 978-1-60327-256-8
DOI: 10.1007/978-1-60327-256-8
Springer New York Dordrecht Heidelberg London

Library of Congress Control Number: 2011925845

Printed on acid-free paper

Humana Press is part of Springer Science+Business Media (www.springer.com)

Dedication

For Justin and his friends, with his parents' deepest hopes that their futures will be more peaceful and healthier

Management of Pediatric Obesity and Diabetes

The twin epidemics of obesity and type 2 diabetes mellitus (T2DM) continue to affect an ever increasing number of children, adolescents, and young adults. The objective of this book is to provide you with practical, comprehensive, and contemporary approaches to the pediatric patient at risk for obesity, T2DM, and related conditions. This is the first guide to integrate basic and clinical sciences for practical approaches to the obese or diabetic pediatric patient. The chapters are sufficiently independent and concise that you can rapidly identify tools for the problem at hand by skipping to a topic of interest. To tailor this volume for a diverse audience of trainees, healthcare professionals, and policy makers, we have focused each chapter on a key clinical issue or mechanism of disease, as outlined by Dr. Bendich on her Series Editor Page.

This volume provides you with clinical paradigms for diagnosis and management of pediatric T2DM and related conditions, while succinctly describing state-of-the-art basic and clinical sciences underlying these problems. You can consider multilevel interventions to prevent and treat obesity and T2DM which are based upon community- and school-based programs (Chapter 6), nutrition (Chapter 11), physical activity (Chapter 7), behavioral modification (Chapter 8), pharmacologic agents (Chapters 12-14), or bariatric surgery (Chapter 9). Although this book focuses on the significant clinical aspects of these epidemics in developed countries, various authors discuss aspects of these problems across all pediatric populations. Finally, this edition reviews secondary causes of T2DM (Chapter 16) and maturity onset diabetes of the young (MODY), a major subset of diabetic patients for whom an explosion of recent research has improved diagnosis and care (Chapter 15).

Over the past three years' gestation for this "baby", I have been blessed not only by all the authors—who gave so generously of their ingenuity and time—but also by outstanding editorial support at Springer as well as the tireless efforts of all pediatric house staff and my faculty colleagues at The University of Tennessee, whose combined support created some time for this editor to complete his tasks. In particular, I wish to thank the following individuals at Springer: Dr. Adrianne Bendich as my muse for her initial invitation to assemble such a volume and her unflagging support; Richard Hruska for his patient encouragement at each reset deadline; and Amanda Quinn and Ian Hayes whose attention to detail ultimately made it easier on the readers' eyes. While each author has diligently researched his/her work, this text is no substitute for an individualized plan of care from the appropriately licensed practitioner(s). If we are fortunate enough to earn the privilege of a second edition, it should discuss telehealth-based interventions (unfortunately omitted here).

This text can be utilized to teach dietary, nursing, graduate, medical, dental, and allied health trainees about staggering problems in pediatrics. We hope this work benefits you by collecting disseminated knowledge in a convenient place. Above all, we hope our ongoing work improves healthcare for all children, adolescents, and young adults. Do find inspiration in the unanswered questions which remain before you as a child advocate.

Robert J. Ferry, Jr., MD, FAAP
Professor of Pediatrics and Chief
Division of Pediatric Endocrinology and Metabolism
Department of Pediatrics
University of Tennessee Health
Science Center at Memphis

Medical Director for Endocrinology
Le Bonheur Children's Hospital
Regional Medical Center of Memphis
St. Jude Children's Research Hospital

Series Editor Page

The great success of the Nutrition and Health Series is the result of the consistent overriding mission of providing health professionals with texts that are essential because each includes: (1) a synthesis of the state of the science, (2) timely, in-depth reviews by the leading researchers in their respective fields, (3) extensive, up-to-date fully annotated reference lists, (4) a detailed index, (5) relevant tables and figures, (6) identification of paradigm shifts and the consequences, (7) virtually no overlap of information between chapters, but targeted, interchapter referrals, (8) suggestions of areas for future research and (9) balanced, data-driven answers to patient as well as health professionals questions which are based upon the totality of evidence rather than the findings of any single study.

The Series volumes are not the outcome of a symposium. Rather, each editor has the potential to examine a chosen area with a broad perspective, both in subject matter as well as in the choice of chapter authors. The editor(s), whose training(s) is (are) both research and practice oriented, have the opportunity to develop a primary objective for their book, define the scope and focus, and then invite the leading authorities to be part of their initiative. The authors are encouraged to provide an overview of the field, discuss their own research and relate the research findings to potential human health consequences. Since each book is developed de novo, the chapters are coordinated so that the resulting volume imparts greater knowledge than the sum of the information contained in the individual chapters.

Management of Pediatric Obesity and Diabetes, edited by Robert J. Ferry, Jr., M.D., clearly exemplifies the goals of the Nutrition and Health Series. Dr. Ferry is an internationally recognized leader in the field of pediatric obesity, currently serving as Professor of Pediatrics and Chief of the Division of Pediatric Endocrinology and Metabolism in the Department of Pediatrics at the University of Tennessee Health Science Center in Memphis, Tennessee. He is also currently serving as the Medical Director for Endocrine Services at Le Bonheur Children's Hospital, St. Jude Children's Research Hospital, and the Regional Medical Center of Memphis. Dr. Ferry has published numerous research articles and currently serves as a member of the Editorial Board of *eMedicineHealth.com*. Dr. Ferry has deployed multiple times as a field, battalion, and brigade surgeon across the US, Italy, and Iraq; he currently holds the rank of lieutenant colonel in the Medical Corps of the U.S. Army National Guard.

Dr. Ferry has organized this volume in three comprehensive sections that provide an in-depth overview of both pediatric obesity and diabetes. The first section includes chapters that define pediatric obesity and diabetes, followed by 12 clinical chapters in these two critical areas. Thus, the first chapters are logically organized to provide the reader with a basic under-standing of the interactions between the latest findings of the role of genet-ics in obesity and the importance of the fetal environment for expression of the genotype based upon the phenotypic characteristics. The genetics of obesity is complex and no single gene will be identified as predictive of most obesity. Studies in monozygotic and dizygotic twins are described in the genetics chapter. Extensive lists of the major genetic loci are included. Discussions of the fat mass and obesity associated gene (*FTO*), leptin and insulin genes, and other relevant genes are reviewed as well. The second chapter outlines the major effectors associated with the fetal origins of obesity. These include maternal obesity, high fat diets of the mother, maternal nutri-ent deprivation (especially micronutrients), smoking, gestational diabetes, and preeclampsia. Research in the fetal origins of obesity has used primates and the chapter includes extensive tables on genetic factors and pathways that affect obesity in baboons. The pancreatic beta-cell is responsible for insulin secretion and the size and number of beta-cells is directly related to childhood obesity and diabetes. Clear, informative explanations concerning the mechanisms that control beta-cells and the consequences of these fac-tors are provided in the next chapter. The final chapter in this section exam-ines the importance of environmental factors in the development of childhood diabetes and includes a detailed review of major epidemiological studies. The data from the National Longitudinal Study of Adolescent Health confirms the seriousness of the rapid rise in childhood obesity and documents the important role of race, ethnicity, and poverty in the current demographics of childhood obesity in the US. Information on the behavioral aspects of eating and the critical importance of the availability, types, and qualities of the fats in the diet is also included.

The second section on the clinical aspects of obesity contains six chapters that address obesity and its comorbidities, treatment options as well as pre-vention strategies. As an example, the chapter on cardiovascular conse-quences of obesity includes both physical as well as biochemical measurements that are used to assess the extent of disease. Additionally, practice opportuni-ties for risk reversal are described using data from major studies in adoles-cents including the Harvard Growth Study and the Bogalusa Heart Study.

Important tables that outline the criteria for assessing the metabolic syndrome in adolescents are included. Separate chapters review the programs that utilize physical activity and exercise approaches, behavioral approaches, and pharmacological approaches. These chapters emphasize the importance of family members, school environment, access to digital assistants and/or computers, and community resources (based on a discussion of 14 successful community-based programs implemented in countries around the world) as determinants of success in stemming the obesity epidemic in children. Detailed tables of studies that have had success are included; the pharmacological approach chapter contains 16 informative tables. Of great value is the inclusion of the unique chapter that describes in detail the surgical interventions available to treat obesity in children and adolescents. This chapter also includes a comprehensive review of the known consequences of surgery including the benefits as well as the risks.

The third section includes six chapters that examine the consequences and treatment of pediatric diabetes. We are reminded in the first chapter that currently, pediatric diabetes is not a nationally reportable disease and therefore the incidence and prevalence are not documented in the U.S. or in most other countries. However, it is clear from epidemiological studies that there has been a precipitous rise in newly diagnosed cases from 3 to 45% in the past 15 years. Although diagnostic criteria are not uniform globally, the most consistent criteria are well described in this chapter, which also includes descriptions of associated physical and biochemical changes from the nondiabetic to the diabetic child. The next chapter is of great value to the practicing physician and health professionals who care for diabetics using insulin. The chapter describes the importance of insulin pumps used for continuous infusion. Criteria for determining who are good candidates, and the management of the patient who uses the pump, are described in detail. The major acute adverse events in childhood Type 1 and which also may be seen in Type 2 childhood diabetes are discussed in the next chapter that describes the critical diagnosis of diabetic ketoacidosis and hyperosmolar nonketotic hyperglycemia. The chapter includes an in-depth description of the differential diagnosis and treatment including laboratory evaluation; flow diagrams and informative tables are included. Nutrition of the diabetic child is of critical importance, yet this is a rapidly developing field. There are recommendations from the American Diabetes Association that are based upon the beneficial effects seen in adults with the diabetes prevention program and also with the DASH diet (Dietary Approaches to Stop Hypertension). The last two chapters in the volume address the complexities of rarer forms of childhood diabetes and include a chapter devoted to maturity onset diabetes of youth (MODY) and a chapter on inherited genetic syndromes and secondary causes of obesity. The two chapters provide valuable information to the clinician and their team that can be very helpful in the diagnosis of young children with complex presentations that include overweight or obesity. Tabulations of diagnostic criteria and genetic syndromes as well as drugs that have been associated with increased weight are included.

This logical sequence of chapters provides the latest information on the current standards of practice for clinicians, related health professionals including the dietician, nurse, pharmacist, physical therapist, behaviorist, psychologist, and others involved in the team effort required for successful treatment of lipid disorders, cardiac and cerebrovascular diseases as well as conditions that adversely affect normal metabolic processes. This comprehensive volume also has great value for academicians involved in the education of graduate students and postdoctoral fellows, medical students, and allied health professionals who plan to interact with pediatric patients with lipid disorders, diabetes as well as those who are overweight or obese.

Cutting edge discussions of the roles of growth factors, hormones, cellular and nuclear receptors, adipose tissue, and all of the cells directly involved in fat metabolism are included in well-organized chapters that put the molecular aspects into clinical perspective. Of great importance, the editor has provided chapters that balance the most technical information with discussions of its importance for clients and patients as well as graduate and medical students, health professionals, and academicians.

There are important chapters that discuss the treatment of obesity, diabetes, and related comorbidities. These include an overview of current treatment options as well as a discussion of future treatments that are already in development. Critical to any weight reduction program is exercise, and there are comprehensive chapters on the role of physical activity, exercise, and nutrition in weight control. The importance of a team approach to the treatment of obesity as a chronic disease is extensively discussed in chapters on community, family and social interactions, lifestyles as well as behavioral modification in the treatment of obesity. Specific treatment modalities are reviewed in separate chapters on nutrition, pharmacotherapies, surgery, combination therapies, and the potential for behavioral interventions. Each of these chapters presents an objective evaluation of the treatment and identifies the positives and negatives that have been seen during clinical studies as well as cumulative data derived from clinical practice.

The volume contains over 100 detailed tables and figures that assist the reader in comprehending the complexities of obesity and diabetes in the pediatric population. The overriding goal of this volume is to provide the health professional with balanced documentation and awareness that their clients'/patients' metabolic conditions are complex states that transcend the simplistic view of just losing a few pounds. Hallmarks of the 16 chapters include bulleted key points at the beginning of each chapter, complete definitions of terms with the abbreviations fully defined for the reader and consistent use of terms between chapters. There are over 1,400 up-to-date references; all chapters include a conclusion to highlight major findings. The volume also contains a highly annotated index.

This important text provides practical, data-driven resources based upon the totality of the evidence to help the reader understand the basics, treatments, and preventive strategies that are involved in the care of obese and diabetic children as well as the potential for prevention of childhood obesity and diabetes. The overarching goal of the editor is to provide fully referenced information to health professionals so they may have a balanced perspective on the value of various treatment options that are available today as well as in the foreseeable future.

In conclusion, Dr. Ferry's *Management of Pediatric Obesity and Diabetes* provides health professionals in many areas of research and practice with the most up-to-date, well referenced, and comprehensive volume on identifying, treating, and preventing the development of chronic, serious metabolic diseases in children. This volume will serve the reader as the most authoritative resource in the field to date and is a very welcome addition to the Nutrition and Health Series.

Adrianne Bendich, PhD, FACN
Series Editor

Contents

PART II   OBESITY: CLINICAL ASSESSMENTS

PART III   DIABETES: CLINICAL ASSESSMENTS

Contributors

RONALD ADKINS, PHD • *Department of Pediatrics, University of Tennessee Health Science Center at Memphis, Le Bonheur Children's Hospital, Memphis, TN, USA*

PETAR ALAUPOVIC, PHD • *Lipid and Lipoprotein Laboratory, Oklahoma Medical Research Foundation, Oklahoma City, OK, USA*

AAYED AL-QAHTANI, MD, FRCSC, FACS, FAAP • *College of Medicine, King Saud University, Riyadh, Saudi Arabia*

LOUISE A. BAUR, MBBS(HONS), BSc(MED), PHD, FRACP • *Discipline of Paediatrics and Child Health, University of Sydney, Clinical School, The Children's Hospital at Westmead, Westmead, Australia*

PIERS R. BLACKETT, MB, CHB • *Diabetes and Endocrinology Section, University of Oklahoma Health Sciences Center, Oklahoma City, OK, USA*

CATHERINE M. CHAMPAGNE, PHD, RD, LDN, FADA • *Pennington Biomedical Research Center, Louisiana State University, Baton Rouge, LA, USA*

DALE CHILDRESS, MD • *Department of Medicine (Endocrinology) and Research Service, Veterans Administration Medical Center of Memphis, Memphis, TN, USA*

KENNETH C. COPELAND, MD • *Diabetes and Endocrinology Section, University of Oklahoma Health Sciences Center, Oklahoma City, OK, USA*

TULAY T. CUSHMAN, PHD • *Novo Nordisk Inc., Princeton, NJ, USA*

FIONA DAVIES, BA (HONS), MPSYCH (APPLIED), PHD • *Department of Psychological Medicine, The Children's Hospital at Westmead, Westmead, Australia*

JUSTIN M. GREGORY, MD • *Department of Pediatrics, University of Tennessee Health Science Center at Memphis, Le Bonheur Children's Hospital, Memphis, TN, USA*

DHANANJAY GUPTA, PhD • *Dhananjay, University of Vermont College of Medicine, Colchester, VT, USA*

PAULA M. HALE, MD • *Novo Nordisk Inc., Princeton, NJ, USA*

DOUGLAS L. HILL, PhD • *Division of Gastroenterology and Nutrition, The Children's Hospital of Philadelphia, Philadelphia, PA, USA*

GENE B. HUBBARD, DVM, MS • *Department of Pathology, The Sam and Ann Barshop Institute for Longevity and Aging Studies, University of Texas Health Science Center at San Antonio, San Antonio, TX, USA*

THOMAS L. JETTON, PhD • *Department of Medicine, Division of Endocrinology, Diabetes and Metabolism, University of Vermont College of Medicine, Colchester, VT, USA*

EDWARD S. KIMBALL, PhD • *Novo Nordisk Inc., Princeton, NJ, USA*

ABBAS E. KITABCHI, PhD, MD • *Department of Medicine, The University of Tennessee Health Science Center, Memphis, TN, USA*

DAWN M. MCNAMEE, MD, PhD • *Department of Pediatrics, University of Tennessee Health Science Center at Memphis, Le Bonheur Children's Hospital, Memphis, TN, USA*

GERRI A. MINSHALL, BBusComm, BA (HONS), MPSYCH (CLINICAL) • *Weight Management Service, The Children's Hospital at Westmead, Westmead, Australia*

AJI NAIR, PhD • *Novo Nordisk Inc., Princeton, NJ, USA*

KATHERINE E. NEUBECKER, MD • *Department of Internal Medicine, University of Texas Southwestern Medical Center, Dallas, TX, USA*

HOOMAN OKTAEI, MD • *Department of Medicine (Endocrinology) and Research Service, Veterans Administration Medical Center of Memphis, Memphis, TN, USA*

KEITH L. PERKINS, MD • *Departments of Pediatrics and Internal Medicine, University of Tennessee Health Science Center at Memphis, Le Bonheur Children's Hospital, Memphis, TN, USA*

MINA PESHAVARIA, PhD • *Medicine–Endocrinology Unit, University of Vermont College of Medicine, Colchester, VT, USA*

PATAMA PONGSUWAN, MD • *Department of Epidemiology and Cancer Control, St. Jude Children's Research Hospital, Memphis, TN, USA*

RABIA REHMAN, MD • *Department of Medicine, Division of Endocrinology, University of Tennessee Health Science Center, Memphis, TN, USA*

NATALIA E. SCHLABRITZ-LOUTSEVICH, MD, PhD • *Department of Obstetrics and Gynecology, University of Tennessee Health Science Center, Memphis, TN, USA*

KATHRYN H. SCHMITZ, PhD, MPH • *Center for Clinical Epidemiology and Biostatistics, University of Pennsylvania School of Medicine, Philadelphia, PA, USA*

REBECCA GUSIC SHAFFER, PhD • *Novo Nordisk Inc., Princeton, NJ, USA*

SHREEPAL M. SHAH, MBBS • *formerly in Division of Pediatric Endocrinology, Department of Pediatrics, The University of Tennessee Health Science Center at Memphis; now at Department of Pediatrics, Louisiana State University Health Science Center, New Orleans, LA, USA*

KEVIN SHORT, PhD • *Diabetes and Endocrinology Section, University of Oklahoma Health Sciences Center, Oklahoma City, OK, USA*

SOLOMON S. SOLOMON, MD • *Departments of Medicine and Pharmacology, University of Tennessee Health Science Center, Memphis, TN, USA and Department of Medicine (Endocrinology) and Research Service, Veterans Administration Medical Center of Memphis, Memphis, TN, USA*

TETYANA L. VASYLYEVA, MD, PhD • *Department of Pediatrics, Nephrology Section, Texas Tech University Health Sciences Center, Amarillo, TX, USA*

DWAIN E. WOODE, MD • *Department of Internal Medicine, The University of Tennessee Health Science Center, Memphis, TN, USA*

BRIAN H. WROTNIAK, PT, PhD • *Center for Clinical Epidemiology and Biostatistics, The Children's Hospital of Philadelphia, University of Pennsylvania School of Medicine, Philadelphia, PA 19104, USA*

Series Editor

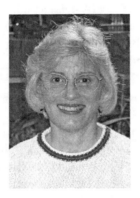

Dr. Adrianne Bendich has recently retired as Director of Medical Affairs at GlaxoSmithKline (GSK) Consumer Healthcare where she was responsible for leading the innovation and medical programs in support of many well-known brands including TUMS and Os-Cal. Dr. Bendich had primary responsibility for GSK's support for the Women's Health Initiative (WHI) intervention study. Prior to joining GSK, Dr. Bendich was at Roche Vitamins Inc. and was involved with the groundbreaking clinical studies showing that folic acid-containing multivitamins significantly reduced major classes of birth defects. Dr. Bendich has co-authored over 100 major clinical research studies in the area of preventive nutrition. Dr Bendich is recognized as a leading authority on antioxidants, nutrition and immunity and pregnancy outcomes, vitamin safety and the cost-effectiveness of vitamin/mineral supplementation.

Dr. Bendich, who is now President of Consultants in Consumer Healthcare LLC, is the editor of ten books including **"Preventive Nutrition: The Comprehensive Guide For Health Professionals, Fourth Edition"** co-edited with Dr. Richard Deckelbaum, and is **Series Editor of "Nutrition and Health"** for Springer/Humana Press (www.springer.com/series/7659). The Series contains 40 published volumes - major new editions in 2010 -2011 include **Vitamin D, Second Edition** edited by Dr. Michael Holick; **"Dietary**

Components and Immune Function" edited by Dr. Ronald Ross Watson, Dr. Sherma Zibadi and Dr. Victor R. Preedy; "Bioactive Compounds and Cancer" edited by Dr. John A. Milner and Dr. Donato F. Romagnolo; "Modern Dietary Fat Intakes in Disease Promotion" edited by Dr. Fabien DeMeester, Dr. Sherma Zibadi, and Dr. Ronald Ross Watson; "Iron Deficiency and Overload" edited by Dr. Shlomo Yehuda and Dr. David Mostofsky; "Nutrition Guide for Physicians" edited by Dr. Edward Wilson, Dr. George A. Bray, Dr. Norman Temple and Dr. Mary Struble; "Nutrition and Metabolism" edited by Dr. Christos Mantzoros and "Fluid and Electrolytes in Pediatrics" edited by Leonard Feld and Dr. Frederick Kaskel. Recent volumes include: "Handbook of Drug-Nutrient Interactions" edited by Dr. Joseph Boullata and Dr. Vincent Armenti; "Probiotics in Pediatric Medicine" edited by Dr. Sonia Michail and Dr. Philip Sherman; "Handbook of Nutrition and Pregnancy" edited by Dr. Carol Lammi-Keefe, Dr. Sarah Couch and Dr. Elliot Philipson; "Nutrition and Rheumatic Disease" edited by Dr. Laura Coleman; "Nutrition and Kidney Disease" edited by Dr. Laura Byham-Grey, Dr. Jerrilynn Burrowes and Dr. Glenn Chertow; "Nutrition and Health in Developing Countries" edited by Dr. Richard Semba and Dr. Martin Bloem; "Calcium in Human Health" edited by Dr. Robert Heaney and Dr. Connie Weaver and "Nutrition and Bone Health" edited by Dr. Michael Holick and Dr. Bess Dawson-Hughes.

Dr. Bendich served as Associate Editor for "Nutrition" the International Journal; served on the Editorial Board of the Journal of Women's Health and Gender-based Medicine, and was a member of the Board of Directors of the American College of Nutrition.

Dr. Bendich was the recipient of the Roche Research Award, is a *Tribute to Women and Industry* Awardee and was a recipient of the Burroughs Wellcome Visiting Professorship in Basic Medical Sciences, 2000-2001. In 2008, Dr. Bendich was given the Council for Responsible Nutrition (CRN) Apple Award in recognition of her many contributions to the scientific understanding of dietary supplements. Dr Bendich holds academic appointments as Adjunct Professor in the Department of Preventive Medicine and Community Health at UMDNJ and has an adjunct appointment at the Institute of Nutrition, Columbia University P&S, and is an Adjunct Research Professor, Rutgers University, Newark Campus. She is listed in Who's Who in American Women.

Volume Editor

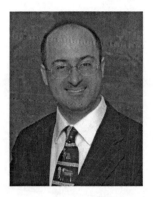

Robert J. Ferry, Jr., MD, FAAP holds full-time appointment as Professor of Pediatrics and Chief for the Division of Pediatric Endocrinology and Metabolism at The University of Tennessee Health Science Center (UTHSC) at Memphis. He directs UTHSC's fellowship training program in pediatric endocrinology and serves as medical director for endocrine services at Le Bonheur Children's Research Hospital and St. Jude Children's Research Hospital in Memphis, Tennessee. Dr. Ferry has received many awards during his professional career. These have included the Clinical Scholar Award of the Pediatric Endocrine Society (formerly the Lawson Wilkins Pediatric Endocrine Society), Research Career Award from the National Institute of Diabetes, Digestive and Kidney Diseases (NIDDK), and two U.S. Army Commendation Medals for service as a physician in Iraq during 2005-06 and 2009. Over the past decade Dr. Ferry has authored or co-authored more than 65 publications, ranging from original peer-reviewed papers to reviews, book chapters, abstracts, and lay articles. He serves on the editorial board of eMedicine Health and holds a reserve commission as lieutenant colonel in the Medical Corps of the Army National Guard.

Part I
Definitions of Pediatric Obesity and Diabetes

1   Genetics of Obesity

Tetyana L. Vasylyeva

Key Points

- Genetic contributions to the clinical risks of obesity or Type 2 diabetes mellitus (T2DM) are multifactorial.
- Rare, inborn errors of adipocyte and lipid metabolism have provided insights, which are clinically relevant to the more common variants of obesity and T2DM.

Keywords: Pediatric, Obesity, Type 2 diabetes mellitus, Genetics

1.1   INTRODUCTION

While it is impossible to overemphasize the importance of diet and exercise on body weight, genetic factors strongly determine a person's predisposition to obesity. Genes regulate intracellular molecular pathways that control energy and nutrient balance as well as hypothalamic pathways that profoundly affect satiety and food intake. Over the past 20 years, population-based linkage analyses and association studies have revealed the processes and genetic loci associated with obesity phenotypes that present in childhood, adolescence, or adulthood. Obesity persisting or presenting shortly after birth typically results from maternal factors (such as uncontrolled gestational diabetes mellitus) but can result from classic Mendelian mutations resulting in monoallelic change of function (homozygous deletion of the leptin gene is the archetype of such disorders) or a range of different genetic defects (such as Beckwith–Wiedemann syndrome). By contrast, the common obesity phenotypes of late childhood, adolescence, or adulthood typically arise from actions and interactions of multiple genes

From: *Nutrition and Health: Management of Pediatric Obesity and Diabetes,*
Edited by: R.J. Ferry, Jr., DOI 10.1007/978-1-60327-256-8_1,
© Springer Science+Business Media, LLC 2011

with environmental factors. Despite an explosion of candidate genes and loci over the past 40 years, no single gene can be recognized as the most clinically significant among its peers, *e.g.*, a gene or locus most predictive of cardiac risks or the progression to clinical diabetes. Indeed, our understanding of the epigenome is just emerging and may ultimately prove more clinically significant than collecting specific bits of the genome. While recognizing the over-riding impact of obesogenic environmental factors in the general pediatric population, this chapter will review genetic contributors that promote obesity.

1.2   MONOZYGOTIC AND DIZYGOTIC TWIN PAIR STUDIES

The characterization of monozygotic (MZ) twin pairs, dizygotic (DZ) twin pairs, and adopted children has strongly established that human obesity is substantially governed by genetic control. Stunkard *et al.* (1986) assessed a sample of 1,974 MZ and 2,097 DZ male twin pairs. Concordance rates for different degrees of excess weight were twice as high for MZ twins as for DZ twins [1], after controlling for environmental factors. Of note, even the physiological regulation of food selection and nutrient intake was more alike with MZ than with DZ twins [2]. Maes *et al.* (1997) found strikingly convergent results for various familial relationships, body mass index (BMI), and other adiposity measures [3]. Their studies suggested that genetic factors could explain 50–90% of the variance in BMI between twins. Parent–offspring and sibling–sibling correlations agreed with BMI heritabilities between 20 and 80%. Data from adoption studies further support the contention that genetic factors account for 20–60% of the variation in BMI. Based on data from more than 25,000 twin pairs and 50,000 biological and adoptive family members, the weighted-mean-correlations were as strong as 74% for MZ twins *vs.* 32% for DZ twins, 25% for siblings, 19% for parent–offspring pairs, and only 6% for adoptive relatives. Even MZ twins reared apart displayed heritability estimates for BMI up to 70% [4, 5]. Among 25,000 pairs of twins born in Sweden, the intrapair correlation for MZ twins reared apart was the most direct estimate of heritability for BMI, calculated as 70% for men and 66% for women [6].

Price and Gottesman (1991) obtained similar results by comparing data on body fat from a cohort of 34 separated MZ pairs with a matched sample of 38 pairs of MZ twins reared together. Their correlation for separated MZ pairs was 61%, and the correlation for MZ pairs living together was 75%. These correlations did not differ significantly, nor did correlations differ between MZ pairs reared apart, when subclassified as having been raised in relatively similar environments. These results, suggesting that both genetic factors and the rearing environment promote accumulation of body fat, have been supported by other adoption studies [7].

Adoption studies have yielded useful information on obesogenic environments because adoptive parents and their adoptive offspring share only environmental sources of variance, whereas children living with their biological parents share both genetic and environmental sources of variance. In 1989 Danish investigators reported their analysis of adoptees separated from their natural parents very early in life, compared with their biological full and half-siblings reared by their natural parents. The adoptees represented four groups who were categorized as either thin, medium weight, overweight, or obese. Weight and height were obtained for 115 full-siblings of 57 adoptees and for 850 half-siblings of 341 adoptees. Full-siblings of overweight and obese adoptees displayed the highest BMI. BMI of the half-siblings showed a consistent but weaker association across the four weight groups of adoptees. The study confirmed that the degree of adiposity of adults living in the same environment can result from genetic factors, whether monoallelic or polyallelic [8].

People with different genetic predispositions inherit factors influencing either energy expenditure (nonobese habitus) or nutrient partitioning (obesity), resulting in different body weights despite similar caloric consumption. Inherited characteristics explain about 40% of the variance in resting metabolic rate, thermic effect of food, and energy cost of low to moderate intensity exercise [9]. When Bouchard *et al.* (1990) overfed 12 male MZ pairs by 1,000 kcal daily for 100 days, they found that the within-pair similarity was strongest with respect to changes in regional fat distribution and the amount of abdominal visceral fat they accumulated [10]. Variance within these pairs was about six-fold lower than between pairs. They concluded that genetic factors were the most likely explanation for the intra-pair similarity in their adaptation to long-term overfeeding and for variations in weight gain and fat distribution between the twin pairs. Genetic factors determine energy storage and the resting expenditure of energy. Similar results were observed with the induction of negative energy balance in identical twin pairs [11]. A significant genetic effect has also been reported related to the level of habitual physical activity [12].

Decades of research effort have focused on the identification of biochemical and molecular markers of energy expenditure and specific genetic loci linked to body weight regulation. In such studies, the first step is to identify the genetic loci with the strongest statistical association with obesity, followed by characterization of the genotype–phenotype relationship and risk factors in order to develop an obesogenic genetic profile.

1.3 GENETIC LOCI IDENTIFIED IN COMMON OBESITY

Many genetic loci for body weight and subphenotypes (such as muscle weight and fat weight) have been mapped. Structural equation modeling has been employed to assess special relationships between genetic loci that influence body weight and different phenotypes. Such studies suggest that body weight control is a composite trait [13]. Farooqi and O'Rahilly recently reviewed the extensive literature linking genes to obesity [14]. Multiple linkage analysis studies across divergent ethnic groups have associated major genes with the variation observed in clinical obesity-related phenotypes. Table 1.1 presents a partial list of the major loci found to be most strongly associated by independent studies. Evidence of linkage from genome-wide scans in obesity was considered significant when log odds ratio (LOD) scores were above 2.0. Bivariate linkage analyses suggest that some genetic regions harbor common major genes with pleiotropic effects [15], such as on 9p22 [bivariate LOD 2.35–3.10] and 13q31 [bivariate LOD 1.96–2.64].

1.4 OBESOGENIC GENES FROM ASSOCIATION STUDIES OF COMMON OBESITY

Genetic association through epidemiology examines genetic variation across a genome. These investigations tend to associate genomic variations with observable traits, *i.e.*, genetic factors larger than single or even linked alleles. Variations which associate strongly would suggest candidate regions of the human genome in which to find obesogenic factors. Ongoing association studies use novel technology to obtain, refine, and analyze these tantalizing data. The main principle of such studies is that by sequencing the actual genomes, genotypes of different individuals can be compared and targeted traits 'that are observed more often than can be readily explained by chance' can be identified. Single nucleotide polymorphisms (SNPs) are single nucleotide variants occurring in a particular nucleotide. SNPs in the same haplotype are inherited together, which allows for "tagging SNPs," instead of measuring every SNP in a haplotype block (Fig. 1.1). Commercial microarrays have been developed with tagging SNPs for genome-wide association studies to allow rapid genotyping and analysis of many cases.

Table 1.2 summarizes data from association analyses to identify genes that influence obesity. Unfortunately, such association studies are always confounded by population stratification, small sample size, ascertainment bias, and publication bias [16]. Moreover, several associations shown in Table 1.2 were unconfirmed by other investigators [17–19]. Genome-wide linkage and association analyses have demonstrated that SNPs within

Table 1.1
Major loci associated with obesity from genome-wide scans

Locus	n and Population	Trait	LOD score	Cardidate genes	Reference
1q31.1-q32.2	245 diabetic and 704 nondia-betic American Indian (tribe unspecified)	BMI	3.7	ADIPOR1	[58]
1p32.2	836 Quebec families	Carbohydrate, lipid, protein intake	2.39		[59]
1p35.2			2.41		
10p15.3			2.72		
2p21	458 Mexican–Americans	Leptin	4.95	GCKR POMC	[46]
3q28	2,280 Northern and Western Europeans	Adiponectin levels	1.70	ADIPOQ	[23]
3q27.3	836 Quebec families	Energy intake as carbohydrate and lipid	2.24 2.0 1.65		[59]
2q13	671 Samoans	Adiponectin	2.05		[15]
4q22		% body fat	2.95		
7p14		% body fat	2.64		
9p22		Abdominal circumference	3.08		
		% body fat serum leptin	2.53		

(continued)

Table 1.1 (continued)

Locus	n and Population	Trait	LOD score	Candidate genes	Reference
13q31	671 Samoans	Serum leptin	2.30		
		% body fat	2.48		
		Abdominal circumference	2.04		
		BMI	2.09		
8p23	2,280 Northern and Western Europeans	Adiponectin levels	3.10		[23]
11q	966 Pima Indians	BMI	3.6		[60]
3q27	2,209 Caucasians	BMI, waist circumference, fasting insulin levels	2.4–3.5	GLUT2 PI3K	[61]
17p12		Leptin	5.0	GLUT4 PPARα	
10p	514 Western Europeans (France)	BMI	4.85	D10S197 D10S611	[47]
18q21	367 Caucasians	BMI	2.42	D18S1155	[36]
Xq24	188 Caucasians (Finnish)	BMI	3.14	DXS6804	

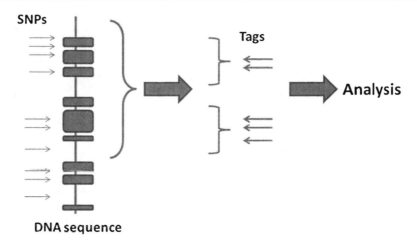

SNPs

Tags

Analysis

DNA sequence

Fig. 1.1. The main principle of a haplotype block "tagging SNPs".

the *ADIPOQ* gene are strongly associated with variations in circulating adiponectin levels. Adiponectin is an adipose-tissue-derived hormone, and its serum levels are negatively correlated with obesity and insulin resistance [20]. Thus, genetic association studies have demonstrated that SNPs +45G15G(T/G) in exon 2 and +276G/T in intron 2 of the *ADIPOQ* gene confer the risk susceptibility to the development of type 2 diabetes, obesity, and diabetic nephropathy [21]. Interestingly, the most recent findings suggest that adiponectin plays a role that goes well beyond its known metabolic function. It could behave as a stem cell factor for several tissues, giving a new perspective for its use as a tool for cell-based therapy of diseased/ injured tissues [22].

CDH1, a gene for cadherin 1 (also called CD324), also influences adiponectin levels [23]. *ADIPOR1* is emerging as a candidate gene for pleiotropic effects on obesity and diabetes susceptibility in humans [24–31]. Distinct *ADIPOR1* SNPs associate with measures of body size, including weight, waist circumference, hip circumference, and BMI. In addition, a gene–gene interaction of *ADIPOR1* and adiponectin was observed with increased overall and abdominal adiposity and higher substrate oxidation. The adiponectin 1 receptor mediates adiponectin effects on fatty acid oxidation and glucose uptake through activation of adenosine 5'-monophosphate-activated protein kinase and peroxisome proliferator-activated receptor (PPAR-α).

The *FTO* gene (fat mass and obesity associated) located on human chromosome 16 has variants correlated with clinical obesity. A recent study correlated *FTO* variants in 38,759 Europeans and other ethnic groups with significant obesity risks [32–34]. Another genome-wide association study,

Table 1.2
List of selected association studies in obesity

Gene	Location	Population	Phenotype	P value	Reference
ADIPOQ	3q28	Northern and Western Europeans	Adiponectin levels	$<10^{-7}$	[23]
rs3774261					
rs6773957					
SOCS3	17q24-17q25	Hispanic Americans	BMI, visceral adipose tissue, waist circumference	0.003–0.017	[62]
rs9914220					
rs9914222					
SLC6A14	Xq24	Finnish (Caucasians)	BMI	0.0007–0.006	[37]
FTO	16q12.2	Sweden (Caucasians)	Adipose mass traits BMI, obesity	<0.001	[63]
rs1121980					
SH2B1	16p11.2				
rs7498665					
MTCH2	11p11.2				
rs4752856					
MC4R	18q22				
rs17782313					
NEGR1	1p31.1				
rs2815752,					
rs10938397					
GNPDA2	4p13				
CHRNA2	8p21	Koreans	Overweight/obesity	0.027	[64]
rs2043063					

with good power, recently identified *FTO* as a strong contributor to both obesity arising in late childhood and adulthood [35].

Fine-mapping in a sample set of 367 obese adults from 166 Finnish families yielded an LOD of 3.48 within the X chromosome. The Xq24 region contains a plausible candidate: the serotonin 2C receptor. Variants of the serotonin 2C receptor predispose mice to obesity and T2DM [36]. Another candidate, SLC6A14, arose from the same Finnish population association study. SLC6A14 encodes an amino acid transporter and may control appetite by regulating tryptophan availability for serotonin synthesis [37]. Chromosomal region linked to obesity, 18q21, flanks the melanocortin 4 receptor (*MC4R*) [38]. *MC4R* attracted strong attention because it is central to the melanocortinergic pathway that controls energy homeostasis. Many missense, nonsense, and frameshift mutations of *MC4R* reduce or eliminate its function, while resulting in an obese phenotype [39–41].

Insulin and the insulin-like growth factors (IGFs) exert major actions on pancreatic β cell development, growth, and maintenance as well as somatic growth and carbohydrate metabolism. A variable nucleotide tandem repeat (VNTR) polymorphism upstream of the insulin gene (*INS*) is associated with varied expression not only of *INS* but also of the nearby *IGF2* gene. Some obese children displayed excess paternal transmission of the class I VNTR alleles, but data are controversial [42, 43]. Children who inherited a class I allele from their fathers (but not those inheriting it from their mothers) displayed increased risk of early-onset obesity. Due to the frequency of class I alleles in the Central European and North African population, this risk is relevant to 65–70% of all infants in this population. Increased *in utero* expression of paternal *INS* or *IGF2* due to this class I *INS* VNTR allele may predispose offspring to excessive postnatal fat deposition [44].

Leptin is a circulating protein released by adipocytes and appears to satisfy the requirements of an afferent signal within a negative feedback loop that regulates fat mass [45]. Clinically, circulating leptin levels closely correlate with an individual's total adiposity. Variations in leptin levels correlate well with genetic markers, with estimates of genetic heritability ranging from 40 to 60% [46, 47]. Farooqi and O'Rahilly first demonstrated how leptin-signaling can play a critical role in the regulation of reproductive and immune function in humans [48]. Leptin remains at the center of a complex network that coordinates changes in nutritional states with other diverse aspects of mammalian biology [46]. Complete loss of leptin production results in a severe congenital obesity phenotype, which largely resolves with administration of exogenous leptin. Apart from these classic clinical reports of rare kindreds with congenital obesity, loci on chromosomes 5cen-q and 2p in a French cohort have been linked to common obesity with altered leptin levels [49].

By a genome-wide scan and multipoint linkage analysis of a Mexican–American cohort, one group used a general pedigree-based variance component approach to identify genes with measurable effects on quantitative variation in leptin levels [50]. A microsatellite polymorphism, D2S1788, mapped to chromosome 2p21 (approximately 74 cM from the tip of the short arm), and showed strong evidence of linkage with serum leptin levels (LOD score 4.95; $P=9\times10^{-7}$). This locus accounted for 47% of the variation in serum leptin levels, with a residual additive genetic component contributing an additional 24%. The region contains several potential candidate genes for obesity, including glucokinase regulatory protein (*GCKR*) and proopiomelanocortin (*POMC*) [46].

POMC is the precursor for several peptide hormones produced by posttranslational processing, some of which are involved in energy homeostasis. These include alpha melanocyte-stimulating hormone (α-MSH), adrenocorticotropic hormone, and β-endorphin. POMC is highly expressed in neuronal cells of the arcuate nucleus, a region of the hypothalamus involved in energy homeostasis [51].

Willer and colleagues recently produced a meta-analysis of 15 genome-wide association studies for BMI ($n>32,000$) and pursued top signals in 14 additional cohorts ($n>59,000$) [52]. They confirmed associations between *FTO* and *MC4R* with BMI and identified six additional loci ($P<5\times10^{-8}$): *TMEM18*, *KCTD15*, *GNPDA2*, *SH2B1*, *MTCH2*, and *NEGR1* (where a 45-kb deletion polymorphism is a candidate causal variant). They emphasized that several of the likely causal genes are highly expressed or known to act in the central nervous system (CNS), which supports the widely recognized role of the CNS for predisposition to obesity [52].

GAD2 encodes for glutamic acid decarboxylase enzyme (*GAD65*) and has been identified as another positional candidate gene for obesity (located on 10p11-12). *GAD2* cropped up as a susceptibility locus for morbid obesity in four independent ethnic populations [53]. *GAD65* catalyzes the formation of gamma-aminobutyric acid, which interacts with neuropeptide Y in the paraventricular nucleus and appears to stimulate food intake [53].

1.5   GENES PROTECTING FROM OBESITY

KLF7 encodes Kruppel-like factor (KLF) 7. *KLF7* is a member of the KLF family of transcription factors, initially shown to play an important role in cellular development and differentiation, and reported to be specifically involved in adipogenesis [54]. In a Danish cohort, with the minor A-allele of rs7568369, protection against obesity was evident (odds ratio (OR)=0.90; 95% confidence interval (CI)=0.84–0.96; $P=0.001$). In studies of quantitative traits ($n = 5,535$), this variant was associated with decreased BMI ($P = 0.002$) and waist circumference ($P = 0.003$) [54].

The I103 allele of *MC4R* can be protective, as confirmed in different populations (LOD = 0.69; 95% CI = 0.50–0.96; $P = 0.03$). Sequencing of *MC4R* revealed three polymorphisms in its noncoding region that displayed strong linkage disequilibrium with V103I. The respective protective effect against obesity implies that *MC4R* variants can produce loss or gain of function [55].

A recent animal study revealed that the loss of *FTO* in mice led to postnatal growth retardation and a significant reduction in adipose tissue and lean body mass [56]. No clinical correlate has been reported to date.

1.6 SINGLE GENE DISORDERS RESULTING IN HUMAN OBESITY

Most single gene disorders causing human obesity can be characterized as heritable neurobehavioral disorders affecting the central control of food intake. Patients with these disorders may also be developmentally impaired or have other developmental abnormalities. Single gene disorders associated with obesity display a Mendelian pattern of inheritance. These disorders include congenital deficiency of leptin (*ob*), the leptin receptor, *POMC*, the *MC4R*, or prohormone convertase 1 (*PC1*). These monoallelic disorders result from classic frameshift, homozygous, or compound heterozygous mutations.

Pleiotropic syndromes associated with obesity include the following (the mutated gene is shown parenthetically): Bardet–Biedl syndrome (*BBS1-8*), Albright's hereditary osteodystrophy (*GNAS1*), fragile X syndrome (unstable expansions of a CGG trinucleotide repeat located in *FMR1*), Borjeson–Forssman–Lehmann syndrome (*PHF6*), Cohen syndrome (*COH1*), Alström syndrome (*ALMS1*), and Ulnar-Mammary syndrome (*TBX3*) among others. Obesity syndromes caused by chromosomal rearrangements include, SIM-1 and WAGR syndrome. For more detailed descriptions of these rare diseases see Chapter 16.

1.7 ROLE OF GENETIC COUNSELING

Advances in genetic technologies raise practical and ethical issues. The positive and negative effects of informing people about the genetic etiology of their obesity have been reviewed [57]. Consultations that included genetic information were superior to consultations without the genetic component, in terms of leading the obese individuals to new insights about their condition (advantage for consultation with genetic information, even

6 months later; $P=0.046$). No negative effects (*e.g.*, loss of self-efficacy/self-control or increase of body weight) were observed [57].

Multiple ongoing studies address environmental influences related to diet and physical activity to evaluate their effectiveness in reducing obesity among youth. Most of the programs are not directed by genetic findings, but known predispositions could encourage early intervention and individualization of treatment plans.

Although the genetics of obesity are challenging, complex, and rapidly changing, the use of genetic information to predict an individual's risk of obesity, need for diet modification, and potential for treatment-response is a step toward improved and individualized early prevention of obesity. Understanding and applying genetics in clinical practice could help children with a predisposition to obesity get earlier referral to a dietitian and get appropriate advice about life style modifications.

1.8   CONCLUSION

The inherited components of obesity are complex and incompletely understood. Everyday, we grow more familiar with emerging molecules with a role in the control of body mass. Although genetic risk cannot yet be modified, recognizing genetic causes can impact clinical therapy. In particular, the clinician must recognize candidates for leptin (recombinant DNA origin) therapy. Individuals at risk of obesity, based on family history or confirmed genetic factors, should be strongly counseled to modify their environment, nutrition, and lifestyle to reduce the impact of obesity and its sequelae.

REFERENCES

1. Stunkard AJ, Foch TT, Hrubec Z (1986) A twin study of human obesity. JAMA 256:51–54
2. Wade J, Milner J, Krondl M (1981) Evidence for a physiological regulation of food selection and nutrient intake in twins. Am J Clin Nutr 34:143–147
3. Maes HH, Neale MC, Eaves LJ (1997) Genetic and environmental factors in relative body weight and human adiposity. Behav Genet 27:325–351
4. Allison DB, Kaprio J, Korkeila M, Koskenvuo M, Neale MC, Hayakawa K (1996) The heritability of body mass index among an international sample of monozygotic twins reared apart. Int J Obes Relat Metab Disord 20:501–506
5. Allison DB, Heshka S, Neale MC, Lykken DT, Heymsfield SB (1994) A genetic analysis of relative weight among 4,020 twin pairs, with an emphasis on sex effects. Health Psychol 13:362–365
6. Stunkard AJ, Harris JR, Pedersen NL, McClearn GE (1990) The body-mass index of twins who have been reared apart. N Engl J Med 322:1483–1487
7. Price RA, Gottesman II (1991) Body fat in identical twins reared apart: roles for genes and environment. Behav Genet 21:1–7

8. Sorensen TI, Price RA, Stunkard AJ, Schulsinger F (1989) Genetics of obesity in adult adoptees and their biological siblings. BMJ 298:87–90

9. Bouchard C, Tremblay A (1990) Genetic effects in human energy expenditure components. Int J Obes 14(Suppl 1):49–55; discussion 55–58

10. Bouchard C, Tremblay A, Despres JP et al. (1990) The response to long-term overfeeding in identical twins. N Engl J Med 322:1477–1482

11. Bouchard C, Tremblay A, Despres JP et al. (1996) Overfeeding in identical twins: 5-year postoverfeeding results. Metabolism 45:1042–1050

12. Samaras K, Kelly PJ, Chiano MN, Spector TD, Campbell LV (1999) Genetic and environmental influences on total-body and central abdominal fat: the effect of physical activity in female twins. Ann Intern Med 130:873–882

13. Brockmann GA, Tsaih SW, Neuschl C, Churchill GA, Li R (2009) Genetic factors contributing to obesity and body weight can act through mechanisms affecting muscle weight, fat weight, or both. Physiol Genomics 36:114–126

14. Farooqi S, O'Rahilly S (2006) Genetics of obesity in humans. Endocr Rev 27: 710–718

15. Dai F, Sun G, Aberg K et al. (2008) A whole genome linkage scan identifies multiple chromosomal regions influencing adiposity-related traits among Samoans. Ann Hum Genet 72:780–792

16. O'Rahilly S, Farooqi IS (2006) Genetics of obesity. Philos Trans R Soc Lond B Biol Sci 361:1095–1105

17. Wiedmann S, Neureuther K, Stark K et al. (2009) Lack of association between a common polymorphism near the INSIG2 gene and BMI, myocardial infarction, and cardiovascular risk factors. Obesity 17:1390–1395

18. Lowe JK, Maller JB, Pe'er I et al. (2009) Genome-wide association studies in an isolated founder population from the Pacific Island of Kosrae. PLoS Genet 5:e1000365

19. Gueorguiev M, Lecoeur C, Meyre D et al. (2009) Association studies on ghrelin and ghrelin receptor gene polymorphisms with obesity. Obesity 17:745–754

20. Liu M, Liu F (2010) Transcriptional and post-translational regulation of adiponectin. Biochem J 425:41–52

21. Gu HF (2009) Biomarkers of adiponectin: plasma protein variation and genomic DNA polymorphisms. Biomark Insights 4:123–133

22. Chiarugi P, Fiaschi T (2010) Adiponectin in health and diseases: from metabolic syndrome to tissue regeneration. Expert Opin Ther Targets 14:193–206

23. Ling H, Waterworth DM, Stirnadel HA et al. (2009) Genome-wide linkage and association analyses to identify genes influencing adiponectin levels: the GEMS study. Obesity 17:737–744

24. Kadowaki T, Yamauchi T, Kubota N, Hara K, Ueki K, Tobe K (2006) Adiponectin and adiponectin receptors in insulin resistance, diabetes, and the metabolic syndrome. J Clin Invest 116:1784–1792

25. Damcott CM, Ott SH, Pollin TI et al. (2005) Genetic variation in adiponectin receptor 1 and adiponectin receptor 2 is associated with type 2 diabetes in the Old Order Amish. Diabetes 54:2245–2250

26. Stefan N, Machicao F, Staiger H et al. (2005) Polymorphisms in the gene encoding adiponectin receptor 1 are associated with insulin resistance and high liver fat. Diabetologia 48:2282–2291

27. Siitonen N, Pulkkinen L, Mager U et al. (2006) Association of sequence variations in the gene encoding adiponectin receptor 1 (ADIPOR1) with body size and insulin levels. The Finnish Diabetes Prevention Study. Diabetologia 49:1795–1805

28. Hara K, Horikoshi M, Kitazato H *et al.* (2005) Absence of an association between the polymorphisms in the genes encoding adiponectin receptors and type 2 diabetes. Diabetologia 48:1307–1314

29. Wang H, Zhang H, Jia Y *et al.* (2004) Adiponectin receptor 1 gene (*ADIPOR1*) as a candidate for type 2 diabetes and insulin resistance. Diabetes 53:2132–2136

30. Vaxillaire M, Dechaume A, Vasseur-Delannoy V *et al.* (2006) Genetic analysis of *ADIPOR1* and *ADIPOR2* candidate polymorphisms for type 2 diabetes in the Caucasian population. Diabetes 55:856–861

31. Loos RJ, Ruchat S, Rankinen T, Tremblay A, Perusse L, Bouchard C (2007) Adiponectin and adiponectin receptor gene variants in relation to resting metabolic rate, respiratory quotient, and adiposity-related phenotypes in the Quebec Family Study. Am J Clin Nutr 85:26–34

32. Frayling TM, Timpson NJ, Weedon MN *et al.* (2007) A common variant in the *FTO* gene is associated with body mass index and predisposes to childhood and adult obesity. Science 316:889–894

33. Chu X, Erdman R, Susek M, *et al.* (2008) Association of morbid obesity with *FTO* and *INSIG2* allelic variants. Arch Surg 143:235–240; discussion 241

34. Tan JT, Dorajoo R, Seielstad M *et al.* (2008) *FTO* variants are associated with obesity in the Chinese and Malay populations in Singapore. Diabetes 57:2851–2857

35. Blakemore AI, Froguel P (2008) Is obesity our genetic legacy? J Clin Endocrinol Metab 93:S51–S56

36. Ohman M, Oksanen L, Kaprio J *et al.* (2000) Genome-wide scan of obesity in Finnish sibpairs reveals linkage to chromosome Xq24. J Clin Endocrinol Metab 85:3183–3190

37. Suviolahti E, Oksanen LJ, Ohman M *et al.* (2003) The *SLC6A14* gene shows evidence of association with obesity. J Clin Invest 112:1762–1772

38. Cody JD, Reveles XT, Hale DE, Lehman D, Coon H, Leach RJ (1999) Haplosufficiency of the melancortin-4 receptor gene in individuals with deletions of 18q. Hum Genet 105:424–427

39. Yeo GS, Lank EJ, Farooqi IS, Keogh J, Challis BG, O'Rahilly S (2003) Mutations in the human melanocortin-4 receptor gene associated with severe familial obesity disrupts receptor function through multiple molecular mechanisms. Hum Mol Genet 12:561–574

40. Rosmond R, Chagnon M, Bouchard C, Bjorntorp P (2001) A missense mutation in the human melanocortin-4 receptor gene in relation to abdominal obesity and salivary corti-sol. Diabetologia 44:1335–1338

41. Hinney A, Hohmann S, Geller F *et al.* (2003) Melanocortin-4 receptor gene: case-control study and transmission disequilibrium test confirm that functionally relevant mutations are compatible with a major gene effect for extreme obesity. J Clin Endocrinol Metab 88:4258–4267

42. Le Fur S, Auffray C, Letourneur F, Cruaud C, Le Stunff C, Bougnères P (2006) Heterogeneity of class I *INS* VNTR allele association with insulin secretion in obese children. Physiol Genomics 25:480–484

43. Bouatia-Naji N, De Graeve F, Brönner G, Lecoeur C, Vatin V, Durand E, Lichtner P, Nguyen TT, Heude B, Weill J, Lévy-Marchal C, Hebebrand J, Froguel P, Meyre D (2008) *INS* VNTR is not associated with childhood obesity in 1,023 families: a family-based study. Obesity 16:1471–1475

44. Le Stunff C, Fallin D, Bougneres P (2001) Paternal transmission of the very common class I *INS* VNTR alleles predisposes to childhood obesity. Nat Genet 29:96–99

45. Friedman JM, Halaas JL (1998) Leptin and the regulation of body weight in mammals. Nature 395:763–770

46. Comuzzie AG, Hixson JE, Almasy L *et al.* (1997) A major quantitative trait locus determining serum leptin levels and fat mass is located on human chromosome 2. Nat Genet 15:273–276
47. Rotimi C, Luke A, Li Z, Compton J, Bowsher R, Cooper R (1997) Heritability of plasma leptin in a population sample of African-American families. Genet Epidemiol 14:255–263
48. Farooqi IS, O'Rahilly S (2009) Leptin: a pivotal regulator of human energy homeostasis. Am J Clin Nutr 89:980S–984S
49. Hager J, Dina C, Francke S *et al.* (1998) A genome-wide scan for human obesity genes reveals a major susceptibility locus on chromosome 10. Nat Genet 20:304–308
50. Martin LJ, Mahaney MC, Almasy L, Hixson JE, Cole SA, MacCluer JW, Jaquish CE, Blangero J, Comuzzie AG (2002) A quantitative trait locus on chromosome 22 for serum leptin levels adjusted for serum testosterone. Obes Res 10:602–607
51. Woods SC, Seeley RJ, Porte D Jr, Schwartz MW (1998) Signals that regulate food intake and energy homeostasis. Science 280:1378–1383
52. Willer CJ, Speliotes EK, Loos RJ *et al.* (2009) Six new loci associated with body mass index highlight a neuronal influence on body weight regulation. Nat Genet 41:25–34
53. Boutin P, Dina C, Vasseur F *et al.* (2003) *GAD2* on chromosome 10p12 is a candidate gene for human obesity. PLoS Biol 1:E68
54. Zobel D, Andreasen C, Burgdorf K *et al.* (2009) Variation in the gene encoding Kruppel-like factor 7 influences body fat: studies of 14, 818 Danes. Eur J Endocrinol 160:603–609
55. Geller F, Reichwald K, Dempfle A *et al.* (2004) Melanocortin-4 receptor gene variant I103 is negatively associated with obesity. Am J Hum Genet 74:572–581
56. Fischer J, Koch L, Emmerling C *et al.* (2009) Inactivation of the *Fto* gene protects from obesity. Nature 458:894–898
57. Rief W, Conradt M, Dierk JM, Rauh E, Schlumberger P, Hinney A, Hebebrand J (2007) Is information on genetic determinants of obesity helpful or harmful for obese people? A randomized clinical trial. J Gen Intern Med 22:1553–1539
58. Franceschini N, Almasy L, MacCluer JW, Göring HH, Cole SA, Diego VP, Laston S, Howard BV, Lee ET, Best LG, Fabsitz RR, North KE (2008) Diabetes-specific genetic effects on obesity traits in American Indian populations: the Strong Heart Family Study. BMC Med Genet 9:90
59. Choquette AC, Lemieux S, Tremblay A *et al.* (2008) Evidence of a quantitative trait locus for energy and macronutrient intakes on chromosome 3q27.3: the Quebec Family Study. Am J Clin Nutr 88:1142–1148
60. Hanson RL, Ehm MG, Pettitt DJ *et al.* (1998) An autosomal genomic scan for loci linked to type II diabetes mellitus and body-mass index in Pima Indians. Am J Hum Genet 63:1130–1138
61. Kissebah AH, Sonnenberg GE, Myklebust J *et al.* (2000) Quantitative trait loci on chromosomes 3 and 17 influence phenotypes of the metabolic syndrome. Proc Natl Acad Sci USA 97:14478–14483
62. Talbert ME, Langefeld CD, Ziegler J *et al.* (2009) Polymorphisms near *SOCS3* are associated with obesity and glucose homeostasis traits in Hispanic Americans from the Insulin Resistance Atherosclerosis Family Study. Hum Genet 125:153–162
63. Renstrom F, Payne F, Nordstrom A *et al.* (2009) Replication and extension of genome-wide association study results for obesity in 4,923 adults from Northern Sweden. Hum Mol Genet 18:1489–1496
64. Kim J (2008) Association of *CHRNA2* polymorphisms with overweight/obesity and clinical characteristics in a Korean population. Clin Chem Lab Med 46:1085–1089

2

Fetal Origins of Obesity and Diabetes

Natalia E. Schlabritz-Loutsevitch, Gene B. Hubbard, and Ronald Adkins

Key Points

- The intrauterine environment creates epigenetic marks, which can increase the lifelong risks of developing obesity or T2DM.
- Maternal obesity during pregnancy can increase the lifelong risks of developing obesity or T2DM.
- Although it remains unknown whether alteration of the intrauterine environment can reduce the lifelong risks of developing obesity and/or T2DM, maternal health during gestation impacts the lifelong health of the offspring.

Keywords: Childhood obesity, Pregnancy, Intrauterine environment, Epigenetic, Animal models

2.1 INTRODUCTION

Obesity is a serious condition that presently affects ~310 million people worldwide. An additional 800 million people in the world are overweight, defined as body mass index (BMI) above the 85‰. Due to its tight association with other features of the metabolic syndrome, obesity represents a major health problem which, if not kept within bounds, threatens to cause tremendous health care costs in the coming years [1].

Obesity is a heterogenic disorder, associated with genetic as well as environmental factors [2, 3]. Genetic factors – such as the common presence of

From: *Nutrition and Health: Management of Pediatric Obesity and Diabetes*,
Edited by: R.J. Ferry, Jr., DOI 10.1007/978-1-60327-256-8_2,
© Springer Science+Business Media, LLC 2011

fat mass and obesity-associated (*FTO*) genotype [4, 5] variants near the *MC4R* gene [6, 7] as well as the rarer primary leptin deficiency and leptin receptor defects [8, 9] – certainly play an important role in the development of the obese phenotype. The lifetime variations in this genotype-associated phenotype have been recognized [7].

The metabolic, physiologic, and genetic mechanisms underlying the clustering of the components of the metabolic syndrome have been studied in adults and children [10–16], but not in the fetus. The maternal *in utero* environment is the first environment to create phenotype from a particular genotype. The consequences of inappropriate intrauterine conditions can persist through the individual's adult life. Indeed, abnormal intrauterine environments have been associated with increased risk for childhood obesity. Such conditions include maternal obesity and a high-fat diet [17, 18], maternal nutrient deprivation [19–21], maternal micronutrient status [22, 23], maternal smoking [24], gestational diabetes mellitus [25, 26], and preeclampsia [27]. Animal experimental models and human population studies have revealed that malnutrition [28], insulin injections [29], and maternal stress (such as injection of endotoxins and immunosuppressants during gestation) also predispose offspring to adult obesity [30–32]. Additionally, developmental exposure to endocrine disruptors has been associated with subsequent development of obesity [33]. Table 2.1 summarizes animal models which address the developmental and genetic aspects of obese offspring. This review will concentrate on maternal obesity as an origin of offspring metabolic disturbances in later life, touching only briefly on the roles that genetics and epigenetics may play in both intrauterine growth retardation (IUGR) and childhood disease risk.

2.2   MATERNAL OBESITY

Maternal obesity, affecting 20.2–34% of all pregnant women [34, 35], remains a major factor influencing the development of obese offspring and metabolic syndrome in later life, as shown by animal experimental models and observed in longitudinal clinical studies [17, 36].

2.3   EFFECT OF MATERNAL OBESITY ON THE OFFSPRING EARLY WEIGHT GAIN IS CHILDHOOD AGE AND SEX DEPENDENT

Children exposed to maternal obesity display higher risk for development of metabolic syndrome and obesity in later life. The gender-specific effect of maternal obesity on the offspring metabolic status has been

Table 2.1
Selected animal models used to study obesity and its developmental programming

Species	Model of obesity	Offspring	Reference
Rodents	*Genetic*		
Mice	*ob/ob*	NA	[128, 129]
Mice	*FTO* mutation		[130]
Mice	Conditional *ob* knock-out from neurons	NA	[131]
Mice	Natural C57BL/6J strain On high-fat diet	NA	[132]
Mice	*5-HT2CRs* knock-out	NA	[133]
Mice	*Ay/a*, ectopic overexpression of the agouti protein	NA	[134, 135]
Mice	*MC4R* knockout mice	NA	[136]
Mice	*db/db*, loss-of-function mutations of leptin receptor genes	NA	[137]
Zucker fatty rats	*fa/fa*, loss-of-function mutations of leptin receptor genes	NA	[138]
Otsuka Long-Evans Tokushima Fatty (OLETF) rat model	Lacks the CCK_1 receptor due to a spontaneous genetic mutation	Fetal macrosomia and childhood onset obesity	[139, 140]
Rodents	*Epigenetic/pregnancy intervention*		
Mice	Natural DBA/2J strain on high-fat diet	Obese	[141]
Mice	Protein restriction		
Outbred CD-1 mice	High perinatal DES dose	Adult onset obesity	[33]
ICR mice	50% global nutrient restriction	Transgenerational passage of late-onset obesity	[142]
C57/BL6 mice	High-fat diet prior to and during pregnancy	Fetal macrosomia	[143]

(continued)

Table 2.1
(continued)

Species	Model of obesity	Offspring	Reference
C57BL/6J mice	Obesogenic diet (16% fat, 33% sugar) for 6 weeks before mating and throughout pregnancy and lactation	Adult-onset obesity	[38]
Mice	Mid- to late-gestation stress	Adult onset obesity	[72]
Sprague–Dawley rats	High-fat diet		[30, 144]
Sprague–Dawley rats	Prolonged consumption of 5.3 kcal/g. high-fat diet	Obesity by day 120 postnatally	[145]
Sprague–Dawley rats	High-fat diet 50%	Weaning–puberty obesity	[146]
Sprague–Dawley rats	Glucose injection at day 11th and 12th of gestation	Fetal macrosomia	[147]
Wistar rats	Fed 30% of global diet	Adult-onset obesity	[148–150]
Rats	Protein restriction; 19 g of protein/100 g of diet	Transgenerational passage of late-onset obesity	[151]
Albino Wistar rats	Isocaloric protein restriction; 10% of casein	Transgenerational passage of obesity of late-onset obesity	[152]
Wistar rats	Dexamethasone exposure duing second half of gestation	Transgenerational passage of late-onset obesity	[153]
Sprague–Dawley rats	Diet containing both n-6 and n-3 PUFA (n-6/n-3 diet) 10 days prior to delivery	Adult onset obesity	[154]
Wistar rats	Dexamethasone injection in pregnancy	Increased fat content in adult male offspring	[155]
Ruminants and other species	*Epigenetic/pregnancy intervention*		
Sheep	50% global nutrient restriction between 28 and 78 days of gestation	Obesity at 4 months of age	[156]
Sheep	Periconceptual somatotropin treatment	Increased weight at birth and at 75 days of life	[157]

Sheep	Propylene glycol administration during second half of gestation	Increased birth weight	[158]
Pigs	Linebred lean (L), linebred obese (O), and reciprocal crossmatings	O fetuses possessed 14% more body fat than L fetuses	[159]
Guinea pigs	Maternal nutrient restriction: 70% *ad libitum* intake from 4 weeks before to midpregnancy, then 90% until day 60 gestation	Early-onset obesity	[160]
Beef heifers	250% of recommended nutrient requirements	Increased birth weight	[161]
Nonhuman primates	*Genetic*		
Gray mouse lemurs	Natural photoperiod-induced obesity	NA	[162]
Baboon	Natural model	Nonobese at birth, increased incidence of stillbirths	[70, 163]
Nonhuman primates	*Epigenetic/pregnancy intervention*		
Rhesus monkeys (*Macaca mulatta*)	High-fat diet		[164]

observed in rodents [37–39] and in humans [40]. However, other population studies have failed to confirm gender-specific differences in the development of childhood obesity. Black children are at greater risk for being overweight than white children, and their overweight phenotype is more likely to develop at a younger age and persist over time [41]. The effects of maternal obesity on maternal and fetal health differ among the various racial groups [42]. Besides ethnic and racial differences, the effect of maternal obesity also depends on fetal gender. Cagnacci *et al.* [43] showed that maternal obesity is associated with a shift of gender ratio toward male offspring. In their longitudinal study, Mamun *et al.* [40] analyzed maternal pregnancy weight gain in association with offspring body composition and cardiovascular system at 21 years of age. They observed significantly more pronounced effect of increased maternal weight gain on male, but not female, offspring. By contrast, studies of Wrotniak *et al.* [44] did not show gender differences in childhood obesity in relation to maternal weight gain and prepregnancy BMI. The first year of life is the most important in terms of subsequent health programming [45], and accelerated weight gain during this period is associated with the increased risk of diabetes development [46]. Interestingly, Botton *et al.* [47] reported that accelerated weight gain in boys during the first 6 months of life is associated with increased lean mass in later life, but not fat mass.

In their comprehensive analysis of existing published databases, Nelson *et al.* [48] recently demonstrated a significant impact of maternal prepregnancy obesity and gestational weight gain on the metabolic status of the offspring. However, the mechanisms by which maternal obesity exerts its unwanted effects on the developing fetus have not yet been established. Several mechanisms have been proposed as causative for the subsequent development of obesity in later life, including fetal macrosomia, fetal insulin resistance, IUGR, appetite programming, fetal inflammatory syndrome, etc.

2.3.1 Maternal Obesity and Fetal Macrosomia

As recorded in the Swedish birth registry, the secular 25–36% increase in maternal BMI over the last decade has translated to an approximately 25% increase in the incidence of newborns large for gestational age (LGA) [49]. LGA is due to a larger amount of fat, but not proteins [50, 51]. Fetal macrosomia is already associated at birth with increased lipolysis and propensity for decreased insulin sensitivity [52, 53]. Fat accumulation in LGA babies is a sensitive marker of fetal status [52].

2.4 MATERNAL OBESITY AND FETAL PANCREATIC FUNCTION AND INSULIN RESISTANCE

Catalano *et al.* [54] showed that children from obese mothers are already developing insulin resistance *in utero*, with female fetuses being more affected than males. Using the sheep model of obesity, Ford *et al.* [55] demonstrated intrauterine damage of fetal pancreatic beta-cells (but not alpha-cells) in animals fed with high-fat diet during pregnancy. Table 2.1 summarizes animal models used to study the effect of maternal obesity.

2.5 MATERNAL OBESITY AND FETAL MONOCYTE ACTIVATION: POSSIBLE MECHANISM OF DEVELOPMENTAL PROGRAMMING

Obesity-related changes in peripheral blood mononuclear cells (PBMC) are central to the chronic inflammation associated with excess of body fat [56, 57]. Maternal obesity in pregnancy is associated with maternal PBMC activation and placental macrophage infiltration [58]. The literature contains extreme cases of fetal inflammatory response syndrome associated with preterm labor and subsequent fetal brain injuries [59, 60]. Intimal fetal monocyte recruitment was increased in fetuses from mothers with hypercholesterolemia [61]. Urashima *et al.* [62] demonstrated that fetal monocytes are capable of synthesizing interleukin (IL)-6, IL-8, and tumor necrosis factor (TNF)-α. However, the number of IL-6- and TNF-α-positive monocytes was significantly smaller compared to adults. By contrast, more fetal than adult monocytes produced IL-8, and the number of IL-8-positive monocytes was positively correlated with gestational age. Macrophages' production of TNF-α. within adipose tissue is associated with obesity [63]. TNF-α. concentration decreased in individuals losing weight. Inflammation precedes metabolic deterioration [64].

2.6 FETAL MONOCYTE ACTIVATION IN A BABOON MODEL OF MATERNAL OBESITY

Nonhuman primates (NHPs) are closely related to the human species and have been used extensively in reproductive studies. One of the most characterized NHP models used to study maternal obesity is the Rhesus macaque. However, Rhesus macaques have certain disadvantages, including a bidiscoid placenta and an immune system with only three IgG subclasses [65, 66]. Another NHP species, the baboon, has been extensively studied as a model for obesity [67, 68]. Increased weight in the baboon has been associated with insulin resistance [69] and stillbirth [70]. These data agree with published human data. Baboon placental structure and development are also very similar to humans [71].

2.7 MATERIAL AND METHODS

2.7.1 Animal Care and Maintenance

All animals were maintained in a social group environment with partly controlled climate conditions, fed, and given water *ad libitum* (LEO5, Purina). Two groups of pregnant female baboons (*Papio* spp.) were selected based on weight and obesity index at delivery by cesarean section at 165 days gestation (G), or 0.9 G (1 G=term=185 days) [72, 73] (Table 2.3). Obesity index (Rh index) was defined as body weight divided by the square of the crown-rump length in another NHP species – rhesus monkeys [74]. We aimed to compare animals that had around a 1.3 incremental increase in the index. This degree of incremental increase was described in obese *vs.* nonobese rhesus monkeys [74]. Rather than BMI, Rh index was used since baboons, like rhesus monkeys, are quadruped animals and display a central type of obesity [69]. In the fetal morphometric studies, ponderal index was calculated as [weight (in g)$\times$100]/[length (in cm^3)] and BMI as [weight (in kg)]/[length (in m^2)]. All procedures were approved by the Animal Care and Use Committee of the Southwest Foundation for Biomedical Research (San Antonio, TX).

2.7.2 FACS Analyses

Blood was collected from fetal umbilical vein and maternal peripheral circulation. Maternal and fetal cells were stained with antibodies (listed in Table 2.2), with and without LPS stimulation for 5 h, and processed on flow cytometer (BD, FACSAria). Numbers of double-positive (*e.g.*, CD14+Notch1+) CD14+ cells were calculated as percentage of CD14+ cells; additional fluorescence intensity was measured.

Table 2.2
List of conjugated antibodies used for this study

CD14	FITC-conjugated	Catalog # 6603262, Beckman Coulter
IL-6 intracellular	PE phycoerythrin (PE)-	Catalog #20655A, BD Pharmingen
TNF-α intracellular	Allophycocyanin (APC)-conjugated	Catalog #340534, Becton Dickinson
Notch-1 receptor	PE-conjugated	Catalog #552768, BD Pharmingen
TIE 2	Phosphorylate form-pe-conjugated	Catalog #5600052, Becton Dickinson

Table 2.3

Morphometric characteristics of baboons enrolled in the study and fetal morphometry from obese and nonobese animals (mean ± SEM) [163]

	Nonobese (n = 4)	Obese (n = 4)
Maternal characteristics		
Prepregnancy weight (kg)	15.7 ± 1.1	18.3 ± 1.6
Prepregnancy Rh index (kg/m^2)	40.6 ± 3.7	53.3 ± 3.3[a]
Postcesarean weight (kg)	15.2 ± 0.7	16.7 ± 1.1
Postcesarean Rh index (kg/m^2)	39.1 ± 3.2	48.7 ± 1.0[a]
Body length (cm)	103.9 ± 2.1	99.0 ± 3.5
Abdominal distance (cm)	20 ± 1.3	22.7 ± 1.5
Femur length (cm)	22 ± 0.9	21.5 ± 1.0
Fetal characteristics		
Heart (g)	4.4 ± 0.6	4.5 ± 0.5
Lungs (g)	23.01 ± 2.94	22.28 ± 3.63
Thymus (g)	3.42 ± 0.34	3.78 ± 0.44
Thyroids (combined) (g)	0.29 ± 0.09	0.31 ± 0.04
Liver (g)	24.93 ± 1.57	25.36 ± 4.85
Spleen (g)	1.61 ± 0.10	1.54 ± 0.15
Pancreas (g)	0.66 ± 0.10	0.56 ± 0.22
Right kidney (g)	2.58 ± 0.17	2.02 ± 0.23
Left kidney (g)	2.53 ± 0.15	1.95 ± 0.23
Brain (g)	80.22 ± 1.54	76.1 ± 6.88
Right adrenal (g)	0.15 ± 0.02	0.14 ± 0.02
Left adrenal (g)	0.19 ± 0.02	0.18 ± 0.02
Pericardial fat (g)	0.35 ± 0.09	0.2 ± 0.07
Right perirenal fat (g)	1.03 ± 0.71	0.31 ± 0.14
Omental fat (g)	1.34 ± 0.64	1.43 ± 1.32
Gall bladder (g)	0.49 ± 0.1	0.3 ± 0.05

[a]$p < 0.05$

2.8   RESULTS

2.8.1   Maternal Morphometry

The Rh index was elevated in the baboons in the obese group by 31% prior to pregnancy and 25% after cesarean section. Obese baboons had seven times the perirenal fat mass (13.9 ± 4.6 g obese *vs.* 1.9 ± 0.4 g control) and nearly double omental fat mass (112.1 ± 32.6 g obese *vs.* 58.3 ± 29.0 g control) ($p < 0.05$). There was a positive correlation of Rh index to maternal leptin levels ($r = 0.87$, $p = 0.004$). However, maternal Rh index was not significantly correlated with maternal omental fat weight or fetal leptin concentrations (data not shown). Combined kidney weight was lower (65.7 ± 2 g *vs.* 72 ± 2 g, respectively) in obese *vs.* nonobese animals ($p < 0.05$).

2.8.2 Fetal Morphometry

Fetal BMI and ponderal index ($p < 0.05$) were higher in the obese group, while fetal weight (810 ± 20 g obese *vs.* 770 ± 70 g control) and organ weights did not differ between the two groups (Table 2.3).

2.8.3 Maternal and Fetal PBMC Transcriptome Analyses

The most significant pathways affected in fetal PBMCs (27 affected of 77 total pathways) were cell adhesion molecules, phosphatidylinositol, m-TOR, and VEGF (Table 2.4). Changes in maternal PBMCs involved ubiquitin-mediated proteolysis, leukocyte transendothelial migration, and insulin signaling (Table 2.4).

2.8.4 Fetal Monocytes Angiogenic and Inflammatory Response in a Baboon Model of Maternal Obesity

Maternal weight directly correlated with TNF-α fluorescence intensity in stimulated fetal monocytes (Fig. 2.1b) ($r = 0.95$, $p < 0.05$). There were no correlations between NOTCH1, TIE-2, and IL-1 expressions and maternal weight.

Table 2.4

Pathways affected by maternal obesity in fetal and maternal peripheral blood mononuclear cells (PBMC) in baboons at the end of gestation [163]

Pathway name (KEGG)	Impact factor	p
Fetal PBMC		
Antigen processing and presentation	42.5	<0.01
Phosphatidylinositol signaling system	22.6	3.6E-9
Pathogenic *Escherichia coli* infection	10.3	3.7E-4
mTOR signaling pathway	10.1	14.7E-4
Epithelial cell signaling in *Helicobacter pylori* infection	8.2	12.6E-3
Ribosome	8.0	3.44E-3
Focal adhesion	7.6	4.4E-3
Compliment and coagulation cascades	7.2	6.0E-3
Leukocyte transendothelial migration	6.4	1.2E-2
Adherent junction	6.4	1.2E-2
Regulation of autophagy	6.3	1.3E-2
Thyroid cancer	6.1	1.6E-2

(continued)

Table 2.4
(continued)

Pathway name (KEGG)	Impact factor	p
Vibrio cholerae infection	6.0	1.8E-2
Pancreatic cancer	5.8	2.0E-2
Proteasome	5.8	2.1E-2
VEGF signaling pathway	5.7	2.3E-2
Chronic myeloid leukemia	5.3	3.2E-2
B cell receptor signaling pathway	5.2	3.3E-2
Regulation of actin cytoskeleton	5.2	3.56E-2
Nonhomologous end-joining	5.1	3.6E-2
Tight junction	5.1	3.7E-2
ErbB signaling pathway	5.1	3.9E-2
Ubiquitin-mediated proteolysis	5.1	3.9E-2
MAPK signaling pathway	5.0	4.1E-2
Nonsmall lung cancer	5.0	4.1E-2
Maternal PBMC		
Ubiquitin-mediated proteolysis	8.3	2.4E-3
Adherent junction	7.3	5.6E-3
Ribosome	6.5	1.1E-2
Basal cell carcinoma	6.5	1.2E-2
Long-term potentiation	6.1	1.5E-2
Gap junction	5.5	1.8E-2
Bladder cancer	5.8	2.1E-2
Amyotrophic lateral sclerosis (ALS)	5.5	2.6E-2
Renal cell carcinoma	5.5	2.7E-2
Leukocyte transendothelial migration	4.9	4.7E-2

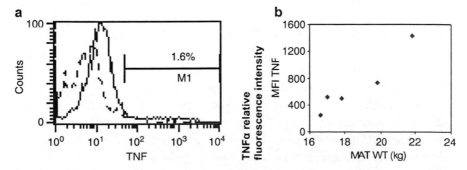

Fig. 2.1. (a) Percentage of baboon fetal monocytes expressing TNF-α after LPS stimulation (10 ng/mL, 5 h). (b) Direct correlation between maternal weight and fluorescence intensity of TNF-α staining (flow cytometry) in baboon fetal monocytes stimulated with LPS (10 ng/mL, 5 h) at the end of gestation ($n=5$; $r=0.95$; $p<0.05$).

2.9   DISCUSSION

The fetal consequences of maternal obesity are controversial. Maternal obesity has been associated with both intrauterine growth restriction and large-for-gestational age (LGA) human fetuses. In our present study, we did not find any changes in fetal weight but we observed an increased ponderal index in fetuses from obese mothers. These minimal morphological changes were associated with significant fetal PBMC response to maternal obesity in our study. Urashima *et al.* [62] showed differences in gene expression between adult and fetal PBMC. In agreement with that data, we found that the response of fetal PBMC included 27 significantly changed pathways, while in mothers ten pathways differed. The major pathway affected in fetus was cell adhesion molecule pathway, while in the mother the most significant pathway affected by maternal obesity was ubiquitin-mediated proteolysis. Vascular endothelial growth factor (VEGF) signaling pathways were significantly upregulated in fetuses from obese animals in our study. VEGF-A is a potent regulator of the integrity, permeability, and proliferation of blood vessels [75]. Increased expression of this pathway might be associated with increased fetal organ capillarization and function. The vascularization of pancreatic islets, for example, is essential for pancreatic function and development [76].

2.10   OTHER FACTORS DURING FETAL DEVELOPMENT CONTRIBUTING TO RISKS OF OBESITY AND DISEASE

2.10.1   *Genetics*

Reduced birth weight is a major risk factor for illness in the neonatal period and throughout life, with the smallest 7.5% of infants accounting for two-thirds of infant deaths [77]. Term infants with low birth weight are at least five times more likely to die in the first year [78] and are second only to premature infants in their rates of early morbidity [79–82] and mortality [83]. Small newborns have an increased risk of several adverse outcomes in childhood, especially cerebral palsy. Through childhood and into adulthood, in conjunction with increased obesity and abdominal fat deposition [84, 121], individuals born small for gestational age (SGA) acquire elevated risk of pregnancy-induced hypertension [85], gestational diabetes [86], essential hypertension [87], type 2 diabetes [88, 89], and cardiovascular disease [90–92].

The cause of the statistically significant and frequently replicated finding of an inverse relationship between birth size and adult predisposition to chronic disease has been heavily debated. The "fetal origins" hypothesis [93] suggests that an inadequate uterine environment (*i.e.*, poor nutrition, placental insufficiency) results in long-term alterations in organ structure, organ function, and hormonal milieu that make the individual more susceptible to disease. An alternative explanation for this association between birth weight and later disease is the existence of genetic factors that both reduce fetal growth and increase predisposition to disease [94, 95]. The "shared genetic etiological factor" hypothesis is supported by a very strong and statistically significant inverse correlation between paternal mortality and offspring birth size – that is only slightly weaker than that between maternal mortality and offspring birth size [96–98], even after adjusting for shared lifestyle risk factors (*i.e.*, smoking) and socioeconomic status. The strong inverse correlation between paternal mortality and birth size indicates that there may be a connection between disease-predisposing genetic variants and reduced fetal size.

Even after adjustment for parental anthropometry, smoking, prenatal care, and education, a man who was SGA is 3.5 times more likely to have an SGA child. A woman who was SGA is 4.7 times more likely to give birth to an SGA child. If both parents were SGA, the risk of an SGA child is 16.3 times greater [99], implying a multiplicative effect. Clausson *et al.* [100] studied the offspring from 2,009 female dizygotic and monozygotic twin pairs and estimated a birth weight heritability of 42%. Svensson *et al.* retrospectively analyzed [101] ~2.2 million Swedish singleton births and reported a maternal genetic component of about 27%, paternal component of about 18%, or a total of about 45%, in excellent agreement with Clausson *et al.* In their study of 3,562 captive macaques that minimized environmental heterogeneity [102], Ha *et al.* estimated a total heritability for birth weight of 51%, with an additive genetic component of 23%. These findings demonstrate a major genetic component to birth weight variation. Consistent with this recent research, SGA births tend both to cluster in families and to recur in successive generations [103–106] even after adjustment for important covariables [107, 108]. Monogenetic forms of obesity, along with its comorbidities, are beyond the scope of this chapter and are covered in depth in Chap. 1 by Dr. Vasylyeva.

2.11   EPIGENETICS

The reversible methylation of cytosines in CpG dinucleotides, particularly in promoter regions, is a mechanism for downregulating gene expression, active for perhaps one-third of human genes [109–111]. At an extreme, DNA methylation is key to the allele-specific silencing of the paternal or maternal allele that occurs in gene imprinting. These methylation marks can operate not only locally (usually called differentially methylated regions (DMRs) but also over distances of a hundred or more kilobases, usually called imprinting control regions (ICRs).

The variably imprinted genes at 11p15 are an excellent demonstration of how altered methylation in different regions of the same locus can exert divergent effects on birth size and disease risk. This region includes the genes for insulin (*INS*), insulin-like growth factor-II (*IGF2*), *H19*, *CDKN1C*, *KCNQ1*, as well as antisense transcripts. Hypomethylation of the *KCNQ1* DMR (called KvDMR1 or ICR2) is observed in over 50% of Beckwith–Wiedemann syndrome (BWS) patients [112], who exhibit large newborn size. By contrast, hypomethylation of the *H19* DMR (called ICR1) is observed in 38–63% of Silver–Russell patients [113–116], who are typically SGA [117]. Even more interestingly, a common haplotype (22% in healthy Caucasians, 35% in BWS patients) within an *IGF2* DMR (called DMR0) is highly correlated with loss of methylation (LOM, or hypomethylation) in BWS at the KvDMR1 located about 550 kb away [118]. Substantial variation exists in the extent of methylation of the DMRs at 11p15, and that variation is highly heritable (0.33–0.35 for *H19* DMR; 0.75–0.80 for *IGF2* DMR), consistent from adolescence through middle age, and highly correlated with single nucleotide polymorphisms [119]. Similarly, genetic factors play a significant role in interindividual variation in *IGF2* DMR methylation levels [120]. Finally, a comparison of DNA methylation between IUGR and normal birth size neonates [121] discovered altered methylation of a promoter for the *HNF4A* gene, mutations within which are strongly associated with increased risk of maturity onset diabetes of the young (MODY, reviewed in Chap. 15 by Rehman *et al.*) [122]. This observation suggests a direct epigenetic link between restricted fetal growth and later risk of insulin resistance or overt diabetes. Comprehensive reviews of animal models of epigenetic influences have been published elsewhere [18, 123–127].

2.12   CONCLUSION

As shown by human population and animal experimental studies, maternal obesity affects development of obesity in later life through different mechanisms. While still a field under intense investigation, these mechanisms can depend upon fetal gender and be present even in the absence of changes in birth weight.

REFERENCES

1. Thompson D, Wolf AM (2001) The medical-care cost burden of obesity. Obes Rev 2:189–197
2. O'Rahilly S, Farooqi IS (2008) Human obesity: a heritable neurobehavioral disorder that is highly sensitive to environmental conditions. Diabetes 57:2905–2910
3. Comuzzie AG, Williams JT, Martin LJ, Blangero J (2001) Searching for genes underlying normal variation in human adiposity. J Mol Med 79:57–70
4. Jonsson A, Franks PW, Palmer CNA, Cecil J, Hetherington M (2009) Obesity, FTO gene variant, and energy intake in children. N Engl J Med 360:1571–1572

5. Frayling TM, Timpson NJ, Weedon MN, Zeggini E, Freathy RM, Lindgren CM, Perry JR, Elliott KS, Lango H, Rayner NW, Shields B, Harries LW, Barrett JC, Ellard S, Groves CJ, Knight B, Patch AM, Ness AR, Ebrahim S, Lawlor DA, Ring SM, Ben-Shlomo Y, Jarvelin MR, Sovio U, Bennett AJ, Melzer D, Ferrucci L, Loos RJ, Barroso I, Wareham NJ, Karpe F, Owen KR, Cardon LR, Walker M, Hitman GA, Palmer CN, Doney AS, Morris AD, Smith GD, Hattersley AT, McCarthy MI (2007) A common variant in the FTO gene is associated with body mass index and predisposes to child-hood and adult obesity. Science 316:889–894

6. Loos RJ, Lindgren CM, Li S, Wheeler E, Zhao JH, Prokopenko I, Inouye M, Freathy RM, Attwood AP, Beckmann JS, Berndt SI; Prostate, Lung, Colorectal, and Ovarian (PLCO) Cancer Screening Trial, Jacobs KB, Chanock SJ, Hayes RB, Bergmann S, Bennett AJ, Bingham SA, Bochud M, Brown M, Cauchi S, Connell JM, Cooper C, Smith GD, Day I, Dina C, De S, Dermitzakis ET, Doney AS, Elliott KS, Elliott P, Evans DM, Sadaf Farooqi I, Froguel P, Ghori J, Groves CJ, Gwilliam R, Hadley D, Hall AS, Hattersley AT, Hebebrand J, Heid IM; KORA, Lamina C, Gieger C, Illig T, Meitinger T, Wichmann HE, Herrera B, Hinney A, Hunt SE, Jarvelin MR, Johnson T, Jolley JD, Karpe F, Keniry A, Khaw KT, Luben RN, Mangino M, Marchini J, McArdle WL, McGinnis R, Meyre D, Munroe PB, Morris AD, Ness AR, Neville MJ, Nica AC, Ong KK, O'Rahilly S, Owen KR, Palmer CN, Papadakis K, Potter S, Pouta A, Qi L; Nurses' Health Study, Randall JC, Rayner NW, Ring SM, Sandhu MS, Scherag A, Sims MA, Song K, Soranzo N, Speliotes EK; Diabetes Genetics Initiative, Syddall HE, Teichmann SA, Timpson NJ, Tobias JH, Uda M; SardiNIA Study, Vogel CI, Wallace C, Waterworth DM, Weedon MN; Wellcome Trust Case Control Consortium, Willer CJ; FUSION, Wraight, Yuan X, Zeggini E, Hirschhorn JN, Strachan DP, Ouwehand WH, Caulfield MJ, Samani NJ, Frayling TM, Vollenweider P, Waeber G, Mooser V, Deloukas P, McCarthy MI, Wareham NJ, Barroso I, Jacobs KB, Chanock SJ, Hayes RB, Lamina C, Gieger C, Illig T, Meitinger T, Wichmann HE, Kraft P, Hankinson SE, Hunter DJ, Hu FB, Lyon HN, Voight BF, Ridderstrale M, Groop L, Scheet P, Sanna S, Abecasis GR, Albai G, Nagaraja R, Schlessinger D, Jackson AU, Tuomilehto J, Collins FS, Boehnke M, Mohlke KL (2008) Common variants near MC4R are associated with fat mass, weight and risk of obesity. Nat Genet 40:768–775

7. Hardy R, Wills A, Wong A, Elks CE, Wareham NJ, Loos RJF, Kuh D, Ong KK (2010) Life course variations in the associations between FTO and MC4R gene variants and body size. Hum Mol Genet 19:545–552

8. Montague CT, Farooqi IS, Whitehead JP, Soos MA, Rau H, Wareham NJ, Sewter CP, Digby JE, Mohammed SN, Hurst JA, Cheetham CH, Earley AR, Barnett AH, Prins JB, O'Rahilly S (1997) Congenital leptin deficiency is associated with severe early-onset obesity in humans. Nature 387:903–908

9. Clement K, Vaisse C, Lahlou N, Cabrol S, Pelloux V, Cassuto D, Gourmelen M, Dina C, Chambaz J, Lacorte JM, Basdevant A, Bougneres P, Lebouc Y, Froguel P, Guy-Grand B (1998) A mutation in the human leptin receptor gene causes obesity and pituitary dys-function. Nature 392:398–401

10. Carmelli D, Cardon LR, Fabsitz R (1994) Clustering of hypertension, diabetes, and obesity in adult male twins: same genes or same environments? Am J Hum Genet 55:566–573

11. Mitchell BD, Kammerer CM, Mahaney MC, Blangero J, Comuzzie AG, Atwood LD, Haffner SM, Stern MP, MacCluer JW (1996) Genetic analysis of the IRS. Pleiotropic effects of genes influencing insulin levels on lipoprotein and obesity measures. Arterioscler Thromb Vasc Biol 16:281–288

12. Hong Y, Pedersen NL, Brismar K, de Faire U (1997) Genetic and environmental architecture of the features of the insulin-resistance syndrome. Am J Hum Genet 60:143–152

13. Arya R, Blangero J, Williams K, Almasy L, Dyer TD, Leach RJ, O'Connell P, Stern MP, Duggirala R (2002) Factors of insulin resistance syndrome-related phenotypes are linked to genetic locations on chromosomes 6 and 7 in non-diabetic Mexican-Americans. Diabetes 51:841–847

14. de Andrade M, Olswold C, Kardia SL, Boerwinkle E, Turner ST (2002) Multivariate linkage analysis using phenotypes related to the insulin resistance-metabolic disorder. 11th Annual Meeting of the International Genetic Epidemiology Society. Genet Epidemiol 23:275

15. Loos RJ, Katzmarzyk PT, Rao DC, Rice T, Leon AS, Skinner JS, Wilmore JH, Rankinen T, Bouchard C (2003) Genome-wide linkage scan for the metabolic syndrome in the HERITAGE Family Study. J Clin Endocrinol Metab 88:5935–5943

16. Butte NF, Comuzzie AG, Cole SA, Mehta NR, Cai G, Tejero M, Bastarrachea R, Smith EO (2005) Quantitative genetic analysis of the metabolic syndrome in Hispanic children. Pediatr Res 58:1243–1248

17. Grattan DR (2008) Programming from maternal obesity: eating too much for two? Endocrinology 149:5345–5347

18. Armitage JA, Taylor PD, Poston L (2005) Experimental models of developmental programming: consequences of exposure to an energy rich diet during development. J Physiol 565:3–8

19. Ravelli G, Stein Z, Susser M (1976) Obesity in young men after famine exposure in utero and early infancy. N Engl J Med 7:349–354

20. Ravelli A, van Der Meulen J, Osmond C, Barker D, Bleker O (1999) Obesity at the age of 50 years in men and women exposed to famine prenatally. Am J Clin Nutr 70:811–816

21. Fernandez-Twinn DS, Ozanne SE (2006) Mechanisms by which poor early growth programs type-2 diabetes, obesity and the metabolic syndrome. Physiol Behav 88:234–243

22. Ward MA, Neville TL, Reed JJ, Taylor JB, Hallford DM, Soto-Navarro SA, Vonnahme KA, Redmer DA, Reynolds LP, Caton JS (2008) Effects of selenium supply and dietary restriction on maternal and fetal metabolic hormones in pregnant ewe lambs online. J Anim Sci 86:1254–1262

23. Mathews F, Yudkin P, Neil A (1999) Influence of maternal nutrition on outcome of pregnancy: prospective cohort study. Br Med J 319:339–343

24. von Kries R, Toschke A, Koletzko B, Slikker W (2002) Maternal smoking during pregnancy and childhood obesity. Am J Epidemiol 156:954–996

25. Reece EA (2010) The fetal and maternal consequences of gestational diabetes mellitus. J Matern Fetal Neonatal Med 23:199–203

26. Vohr BR, Boney CM (2008) Gestational diabetes: the forerunner for the development of maternal and childhood obesity and metabolic syndrome? J Matern Fetal Neonatal Med 21:149–157

27. Ogland B, Vatten LJ, Romundstad PR, Nilsen ST, Forman MR (2009) Pubertal anthropometry in sons and daughters of women with preeclamptic or normotensive pregnancies. Arch Dis Child 94:855–859

28. Jones AP, Simson EL, Friedman MI (1984) Gestational undernutrition and the development of obesity in rats. J Nutr 114:1484–1492

29. Jones AP, Olster DH, States B (1996) Maternal insulin manipulations in rats organize body weight and noradrenergic innervation of the hypothalamus in gonadally intact male offspring. Brain Res Dev Brain Res 97:16–21

30. Levin BE (2006) Metabolic imprinting: critical impact of the perinatal environment on the regulation of energy homeostasis. Philos Trans R Soc Lond B Biol Sci 361:1107–1121

31. Levin BE (2009) Synergy of nature and nurture in the development of childhood obesity. Int J Obes (Lond) 33:S53–S56
32. Levin BE (2010) Interaction of perinatal and pre-pubertal factors with genetic predisposition in the development of neural pathways involved in the regulation of energy homeostasis. Brain Res 1350:10–17
33. Newbold RR, Padilla-Banks E, Snyder RJ, Phillips TM, Jefferson WN (2007) Developmental exposure to endocrine disruptors and the obesity epidemic. Reprod Toxicol 23:290–296
34. Callaway LK, Prins JB, Chang AM, McIntyre HD (2006) The prevalence and impact of overweight and obesity in an Australian obstetric population. Med J Aust 184:56–59
35. Manson JE, Willett WC, Stampfer MJ, Colditz GA, Hunter DJ, Hankinson SE, Hennekens CH, Speizer FE (1995) Body weight and mortality among women. N Engl J Med 333:677–685
36. Knight B, Shields BM, Hill A, Powell RJ, Wright D, Hattersley AT (2007) The impact of maternal glycemia and obesity on early postnatal growth in a nondiabetic Caucasian population. Diab Care 30:777–783
37. Shankar K, Harrell A, Liu X, Gilchrist JM, Ronis MJJ, Badger TM (2008) Maternal obesity at conception programs obesity in the offspring. Am J Physiol Regul Integr Comp Physiol 294:R528–R538
38. Samuelsson A-M, Matthews PA, Argenton M, Christie MA, McConnell JM, Jansen EHJM, Piersma AH, Ozanne SE, Fernandez-Twinn D, Remacle C, Rowlerson A, Poston L, Taylor PD (2008) Diet-induced obesity in female mice leads to offspring hyperphagia, adiposity, hypertension, and insulin resistance: a novel murine model of developmental programming. Hypertension 51:383–392
39. Samuelsson A-M, Morris A, Igosheva N, Kirk SL, Pombo JMC, Coen CW, Poston L, Taylor PD (2010) Evidence for sympathetic origins of hypertension in juvenile offspring of obese rats. Hypertension 55:76–82
40. Mamun AA, O'Callaghan M, Callaway L, Williams G, Najman J, Lawlor DA (2009) Associations of gestational weight gain with offspring body mass index and blood pressure at 21 years of age. Evidence from a birth cohort study. Circulation 119:1720–1727
41. Salsberry PJ, Reagan PB (2005) Dynamics of early childhood overweight. Pediatrics 116:1329–1338
42. Rosenberg TJ, Garbers S, Lipkind H, Chiasson MA (2005) Maternal obesity and diabetes as risk factors for adverse pregnancy outcomes: differences among 4 racial/ethnic groups. Am J Public Health 95:1544–1551
43. Cagnacci A, Renzi A, Arangino S, Alessandrini C, Volpe A (2004) Influences of maternal weight on the secondary sex ratio of human offspring. Hum Reprod 19:442–444
44. Wrotniak BH, Shults J, Butts S, Stettler N (2008) Gestational weight gain and risk of overweight in the offspring at age 7 years in a multicenter, multiethnic cohort study. Am J Clin Nutr 87:1818–1824
45. Gillman MW (2008) The first months of life: a critical period for development of obesity. Am J Clin Nutr 87:1587–1589
46. Harder T, Roepke K, Diller N, Stechling Y, Dudenhausen JW, Plagemann A (2009) Birth weight, early weight gain, and subsequent risk of type 1 diabetes: systematic review and meta-analysis. Am J Epidemiol 169:1428–1436
47. Botton J, Heude B, Maccario J, Ducimetière P, Charles M-A (2008) Postnatal weight and height growth velocities at different ages between birth and 5 y and body composition in adolescent boys and girls. Am J Clin Nutr 87:1760–1768
48. Nelson SM, Matthews P, Poston L (2010) Maternal metabolism and obesity: modifiable determinants of pregnancy outcome. Hum Reprod Update 16:255–275

49. Surkan PJ, Hsieh CC, Johansson ALV, Dickman PW, Cnattingius S (2004) Reasons for increasing trends in large for gestational age births. Obstet Gynecol 104:720–726

50. Sewell MF, Huston-Presley L, Super DM, Catalano P (2006) Increased neonatal fat mass, not lean body mass, is associated with maternal obesity. Am J Obstet Gynecol 195:1100–1103

51. Durnwald C, Huston-Presley L, Amini S, Catalano P (2004) Evaluation of body composition of large-for-gestational-age infants of women with gestational diabetes mellitus compared with women with normal glucose tolerance levels. Am J Obstet Gynecol 191:804–808

52. Ahlsson FSE, Diderholm B, Ewald U, Gustafsson J (2007) Lipolysis and insulin sensitivity at birth in infants who are large for gestational age. Pediatrics 120:958–965

53. Dyer JS, Rosenfeld CR, Rice J, Rice M, Hardin DS (2007) Insulin resistance in Hispanic large-for gestational-age neonates at birth. J Clin Endocrinol Metab 92:3836–3843

54. Catalano PM, Presley L, Minium J, Hauguel-de Mouzon S (2009) Fetuses of obese mothers develop insulin resistance in utero. Diab Care 32:1076–1080

55. Ford SP, Zhang L, Zhu M, Miller MM, Smith DT, Hess BW, Moss GE, Nathanielsz PW, Nijland MJ (2009) Maternal obesity accelerates fetal pancreatic beta-cell but not alpha-cell development in sheep: prenatal consequences. Am J Physiol Regul Integr Comp Physiol 297:R835–R843

56. Fontana L, Eagon JC, Colonna M, Klein S (2007) Impaired mononuclear cell immune function in extreme obesity is corrected by weight loss. Rejuvenation Res 10:41–46

57. Ghanim H, Aljada A, Hofmeyer D, Syed T, Mohanty P, Dandona P (2004) Circulating mononuclear cells in the obese are in a proinflammatory state. Circulation 110:1564–1571

58. Challier JC, Basu S, Bintein T, Minium J, Hotmire K, Catalano PM, Hauguel-de Mouzon S (2008) Obesity in pregnancy stimulates macrophage accumulation and inflammation in the placenta. Placenta 29:274–281

59. Romero R, Gomez R, Ghezzi F, Yoon BH, Mazor M, Edwin SS, Berry SM (1998) A fetal systemic inflammatory response is followed by the spontaneous onset of preterm parturition. Am J Obstet Gynecol 179:186–193

60. Romero R, Maymon E, Pacora P, Gomez R, Mazor M, Yoon BH, Berry SM (2000) Further observations on the fetal inflammatory response syndrome: A potential homeostatic role for the soluble receptors of tumor necrosis factor [alpha]. Am J Obstet Gynecol 183:1070–1077

61. Napoli C, D'Armiento FP, Mancini FP, Postiglione A, Witztum JL, Palumbo G, Palinski W (1997) Fatty streak formation occurs in human fetal aortas and is greatly enhanced by maternal hypercholesterolemia. Intimal accumulation of low density lipoprotein and its oxidation precede monocyte recruitment into early atherosclerotic lesions. J Clin Invest 100:2680–2690

62. Urashima M, Sakuma M, Teramoto S, Fuyama Y, Eto Y, Kondo K, Tanaka T (2005) Gene expression profiles of peripheral and cord blood mononuclear cells altered by thymic stromal lymphopoietin. Pediatr Res 57:563–569

63. de Ferranti S, Mozaffarian D (2008) The perfect storm: obesity, adipocyte dysfunction, and metabolic consequences. Clin Chem 54:945–955

64. Hotamisligil GS (2008) Inflammation and endoplasmic reticulum stress in obesity and diabetes. Int J Obes (Lond) 32:S52–S54

65. Wooding P, Burton G (eds) (2008) Comparative placentation: structures, functions and evolution. Springer, Berlin, p 302

66. Kim KH, Park MK, Peeters CC, Poolman JT, Shearer MH, Kennedy RC, Nahm MH (1994) Comparison of non-human primate antibodies against *Haemophilus influenza*

type b polysaccharide with human antibodies in oligoclonality and *in vivo* protective potency. Infect Immun 62:2426–2431

67. Altmann J, Schoeller D, Altmann SA, Muruthi P, Sapolsky RM (1993) Body size and fatness of free-living baboons reflect food availability and activity levels. Am J Primatol 30:149–161

68. Comuzzie AG, Cole SA, Martin L, Carey KD, Mahaney MC, Blangero J (2003) The baboon as a nonhuman primate model for the study of the genetics of obesity. Obes Res 11:75–80

69. Chavez AO, Lopez-Alvarenga JC, Tejero ME, Triplitt C, Bastarrachea RA, Sriwijitkamol A, Tantiwong P, Voruganti VS, Musi N, Comuzzie AG, DeFronzo RA, Folli F (2008) Physiological and molecular determinants of insulin action in the baboon. Diabetes 57:899–908

70. Schlabritz-Loutsevitch NE, Moore CM, Lopez-Alvarenga JC, Dunn BG, Dudley D, Hubbard GB (2008) The baboon model (*Papio hamadryas*) of fetal loss: maternal weight, age, reproductive history and pregnancy outcome. J Med Primatol 37:337–345

71. Enders AC, Lantz KC, Peterson PE, Hendrickx AG (1997) From blastocyst to placenta: the morphology of implantation in the baboon. Hum Reprod Update 3:561

72. Kriewaldt FN, Hendrickx AG (1968) Reproductive parameters in the baboon. Lab Anim Care 18:361–370

73. Beehner JC, Nguyen N, Wango EO, Alberts SC, Altmann J (2006) The endocrinology of pregnancy and fetal loss in wild baboons. Horm Behav 49:688–699

74. Jen KL, Hansen BC, Metzger BL (1985) Adiposity, anthropometric measures, and plasma insulin levels of rhesus monkeys. Int J Obes 9:213–224

75. Ferrara N, Smith DT (1997) The biology of vascular endothelial growth factor. Endocr Rev 18:4–25

76. Lammert E, Cleaver O, Melton D (2001) Induction of pancreatic differentiation by signals from blood vessels. Science 294:564–567

77. MacDorman MF, Atkinson JO (1999) Infant mortality statistics from the 1997 period linked birth/infant death data set. Natl Vital Stat Rep 47:1–23

78. McIntire DD, Bloom SL, Casey BM, Leveno KJ (1999) Birth weight in relation to morbidity and mortality among newborn infants. N Engl J Med 340:1234–1238

79. Hay WW Jr, Catz CS, Grave GD, Yaffe SJ (1997) Workshop summary: fetal growth: its regulation and disorders. Pediatrics 99:585–591

80. O'Keeffe MJ, O'Callaghan M, Williams GM, Najman JM, Bor W (2003) Learning, cognitive, and attentional problems in adolescents born small for gestational age. Pediatrics 112:301–307

81. Jelliffe-Pawlowski LL, Hansen RL (2004) Neurodevelopmental outcome at 8 months and 4 years among infants born full-term small-for-gestational-age. J Perinatol 24:505–514

82. Lundgren M, Cnattingius S, Jonsson B, Tuvemo T (2004) Intellectual performance in young adult males born small for gestational age. Growth Horm IGF Res 14(Suppl A):7–8

83. Bernstein I, Gabbe SG (1989) Intrauterine growth retardation. In: Gabbe SG, Niebyl JR, Simpson JL, Annas GJ (eds) Obstetrics: normal and problem pregnancies, 3rd edn. Churchill Livingstone, New York, pp 863–886

84. Meas T, Deghmoun S, Armoogum P, Alberti C, Levy-Marchal C (2008) Consequences of being born small for gestational age on body composition: an 8-year follow-up study. J Clin Endocrinol Metab 93:3804–3809

85. Innes KE, Byers TE, Marshall JA, Baron A, Orleans M, Hamman RF (2003) Association of a woman's own birth weight with her subsequent risk for pregnancy-induced hypertension. Am J Epidemiol 158:861–870

86. Innes KE, Byers TE, Marshall JA, Baron A, Orleans M, Hamman RF (2002) Association of a woman's own birth weight with subsequent risk for gestational diabetes. JAMA 287:2534–2541

87. Frontini MG, Srinivasan SR, Xu J, Berenson GS (2004) Low birth weight and longitudinal trends of cardiovascular risk factor variables from childhood to adolescence: the Bogalusa heart study. BMC Pediatr 4:22

88. Rich-Edwards JW, Colditz GA, Stampfer MJ et al. (1999) Birthweight and the risk for type 2 diabetes mellitus in adult women. Ann Intern Med 130:278–284

89. Lithell HO, McKeigue PM, Berglund L, Mohsen R, Lithell UB, Leon DA (1996) Relation of size at birth to non-insulin dependent diabetes and insulin concentrations in men aged 50-60 years. BMJ 312:406–410

90. Lawlor DA, Ronalds G, Clark H, Smith GD, Leon DA (2005) Birth weight is inversely associated with incident coronary heart disease and stroke among individuals born in the 1950s: findings from the Aberdeen children of the 1950s prospective cohort study. Circulation 112:1414–1418

91. Huxley R, Neil A, Collins R (2002) Unravelling the fetal origins hypothesis: is there really an inverse association between birthweight and subsequent blood pressure? Lancet 360:659–665

92. Huxley R, Owen CG, Whincup PH, Cook DG, Colman S, Collins R (2004) Birth weight and subsequent cholesterol levels: exploration of the "fetal origins" hypothesis. JAMA 292:2755–2764

93. Barker DJ (1998) Mother, babies, and health in later life. Churchill Livingstone, London

94. Basso O, Wilcox AJ, Weinberg CR (2006) Birth weight and mortality: causality or confounding? Am J Epidemiol 164:303–311

95. Schisterman EF, Hernandez-Diaz S (2006) Invited commentary: simple models for a complicated reality. Am J Epidemiol 164:312–314

96. Smith GD, Sterne J, Tynelius P, Lawlor DA, Rasmussen F (2005) Birth weight of offspring and subsequent cardiovascular mortality of the parents. Epidemiology 16:563–569

97. Andersen AM, Osler M (2004) Birth dimensions, parental mortality, and mortality in early adult age: a cohort study of Danish men born in 1953. Int J Epidemiol 33:92–99

98. Friedlander Y, Paltiel O, Manor O, Deutsch L, Yanetz R, Calderon-Margalit R, Siscovick DS, Harlap S (2007) Birthweight of offspring and mortality of parents: The Jerusalem Perinatal Study Cohort. Ann Epidemiol 17:914–922

99. Jaquet D, Swaminathan S, Alexander GR, Abajian C (2005) Significant paternal contribution to the risk of small for gestational age. BJOG 112:153–159

100. Clausson B, Lichtenstein P, Cnattingius S (2000) Genetic influence on birthweight and gestational length determined by studies in offspring of twins. BJOG 107:375–381

101. Svensson AC, Pawitan Y, Cnattingius S, Reilly M, Lichtenstein P (2006) Familial aggregation of small-for-gestational-age births: the importance of fetal genetic effects. Am J Obstet Gynecol 194:475–479

102. Ha JC, Ha RR, Almasy L, Dyke B (2002) Genetics and caging type affect birth weight in captive pigtailed macaques (*Macaca nemestrina*). Am J Primatol 56:207–213

103. Magnus P, Bakketeig LS, Hoffman H (1997) Birth weight of relatives by maternal tendency to repeat small-for-gestational-age (SGA) births in successive pregnancies. Acta Obstet Gynecol Scand Suppl 165:35–38

104. Klebanoff MA, Meirik O, Berendes HW (1989) Second-generation consequences of small-for-dates birth. Pediatrics 84:343–347

105. Wang X, Zuckerman B, Coffman GA, Corwin MJ (1995) Familial aggregation of low birth weight among whites and blacks in the United States. N Engl J Med 333(26):1744–1749

106. Strauss RS, Dietz WH (1998) Growth and development of term children born with low birth weight: effects of genetic and environmental factors. J Pediatr 133:67–72
107. Selling KE, Carstensen J, Finnstrom O, Sydsjo G (2006) Intergenerational effects of preterm birth and reduced intrauterine growth: a population-based study of Swedish mother-offspring pairs. BJOG 113:430–440
108. La Batide-Alanore A, Tregouet DA, Jaquet D, Bouyer J, Tiret L (2002) Familial aggregation of fetal growth restriction in a French cohort of 7,822 term births between 1971 and 1985. Am J Epidemiol 156:180–187
109. Eckhardt F, Lewin J, Cortese R, Rakyan VK, Attwood J, Burger M, Burton J, Cox TV, Davies R, Down TA, Haefliger C, Horton R, Howe K, Jackson DK, Kunde J, Koenig C, Liddle J, Niblett D, Otto T, Pettett R, Seemann S, Thompson C, West T, Rogers J, Olek A, Berlin K, Beck S (2006) DNA methylation profiling of human chromosomes 6, 20 and 22. Nat Genet 38:1378–1385
110. Rakyan VK, Hildmann T, Novik KL, Lewin J, Tost J, Cox AV, Andrews TD, Howe KL, Otto T, Olek A, Fischer J, Gut IG, Berlin K, Beck S (2004) DNA methylation profiling of the human major histocompatibility complex: a pilot study for the human epigenome project. PLoS Biol 2:e405
111. Song F, Smith JF, Kimura MT, Morrow AD, Matsuyama T, Nagase H, Held WA (2005) Association of tissue-specific differentially methylated regions (TDMs) with differential gene expression. Proc Natl Acad Sci USA 102:3336–3341
112. Enklaar T, Zabel BU, Prawitt D (2006) Beckwith–Wiedemann syndrome: multiple molecular mechanisms. Expert Rev Mol Med 8:1–19
113. Gicquel C, Rossignol S, Cabrol S, Houang M, Steunou V, Barbu V, Danton F, Thibaud N, Le Merrer M, Burglen L, Bertrand AM, Netchine I, Le Bouc Y (2005) Epimutation of the telomeric imprinting center region on chromosome 11p15 in Silver-Russell syndrome. Nat Genet 37(9):1003–1007
114. Bliek J, Terhal P, van den Bogaard MJ, Maas S, Hamel B, Salieb-Beugelaar G, Simon M, Letteboer T, van der Smagt J, Kroes H, Mannens M (2006) Hypomethylation of the *H19* gene causes not only Silver-Russell syndrome (SRS) but also isolated asymmetry or an SRS-like phenotype. Am J Hum Genet 78:604–614
115. Eggermann T, Schönherr N, Eggermann K, Buiting K, Ranke MB, Wollmann HA, Binder G (2008) Use of multiplex ligation-dependent probe amplification increases the detection rate for 11p15 epigenetic alterations in Silver-Russell syndrome. Clin Genet 73:79–84
116. Netchine I, Rossignol S, Dufourg MN, Azzi S, Rousseau A, Perin L, Houang M, Steunou V, Esteva B, Thibaud N, Demay MC, Danton F, Petriczko E, Bertrand AM, Heinrichs C, Carel JC, Loeuille GA, Pinto G, Jacquemont ML, Gicquel C, Cabrol S, Le Bouc Y (2007) 11p15 ICR1 loss of methylation is a common and specific cause of typical Russell-Silver syndrome: clinical scoring system and epigenetic-phenotypic correlations. J Clin Endocrinol Metab 92:3148–3154
117. Eggermann T, Eggermann K, Schonherr N (2008) Growth retardation versus overgrowth: Silver-Russell syndrome is genetically opposite to Beckwith-Wiedemann syndrome. Trends Genet 24:195–204
118. Murrell A, Heeson S, Cooper WN, Douglas E, Apostolidou S, Moore GE, Maher ER, Reik W (2004) An association between variants in the *IGF2* gene and Beckwith-Wiedemann syndrome: interaction between genotype and epigenotype. Hum Mol Genet 13:247–255
119. Heijmans BT, Kremer D, Tobi EW, Boomsma DI, Slagboom PE (2007) Heritable rather than age-related environmental and stochastic factors dominate variation in DNA methylation of the human *IGF2/H19* locus. Hum Mol Genet 16:547–554

120. Sandovici I, Leppert M, Hawk PR, Suarez A, Linares Y, Sapienza C (2003) Familial aggregation of abnormal methylation of parental alleles at the *IGF2/H19* and *IGF2R* differentially methylated regions. Hum Mol Genet 12:1569–1578

121. Einstein F, Thompson RF, Bhagat TD, Fazzari MJ, Verma A, Barzilai N, Greally JM (2010) Cytosine methylation dysregulation in neonates following intrauterine growth restriction. PLoS One 5:e8887

122. Yamagata K, Furuta H, Oda N, Kaisaki PJ, Menzel S, Cox NJ, Fajans SS, Signorini S, Stoffel M, Bell GI (1996) Mutations in the hepatocyte nuclear factor-4α gene in maturity-onset diabetes of the young (MODY1). Nature 384:458–460

123. Casper RS, Sullivan EL, Tecott L (2008) Relevance of animal models to human eating disorders and obesity. Psychopharmacology 199:0033–3158

124. Bocock PN, Aagaard-Tillery KM (2009) Animal models of epigenetic inheritance. Semin Reprod Med 27:369–379

125. Wu G, Bazer FW, Wallace JM, Spencer TE (2006) Intrauterine growth retardation: implications for the animal science. J Anim Sci 84:2316–2337

126. Taylor PD, Poston L (2006) Developmental programming of obesity in mammals. Exp Physiol 92:287–298

127. Barry JS, Anthony RV (2008) The pregnant sheep as a model for human pregnancy. Theriogenology 69:55–67

128. Friedman JM, Leibel RL, Siegel DS, Walsh J, Bahary N (1991) Molecular mapping of the mouse *ob* mutation. Genomics 11:1054–1062

129. Zhang Y, Proenca R, Maffei M, Barone M, Leopold L, Friedman JM (1994) Positional cloning of the mouse obese gene and its human homologue. Nature 372:425–432

130. Church C, Lee S, Bagg EA, McTaggart JS, Deacon R, Gerken T, Lee A, Moir L, Mecinović J, Quwailid MM, Schofield CJ, Ashcroft FM, Cox RD (2009) A mouse model for the metabolic effects of the human fat mass and obesity associated *FTO* gene. PLoS Genet 5:e1000599

131. Cohen P, Zhao C, Cai X, Montez JM, Rohani SC, Feinstein P, Mombaerts P, Friedman JM (2001) Selective deletion of leptin receptor in neurons leads to obesity. J Clin Invest 108:1113–1121

132. Surwit RS, Feinglos MN, Rodin J, Sutherland A, Petro AE, Opara EC, Kuhn CM, Rebuffe-Scrive M (1995) Differential effects of fat and sucrose on the development of obesity and diabetes in C57BL/6J and A/J mice. Metabolism 44:645–651

133. Tecott LH, Sun LM, Akana SF, Strack AM, Lowenstein DH, Dallman MF, Julius D (1995) Eating disorder and epilepsy in mice lacking 5-HT2c serotonin receptors. Nature 374:542–546

134. Miltenberger RJ, Mynatt RL, Wilkinson JE, Woychik RP (1997) The role of the agouti gene in the yellow obese syndrome. J Nutr 127:1902S–1907S

135. Salton SR, Hahm S, Mizuno TM (2000) Of mice and MEN: what transgenic models tell us about hypothalamic control of energy balance. Neuron 25:265–268

136. Huszar D, Lynch CA, Fairchild-Huntress V, Dunmore JH, Fang Q, Berkemeier LR, Gu W, Kesterson RA, Boston BA, Cone RD, Smith FJ, Campfield LA, Burn P, Lee F (1997) Targeted disruption of the melanocortin-4 receptor results in obesity in mice. Cell 88:131–141

137. Elmquist JK, Elias CF, Saper CB (1999) From lesions to leptin: hypothalamic control of food intake and body weight. Neuron 22:221–232

138. Schroeder M, Zagoory-Sharon O, Lavi-Avnon Y, Moran TH, Weller A (2006) Weight gain and maternal behavior in CCK1 deficient rats. Physiol Behav 89:402–409

139. Schroeder M, Shbiro L, Zagoory-Sharon O, Moran TH, Weller A (2009) Toward an animal model of childhood-onset obesity: follow-up of OLETF rats during pregnancy and lactation. Am J Physiol Regul Integr Comp Physiol 296:R224–R232

140. Alexander J, Chang GQ, Dourmashkin JT, Leibowitz SF (2006) Distinct phenotypes of obesity-prone AKR/J, DBA2J and C57BL/6J mice compared to control strains. Int J Obes (Lond) 30:50–59

141. Jimenez-Chillaron JC, Isganaitis E, Charalambous M, Gesta S, Pentinat-Pelegrin T, Faucette RR, Otis JP, Chow A, Diaz R, Ferguson-Smith A, Patti ME (2009) Intergenerational transmission of glucose intolerance and obesity by in utero undernutrition in mice. Diabetes 58:460–468

142. Jones HN, Woollett LA, Barbour N, Prasad PD, Powell TL, Jansson T (2009) High-fat diet before and during pregnancy causes marked up-regulation of placental nutrient transport and fetal overgrowth in C57/BL6 mice. FASEB J 23:271–278

143. Mueller BR, Bale TL (2006) Impact of prenatal stress on long term body weight is dependent on timing and maternal sensitivity. Physiol Behav 88:605–614

144. Levin BE (1999) Obesity-prone and -resistant rats differ in their brain [³H] paramino-clonidine binding. Brain Res 512:54–59

145. Srinivasan M, Katewa SD, Palaniyappan A, Pandya JD, Patel MS (2006) Maternal high-fat diet consumption results in fetal malprogramming predisposing to the onset of metabolic syndrome-like phenotype in adulthood. Am J Physiol Endocrinol Metab 291:E792–E799

146. Chang G-Q, Gaysinskaya V, Karatayev O, Leibowitz S-F (2008) Maternal high-fat diet and fetal programming: increased proliferation of hypothalamic peptide-producing neurons that increase risk for overeating and obesity. J Neurosci 28:12107–12119

147. Ericsson A, Säljö K, Sjöstrand E, Jansson N, Prasad PD, Powell TL, Jansson T (2007) Brief hyperglycaemia in the early pregnant rat increasing fetal weight at term by stimulating placental growth and affecting placental nutrient transport. J Physiol 581:1323–1332

148. Vickers MH, Breier BH, Cutfield WS, Hofman PL, Gluckman PD (2000) Fetal origins of hyperphagia, obesity, and hypertension and postnatal amplification by hypercaloric nutrition. Am J Physiol Endocrinol Metab 279:E83–E87

149. Gluckman PD, Lillycrop KA, Vickers MH, Pleasants AB, Phillips ES, Beedle AS, Burdge GC, Hanson MA (2007) Metabolic plasticity during mammalian development is directionally dependent on early nutritional status. Proc Natl Acad Sci USA 104:12796–12800

150. Morris TJ, Vickers M, Gluckman P, Gilmour S, Affara N (2009) Transcriptional profiling of rats subjected to gestational undernourishment: implications for the developmental variations in metabolic traits. PLoS One 4:e7271

151. Pinheiro AR, Salvucci ID, Aguila MB, Mandarim-de-Lacerda CA (2008) Protein restriction during gestation and/or lactation causes adverse transgenerational effects on biometry and glucose metabolism in F1 and F2 progenies of rats. Clin Sci (Lond) 114:381–392

152. Zambrano E, Bautista CJ, Deás M, Martínez-Samayoa PM, González-Zamorano M, Ledesma H, Morales J, Larrea F, Nathanielsz PW (2006) A low maternal protein diet during pregnancy and lactation has sex- and window of exposure-specific effects on offspring growth and food intake, glucose metabolism and serum leptin in the rat. J Physiol 15:221–230

153. Drake AJ, Walker BR, Seckl JR (2005) Intergenerational consequences of fetal programming by in utero exposure to glucocorticoids in rats. Am J Physiol Regul Integr Comp Physiol 288:R34–R38

154. Korotkova M, Gabrielsson BG, Holmäng A, Larsson B-M, Hanson LÅ, Strandvik B (2005) Gender-related long-term effects in adult rats by perinatal dietary ratio of n-6/n-3 fatty acids. Am J Physiol Regul Integr Physiol 288:R575–R579

155. Franko KL, Forhead AJ, Fowden AL (2010) Differential effects of prenatal stress and glucocorticoid administration on postnatal growth and glucose metabolism in rats. J Endocrinol 204:319–329

156. Ford SP, Hess BW, Schwope MM, Nijland MJ, Gilbert JS, Vonnahme KA, Means WJ, Han H, Nathanielsz PW (2007) Maternal undernutrition during early to mid-gestation in the ewe results in altered growth, adiposity, and glucose tolerance in male offspring. J Anim Sci 85:1285–1294

157. Costine BA, Inskeep EK, Wilson ME (2005) Growth hormone at breeding modifies conceptus development and postnatal growth in sheep. J Anim Sci 83:810–815

158. Smith NA, McAuliffe FM, Quinn K, Lonergan P, Evansa ACO (2009) Transient high glycaemic intake in the last trimester of pregnancy increases offspring birthweight and postnatal growth rate in sheep: a randomised control trial. BJOG 116:975–983

159. Campion DR, Hausman GJ, Stone RT, Klindt J (1988) Influence of maternal obesity on fetal development in pigs. J Anim Sci 66:28–33

160. Kind KL, Clifton PM, Grant PA, Owens PC, Sohlstrom A, Robinson RCT, JS OJA (2003) Effect of maternal feed restriction during pregnancy on glucose tolerance in the adult guinea pig. Am J Physiol Regul Integr Comp Physiol 284:R140–R152

161. Sullivan TM, Micke GC, Perkins N, Martin GB, Wallace CR, Gatford KL, Owens JA, Perry VEA (2009) Dietary protein during gestation affects maternal insulin-like growth factor insulin-like growth factor binding protein, leptin concentrations, and fetal growth in heifers. J Anim Sci 87:3304–3316

162. Génin F, Perret M (2000) Photoperiod-induced changes in energy balance in gray mouse lemurs. Physiol Behav 71:315–321

163. Farley D, Tejero ME, Comuzzie AG, Higgins PB, Cox L, Werner SL, Jenkins SL, Li C, Choi J, Dick EJ Jr, Hubbard GB, Frost P, Dudley DJ, Ballesteros B, Wu G, Nathanielsz PW, Schlabritz-Loutsevitch NE (2009) Feto-placental adaptations to maternal obesity in the baboon. Placenta 30:752–760

164. Sullivan EL, Koegler FH, Cameron JL (2006) Individual differences in physical activity are closely associated with changes in body weight in adult female rhesus monkeys (*Macaca mulatta*). Am J Physiol Regul Integr Comp Physiol 291:R633–R642

3   β-Cell Growth Mechanisms

Thomas L. Jetton, Dhananjay Gupta, and Mina Peshavaria

Key Points

- Specific pathways continue to emerge, which regulate beta-cell differentiation and growth.
- Possible therapeutic targets are under intense study as part of broader strategies to develop replenishable sources of endocrine cells.

Keywords: β-Cell, Growth factor, Adaptation, Insulin signaling, Pathway

Abbreviations

Akt	Akt/PKB (protein kinase B)
AMPK	cAMP-activated protein kinase
BCM	β-cell mass
CREB	cAMP response element binding protein
EGFR	Epidermal growth factor receptor
GIPR	Glucose-dependent insulinotropic peptide receptor
GLP-1R	Glucagon-like peptide-1 receptor
GPCR	G-protein-coupled receptor
IGF-1R	Insulin-like growth factor-1 receptor
IR	Insulin receptor
Irs2	Insulin receptor substrate-2
mTOR	Mammalian target of rapamycin

From: *Nutrition and Health: Management of Pediatric Obesity and Diabetes*,
Edited by: R.J. Ferry, Jr., DOI 10.1007/978-1-60327-256-8_3,
© Springer Science+Business Media, LLC 2011

Pdx1   Pancreatic/duodenal homeobox-1
PI3K   Phosphoinositide-3-kinase
ZF   Zucker fatty rat
ZDF   Zucker diabetic fatty rat

3.1   INTRODUCTION

3.1.1   *β-Cell Mass Maintenance: A Dynamic Balance of Several Parameters*

From what we have learned from rodent models over the years, the steady state β-cell mass (BCM) is determined by a balance of several factors [1] (Fig. 3.1). These include mechanisms to increase net β-cell growth: proliferation of existing β-cells, new cell development from progenitors (neogenesis), and individual cell growth. Equally important to BCM homeostasis are the processes that reduce mass that include cell death (primarily apoptosis) and clearance (by phagocytosis), and individual cell shrinkage (hypotrophy). In mice, proliferation apparently occurs randomly in the β-cell population; therefore, β-cells of a particular islet are at different ages, but most are at least several months old [2, 3]. β-cells of an individual islet are not necessarily clones [4], but are aggregates of clonal cells. Most β-cells in the adult pancreas are "quiescent" with respect to the cell cycle (G_0, in interphase), but remain highly active by synthesizing and secreting insulin. A few β-cells enter the cell cycle and

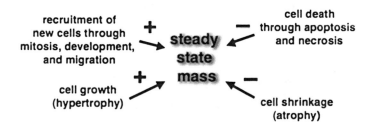

Fig. 3.1. Steady state β-cell mass is controlled by several factors.

may divide, while others are fated to undergo senescence and apoptosis. A constant balance of β-cell proliferation, neogenesis, individual cell growth, and death and clearance is vital to sustain normal BCM and maintain blood glucose homeostasis based on the prevailing insulin requirements of the body.

A comprehensive picture of the physiological regulation of BCM is not yet available and reflects the complexity and evolution of glucose homeostatic control. Although a myriad of factors are known to influence β-cell growth, the prime signaling pathway in the β-cell that mediates growth and survival is thought to be the core insulin-signaling cascade involving insulin receptor substrate-2 (Irs2), PI3-kinase, Akt, and several downstream targets of Akt. Unfortunately, a definitive scheme of the physiological integration of hormonal, growth factor, nutrient, and neural pathways of BCM regulation will be several years away.

3.2   MEASURING β-CELL GROWTH PARAMETERS

3.2.1   β- Cell Mass

BCM is not an actual weight of the islet β-cells, but a useful index derived from morphometric methods that serves as the standard for comparing relative β-cell accumulation in animal models [1, 5] and humans [6, 7]. These values are based on the product of the total mass or volume of the pancreas (therefore generally requiring necropsied pancreas, or computed tomography in humans) and the relative β-cell fractional volume, or the proportional microscopic surface area in histologic sections of the insulin immunostained area over the total pancreas area. This entails point-counting morphometry [8, 9], or a derivative known as volume-weighted mean islet volume [10], or computer-based planimetric measurements [11]. A less powerful, but popular surrogate, measurement for BCM is fractional β-cell surface area (relative β-cell volume). However, this approach is limited due to the fact that many animal models of β-cell growth exhibit changes in total pancreas mass that necessarily impact BCM values. Since islets are not equally distributed throughout the pancreas, multiple sections at regular intervals throughout the pancreas must be screened to obtain accurate, unbiased morphometric data.

3.2.2   Proliferation

Proliferation, or cell division, is by far the best-studied β-cell growth parameter and is widely considered to play the predominant role in postnatal β-cell growth [12, 13]. β-cell mitosis is more active in the first couple of weeks of life and progressively wanes thereafter [5]. β-cells are recognized as being a tissue with slow turnover, so generally >1,000 β-cells must be counted on histologic sections for meaningful proliferation rates or frequencies. Traditionally, labeled thymidine analogs (*e.g.*, bromodeoxyuridine, BrdU) are used to trace DNA synthesis ("S" phase) by *in vivo* pulse/chasing followed by tissue fixation and BrdU immunohistochemistry and insulin costaining. Rates of DNA synthesis (via uridine incorporation) can be calculated based on the pulse duration, but these values do not always correlate with genuine cell proliferation and, therefore, are prone to overestimation. Alternatively, β-cell proliferation frequency is often measured using immunohistochemistry probing for specific cell cycle-specific nuclear antigens such as Ki-67, PCNA, or phospho-histone 3.

3.2.3   Neogenesis

β-cell neogenesis is the differentiation of β-cells from non-β cell pancreatic sources, usually exocrine tissue [14, 15]. This process is generally thought to be most active in the late fetal stage through the first few weeks of life in rodents [1]. The physiological impact of neogenesis in physiological adaptation has been challenged in mice [12, 16, 17]. However, in rats [18–20], pigs [21], and humans [6, 22], β-cell adaptive growth contributed by neogenesis may be substantial. Past studies have indirectly calculated the contribution of neogenesis using a mathematical formula based on BCM and the proliferation rate [23]. More commonly, neogenesis frequency can be estimated by counting β-cell clusters below a certain arbitrary size or cell number in histologic sections. These clusters are often associated with ducts of all sizes but can be embedded in acini as well [11, 20, 24]. There is no universal agreement as to the distinction between β-cell clusters (*presumably* newly formed) and very small islets. Furthermore, the functional capacity of these small clusters *in vivo* is not known, as they have largely evaded biochemical characterization due to their difficulty in isolation and purification. Clusters and small islets can be measured and ranked according to their surface area using computer-based morphometry to gain insight into potential trends of new β-cell development [20, 25]. Importantly, although the contribution of small β-cell clusters to the total BCM in the adult rodent is miniscule, a transient surge in the prevalence of these clusters suggests that neogenesis contributes to adaptive β-cell growth. However, it must be emphasized that the presence or increased frequency of these clusters does not *prove* neogenesis. Definitive evidence for whether single β-cells and small clusters contribute to larger islets, or rather persist as small clusters, awaits lineage marking strategies in tissue explants *ex vivo* with real-time imaging capabilities.

3.2.4 β-Cell Size

Individual β-cell growth, or hypertrophy, is a well-established means of increasing BCM [1]. Past studies have coarsely estimated changes in β-cell size based on the quotient of total β-cell surface area of a given islet divided by the number of β-cell nuclei. Although flow cytometric methods exist for cell size/volume analyses [26], a more convenient method is to measure the average individual β-cell surface area in several islets in confocal microscope-imaged histologic sections of pancreas using β-cell membrane immunostaining (*i.e.*, GLUT2, β-catenin, pan-cadherin) in conjunction with insulin costaining. Geometric considerations dictate that average β-cell surface area values alone underestimate actual β-cell size when cell volumes are considered.

3.2.5 β-Cell Death and Clearance

β-cell death entails both apoptosis and necrosis, comprising the prime mechanism for normal β-cell turnover, but also loss of BCM during progressive diabetes. Similar to the calculations for neogenesis, a formula has also been devised to estimate the contribution of β-cell loss [23]. A range of biochemical, immunological, and molecular biology methods are used to detect β-cell death. Common *in situ* methods for microscopic sections to detect apoptosis, the most prevalent mechanism of β-cell death, include the "TUNEL" assay, activated (cleaved) caspase-3 immunostaining, and a host of DNA-binding dyes to visualize nuclear apoptotic bodies such as hematoxylin, propidium iodide, and Hoechst/DAPI. In adult rodent models of β-cell growth, direct detection of apoptotic cells is rare; therefore, useful measurements of apoptotic frequencies generally require analysis of several thousand β-cells or flow cytometric analysis. This pitfall in the *in vivo* detection is likely due to efficient scavenging of apoptotic bodies in islets [27]. A more useful approach has been to address apoptosis in these models in terms of survival or apoptosis potential based on the preponderance of the expression and activity of prosurvival or proapoptotic molecules.

3.3 β-CELL MASS COMPENSATION

The pancreatic β-cell in rodents has a tremendous capacity to compensate in response to physiological and pathophysiological changes in tissue insulin demands. A key feature of these adaptive responses is the ability of the BCM to be dynamically regulated by altering the balance of the aforementioned factors. For instance, BCM is normally maintained proportional to body size [28]. It increases during obesity and pregnancy [1, 23, 27] and regresses in the mother postpartum [27] to adjust to the decreased insulin requirements. In animal models, the relative importance of β-cell proliferation, neogenesis, and individual cell growth likely depends on the physiological mechanism underlying the increased insulin demands, or the particular experimental conditions provoking the β-cell growth response. An important limitation in many of these studies is the reliance on relatively young adult animal models with enhanced regenerative capacity that may not reflect the patterns in older individuals.

3.3.1   Impact of Proliferation vs. Neogenesis

In humans, the contribution of β-cell proliferation *vs.* nonproliferative growth mechanisms is unknown [7]. However, several recent studies in both genetically "normal" and genetically manipulated mouse models suggest that proliferation from preexisting β cells is the predominant β-cell growth mechanism in the adult [12, 13, 16]. In fact, the process of postnatal islet neogenesis has become a controversial subject due to reports in adult mice questioning its occurrence, the lack of a consensus on the identity of the progenitor cell(s), and its elusive physiological impact. Furthermore, the presence of small endocrine cell clusters alone does not prove their nascence. However, their heightened prevalence, such as their transient increased frequency following an experimental growth stimulus (Fig. 3.2), does suggest a role in islet formation and adaptive β-cell growth. Importantly,

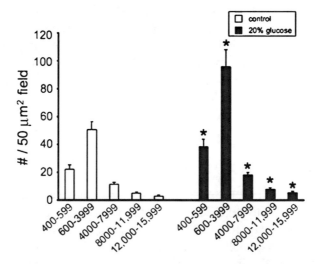

Fig. 3.2. β-cell cluster analysis in 48 h normoglycemic glucose-infused rats. Significant increases (*; $P<0.01$) in the prevalence of all size categories were observed. Size classes in μm^2. Entire range was ~23–143 μm^2 diameter (adapted from Jetton *et al.* [20]).

there are histological indications that the process occurs in adult humans by the presence of small β-cell clusters [19], even in elderly type 1 diabetes patients [29, 30]. It has been estimated that these clusters may constitute as much as 15–20% of the BCM humans [22]. In various rodent models of adaptive β-cell growth and regeneration, neogenesis may contribute substantially to the enhanced BCM [20, 25]. Surprisingly, chronically glucose-infused rats exhibit significantly enhanced BCM without any detectable increases in β-cell proliferation [20, 24, 31]. Although the actual source of the progenitors and the physiological impact of neogenesis in the adult pancreas awaits further scrutiny by careful cell lineage tracing analyses (see below), neogenesis and proliferation most probably occur in sequence since the growth of β-cell clusters into islets would necessarily entail proliferation, but this has not been directly demonstrated. In fact, proliferation of single β-cells and the smallest β-cell clusters in Sprague-Dawley rats [20] and C57Bl6 mice (Jetton and Peshavaria, unpublished) are rare. In adult mice, β-cells of small islets apparently proliferate at the same slow rate as those of bigger islets [2].

3.3.2 Importance of Neogenesis During Development

The environmental and nutritional status of the mother can play roles in diabetes susceptibility later in life and can manifest as reduced BCM and *Pdx-1* expression that leads to reduced proliferation and/or neogenesis (reviewed by [32]). Paradoxically, it has also been reported that undernutrition in the last few days of gestation in rats stimulates an increased BCM as the result of enhanced insulin-like growth factor-1 receptor (IGF1R) and Irs2 signaling [33]. Islet cluster proliferation and β-cell maturation during fetal and neonatal life in mice are dependent on β-cell *PERK* expression, a key protein of the unfolded protein response [34], but whether it has similar functions in adult β-cell neogenesis is unknown. The well-studied Goto-Kakizaki rat exhibits a heritable form of diabetes that is, in part, caused by reduced β-cell number due to decreased neogenesis in the fetal period [35]. Hence, perturbed fetal and neonatal neogenesis can predispose an individual to diabetes.

A useful consideration in studies of β-cell differentiation in the postnatal animal has been to address the extent to which the pancreatic endocrine cell developmental pathway recapitulates the well-described pattern during embryogenesis. The basic plan of pancreatogenesis entails a sort of branching morphogenesis of dividing duct-like epithelial cells that express high levels of the key pancreas-specific transcription factor pancreatic/duodenal homeobox-1 (*Pdx1*) [36]. Subsequently, a subpopulation of Pdx1+ cells expresses insulin and other islet hormones while Pdx1 levels progressively decrease in cells of the developing ducts and acini. The complex ontogeny of the islet endocrine cells is well elucidated, and involves a hierarchal sequence of the expression of key transcription factors in Pdx1+ epithelial precursors (reviewed by [37, 38]). This primal pattern appears to be partially reiterated following certain regeneration stimuli in adult animals including the well-studied 90% partial pancreatectomy (Px) rat model [18] where transient ductal proliferation was followed by strong Pdx1 expression in those same cells [39], although it is not clear how many of the Pdx1+ cells differentiate into endocrine cells and assemble into definitive islets. A compelling study using cell lineage tracing [40] has employed engineered mice subjected to a regeneration/injury stimulus by a partial pancreatic duct ligation, which demonstrated the activation of duct-borne neurogenin-3 (Ngn3)+ precursors cells. Significantly, Ngn3, a neuroendocrine transcription factor required for the establishment of all endocrine cell lineages during embryogenesis [41], is also essential for the neogenesis-driven BCM increase in this model [40]. Conversely, it has also been reported that *Ngn3* expression was not reinstated during β-cell regeneration in mice due to injury following a 50% Px [42]. In glucose-infused rats whereby normoglycemia was maintained, increased expression of factors Pax6 and Pdx1 was observed among the duct epithelium that correlated with significant increases in the numbers of endocrine cell clusters [20]. Using a conditional gene knockout strategy whereby inactivation can be precisely controlled in adult mice, Holland *et al.* [43] determined that Pdx1 is essential for maintaining BCM and for driving β-cell regeneration from the duct epithelium. Hence, new β-cell development in the adult rodent entails the expression of some of the key developmental transcription factors important for β-cell differentiation from exocrine-borne precursors.

3.3.3   Impact of Individual β-Cell Growth and Enhanced Survival

β-cell growth by hypertrophy is a well-recognized mechanism contributing to BCM during regeneration following Px [1, 5], following substrate oversupply by glucose infusion [20, 43], and in response to prolonged insulin resistance [1, 11]. Transgenic/knockout mouse models also demonstrate enhanced β-cell size due to Akt1 overexpression [44] as well as a leptin receptor deficiency [45], whereas a global p70$^{S6\text{-kinase1}}$ gene inactivation leads to significantly smaller β-cells [46] as does its respective target ribosomal protein S6 [47].

Due to the difficulty in detecting apoptotic cells *in vivo* in β-cell growth models, many studies have correlated the increased expression or activity of prosurvival factors with the downregulation of genes with proapoptotic roles and their decreased activity. Several of these factors are components in the insulin-signaling pathway, substrates of Akt/PKB, and members of the *Bcl2* gene family (see below). Since individual cell growth and control of apoptosis are inextricably linked to cell cycle regulation and nutrient availability, it is presently not feasible to determine the contribution of cell size and survival potential to BCM in currently available animal models.

3.4 REGULATION OF β-CELL GROWTH: THE IMPORTANCE OF THE INSULIN SIGNALING PATHWAY

3.4.1 The Key Players

The preponderance of data thus far strongly suggests that the core components of the insulin-signaling pathway play pivotal roles in the regulation of BCM by controlling proliferation, cell growth, survival, and differentiation (Fig. 3.3). Impinging on this central pathway are signaling inputs from gluco-incretins, nutrients, the CNS, and modulation by a host of other hormonal and growth factor signaling cascades. Of the three known insulin receptor-family tyrosine kinases on the surfaces of adult β-cells—insulin receptor [48–51], insulin receptor-related receptor [52], and IGF receptors [53]—the insulin receptor is most crucial in mediating β-cell compensatory growth and proliferation [54].

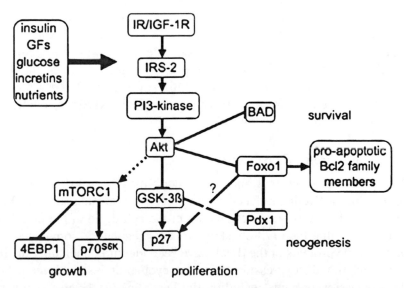

Fig. 3.3. Core β-cell insulin signaling components governing β-cell growth and survival. Stimulation through IRS-2 leads to increased Akt activity and subsequent activation (↓) or inhibition (⊥) of several key downstream targets that mediate increased β-cell size, increased proliferation, increased neogenesis, and enhanced survival.

Signaling through the IGF-1R, especially at the level of the pancreatic ducts, may be important as well [55]. Landmark studies of both a single gene (*irs2*) [56] and double gene-knockout mice (*irs2* and *igf-1r*) [55], investigating the impact of the insulin-signaling cascade, have identified a critical role for Irs2 in compensatory β-cell expansion. The double mutant develops insulin resistance and severe diabetes due to a deficient β-cell growth response. It has been established that the cAMP response element binding protein (CREB) in β-cells controls *irs2* transcription and β-cell survival [57]. Irs2 protein levels are dynamically regulated in the β-cell [58], suggesting that signaling flux through this molecule is integral for adjusting BCM. Irs2 also mediates the BCM effects of glucoincretin signaling [59]. Accordingly, the glucagon-like peptide-1 receptor (GLP-1R) agonist exendin-4 improves β-cell function, growth, and survival through enhanced insulin-signaling [60] (see below). A strong functional link between Irs2 and Pdx1 has been demonstrated by transgenic overexpression of Pdx1 that can normalize islet mass and function in *irs2* knockout mice [61]. It appears that the functional connection between adaptive β-cell growth and this signaling cascade likely involves the interaction of factors controlling *pdx1* transcription with the forkhead transcription factor Foxo1 [62]. This may involve competition of Foxo1 with binding sites for Foxa2 on the *Pdx1* promoter.

The core insulin-signaling intermediates, PI3-kinase [63, 64] and Akt [65], have been implicated in regulating β-cell proliferation through IGF1R stimulation, although they can also function in other growth factor cascades to mediate a variety of biological functions. Transgenic overexpression of activated Akt in β-cells results in increased islet mass, and enhanced β-cell survival and hypertrophy [44, 66], with p70[S6-kinase1] playing an essential role in compensatory β-cell size modulation [46]. A β-cell Akt2 knockout study established that this isoform is likely the principal Akt-kinase controlling BCM compensation and survival [67].

3.4.2   Regulation of Proliferation

β-cell turnover in normal middle age adult mice [2] and humans [7] is extremely low, reflecting reduced rates of proliferation and apoptosis. From a consensus of studies on the regulation of the cell cycle of the β-cell [68, 69], it appears that the G_1/S checkpoint exerts regulatory dominance. The chief cell cycle proteins of the β-cell have been identified including the E2F factors regulating the expression of key cell cycle proteins, the principal cell cycle progression proteins including the D-cyclins (especially cyclin D2) [12, 70], cyclin-dependent kinase-4 [71–73], pRb (retinoblastoma protein) [74, 75], the tumor suppressor p53, and the CIP/KIP class of cdk inhibitors (especially p21Cip and p27Kip1 [72, 76–82]).

As evidenced from numerous recent studies in transgenic and gene knockout mice (PTEN [83, 84] and many others), PI3-kinase/Akt signaling in β-cells plays pivotal roles in cell cycle regulation, but key downstream molecules and the nature of their interplay are still being defined. Whereas the insulin signaling pathway in mice regulates β-cell proliferation by the activation of cdk4, cyclins D1 and D2, and p21 [72], the latter protein, regarded as a cell cycle inhibitor, is paradoxically increased in β-cells by the mitogens HGF, lactogenic hormones, and PTHrP [69]. Cyclin D levels are controlled by the GSK3β-ubiquitin-proteosomal degradation pathway, and are increased upon insulin/growth factor stimulation due to enhanced Akt signaling and the corresponding inhibition of GSK3β activity [85]. Both p21 and p27 have complex roles in cell cycle regulation in general as they also can function as nuclear chaperones, promote cdk-cyclin binding, and are direct targets of Akt kinase [85]. Whether they perform these other functions in β-cells remains to be clarified.

The cell cycle inhibitor p27 maintains control of β-cell proliferation in mice under metabolic stress but also appears to play a major role during the increased β-cell proliferation observed during fetal development and the neonatal period [80, 81]. The importance of p27 in the β-cell is underscored by its tight regulation at several levels. Whereas p27 transcription is controlled by Foxo1 in non-β-cells [86], the transcriptional regulator menin governs the expression of β-cell p27 epigenetically during pregnancy and gestational diabetes [87]. Regulation of p27 protein levels by the SCF ubiquitin ligase complex component, Skp2, is crucial for compensatory β-cell growth [82]. In turn, Skp2 gene expression may be positively regulated by PI3-kinase/Akt signaling [85]. p27 can also be regulated by nuclear to cytoplasmic translocation in the rapidly growing β-cells of young insulin-resistant Zucker rat (Fig. 3.4) (Jetton and Peshavaria, unpublished observations). Hence, multilevel regulation of β-cell p27 is likely critical for cell cycle progression and proliferation in response to growth factor, nutrient, and metabolic stimuli.

3.4.3   Regulation of Neogenesis

Whereas a range of growth factors, hormones, and nutrients stimulate β-cell proliferation, little is known of the factors that may specifically induce neogenesis. This is largely due to the fact that enhanced proliferation of pre-existing β-cells is nearly universal and dominates in adult β-cell growth models. However, chronic vascular infusion studies in normal rats, but not mice [88], shed some insight into factors contributing to new β-cell differentiation in the adult. Insulin infusion in rats under euglycemic conditions is reported to stimulate new β-cell generation from exocrine tissue [89].

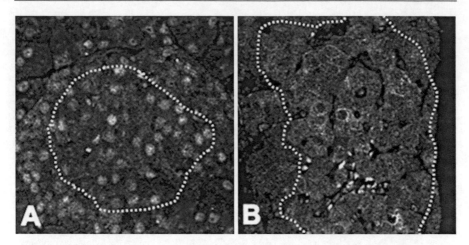

Fig. 3.4. P27^{kip1} localization in representative islet β-cells from young Zucker rats. (**a**) 28-day-old Zucker lean. (**b**) 28-day-old Zucker fatty. β-cell area is designated by *dashed line*. Note the striking difference in the localization patterns of p27^{kip1}, which likely correlates with their observed proliferation differences.

Glucose infusions under both hyperglycemic/hyperinsulinemic conditions [24, 31, 90] and euglycemic/transiently hyperinsulinemic conditions [20] exhibit an increased frequency of β-cell clusters and small islets. In the euglycemic Zucker fatty (ZF) rats, enhanced β-cell neogenesis commences following the onset of lifelong hyperinsulinemia in the postweaning period and is maintained throughout adulthood [11]. Hence, the primary neogenic stimulus for each of these models appears to be heightened plasma insulin levels. Since neogenesis in these rat models appears to occur randomly in exocrine pancreas originating from the duct epithelium, acini, and even the centroacinar region, it would seem that the β-cell progenitors in this model are likely scattered throughout the pancreas. However, the precise identity of the endocrine precursors is unknown. Whether these progenitors may be equally developmentally competent and thus rely on paracrine signals or, instead, might be specialized insulin and/or glucose sensitive cells remains to be elucidated. The latter contention is supported by observations in rats [11, 20, 91] and mice [25] under β-cell growth stimulating conditions where high concentrations of activated (phosphorylated Akt) have been localized to specific islet hormone-negative cells among the exocrine tissue. Furthermore, strong nuclear Pdx1 immunoreactivity is observed in these same cells suggesting a role for Akt signaling in Pdx1 expression and their maturation into functional β-cells. Recent findings highlight the role of the insulin-signaling pathway not only in the regulation of *pdx1* expression (by Foxo1) but also by controlling Pdx1 protein stability. The Akt target GSK3β has been demonstrated to phosphorylate Pdx1, marking it for proteasomal degradation [92, 93]. Hence, GSK3β plays an important role in BCM regulation and function (see below).

It is conceivable that glucose and its metabolism may provide signals for new β-cell development. It has recently been shown [94] that glucose signaling via the β-cell glucose sensor glucokinase and Irs2 are required for BCM adaptation to metabolic stress in mice. Although the glucose effects were thought to manifest through enhanced β-cell proliferation, the potential influence of this sort of glucose signaling on neogenesis is not known. Nonetheless, the β-cell isoform of glucokinase is expressed in certain rare pancreatic duct cells in mice that are islet hormone-negative [95] and lack Pdx1 expression [96]. In the duct epithelium of rodents following a 60% Px [91] as well in glucose-infused rats [20], Irs2 and activated Akt levels are consistently increased, and both models exhibit significantly enhanced neogenesis. Thus, glucokinase might have a role in endocrine cell differentiation from ducts. Future studies are warranted to resolve whether nutrient signaling, such as that mediated by "β-cell glucokinase" [97], may play a role in new β-cell development.

3.4.4 Cell Growth

Individual β-cell growth has been widely studied and involves integration of nutrient (glucose and amino acids), glucoincretin, and growth factor signals by mammalian target of rapamycin (mTOR), in turn, increasing protein synthesis [98–100]. As in other cell types, β-cell growth in response to growth factor stimulation is mediated by the PI3-kinase/Akt module that, in turn, regulates mTOR activity, with p70[S6-kinase] and 4EBP1 (the eIF4E binding protein) as terminal intermediates promoting mRNA translation. These molecules are important not only for increasing β-cell volume and insulin secretion potential but also indispensable for synthesizing the cell cycle proteins necessary for cycle entry and progression and, thus, proliferation.

3.4.5 Cell Survival

The contribution of the integrated mechanisms that counter apoptosis toward BCM maintenance and growth are probably underestimated due to inherent β-cell heterogeneity and the pitfalls in detecting cell death *in situ*. Furthermore, as alluded to previously, apoptosis is tightly linked to cell cycle regulation, and rapidly dividing cells appear to be vulnerable to apoptotic death. The PI3-kinase/Irs2/Akt pathway performs a pivotal role in mediating the balance between β-cell survival and apoptosis with integration of glucoincretin, nutrient, and growth factor signaling modules. The essential mediators of mitochondrial-driven apoptosis are members of the Bcl2 family whose expression and activity are controlled by Akt. A principal direct target of Akt in the β-cell is the proapoptotic factor BAD [101] whose action is inhibited by Akt phosphorylation [102]. Hence, in models of β-cell growth, BAD gene expression levels are reduced [20] and phosphorylated BAD is increased [11]. BAD reversibly associates with Bcl2, a principal prosurvival factor that is upregulated during β-cell growth [11]. However, BAD appears to have roles in the β-cell other than apoptosis since it can reversibly complex with glucokinase [103] and thus affects β-cell function. Bcl2 levels in β-cell may also be regulated by Akt in a CREB-dependent manner similar to what has been reported in neurons [104]. The related proapoptotic protein, BAX, is negatively regulated by CREB/Irs2/PI3-kinase/Akt signaling via its inhibition of the transcriptional regulator, Foxo1 [105]. Although caspases can be direct targets of Akt, their potential regulation by the insulin-signaling pathway in the β-cell is obscure. Caspase 8 has recently been found to mediate β-cell apoptosis in mouse models of type 1 and type 2 diabetes, but it also has an important, but undefined role in normal BCM maintenance, possibly even countering apoptosis, where it integrates with CREB/Irs2/PI3-kinase/Akt pathway [106]. Increased β-cell CREB activity through G-protein-coupled receptor (GPCR)-incretin activation (GLP-1R and glucose-dependent insulinotropic peptide receptor [GIPR]), and its subsequent signaling through the Irs2/Akt system, appears to be a major pathway for enhancing β-cell survival. Inhibition of Foxo1 activity by Akt signaling in the β-cell leads to growth and survival. Accordingly, the Foxo1 target and critical β-cell factor Pdx1 has also been ascribed roles in countering apoptosis [107].

3.5 FURTHER FINE-TUNING β-CELL GROWTH AND SURVIVAL

3.5.1 The Role of Glucoincretins

The intestinal glucoincretins, GLP-1 and GIP, are secreted in response to nutrient ingestion and play essential roles in energy metabolism and modulating BCM [60]. Studies of incretin receptor knockout mice and the use of pharmacological agents have demonstrated that the glucoincretins augment insulin secretion, lower blood glucose levels, and regulate satiety, gastric emptying and body weight [108–115]. Importantly, GLP-1 secretion and GIP action are impaired in diabetic patients suggesting roles in the pathogenesis of the disease [116].

A growing consensus affirms that GLP-1 enhances BCM through growth, proliferation, neogenesis, and survival mechanisms [57, 59, 64, 117–120]. In several diabetic rodent models, BCM was augmented by GLP-1 and GLP-1R agonists [121–123]. In the 90% Px and the neonatal STZ rat models, the GLP-1R agonist exendin-4 enhanced BCM through increased β-cell proliferation and neogenesis [124–126]. GIPR may also play a role in BCM regulation [104, 105]. Whereas adult Zucker diabetic fatty rats (ZDFs) exhibited impaired β-cell GIPR signaling [105, 127], post-weaning normoglycemic/hyperinsulinemic ZF rats exhibit increased β-cell GIPR levels correlating with enhanced β-cell growth (Jetton and Peshavaria, unpublished data).

GLP-1 enhances β-cell growth mechanisms through multiple pathways that intersect with the PI3K/Irs-2/Akt pathway [60, 118]. Through transactivation of epidermal growth factor receptor (EGFR), GLP-1R agonists stimulate β-cell proliferation and growth through PI3-kinase concomitant with Akt and/or PKCζ activation [120, 128]. In this network, activation of cAMP/PKA, phosphoinositide-3-kinase (PI3K), and MAPK pathways are also elicited [60, 118]. Key terminal effects of these GLP-1R pathways appear to be mediated via Pdx1 induction [64, 129–132] and Foxo1 inhibition [119]. Accordingly, GLP-1R activation from exendin-4 treatment in β-cell *pdx1*⁻/⁻ mice was unable to promote β-cell proliferation and inhibit apoptosis [133]. Like IR/IGF-1R signaling, incretin receptor signaling converges on Akt and stimulates β-cell growth and proliferation by the suppression of Foxo1 activity through its nuclear exclusion, in turn, increasing Pdx1 and Foxa2 levels [62, 119]. Similarly, GIP also mediates β-cell survival through Foxo1 inactivation and decreased BAX levels [105, 134].

β-cell survival effects of GLP-1R activity are also mediated through the activation of cAMP/PKA and CREB phosphorylation leading to increased Irs2 levels and Akt activation [57]. In general, this signaling pathway appears to result in attenuated levels of the proapoptotic factors caspase-3 and thioredoxin-interacting protein, but enhanced levels of survival factors Bcl2, Bcl$_{xL}$, and NFκB [135]. Exendin-4 functions to curtail ER-associated β-cell death by inducing ATF-4 levels in a PKA-dependent manner, promoting β-cell survival [134].

3.5.2 Nutrient and Glucose Signaling Pathways Regulating β-Cell Growth

The most widely studied nutrient affecting β-cell growth, proliferation, and function is glucose. Among the different islet cell types, it is principally the β-cells that undergo accelerated replication in response to hyperglycemia. Although it is firmly established that glucose can stimulate β-cell proliferation *in vitro*, the importance of glucose as a regulator of BCM was first suggested by the observation that hyperglycemic rats infused with glucose for 4 days developed an increased BCM [9]. Although this was attributed to β-cell proliferation and hypertrophy, a milder glucose infusion that maintained normoglycemia resulted in no detectable change in proliferation, despite an increase in BCM in the initial 48 h period largely due to enhanced neogenesis [20]. Furthermore, new β-cell development in this model correlated with enhanced Akt signaling activity and Pdx-1 expression [20]. By contrast, glucose-infused mice with a comparable glucose dosage exhibit a several-fold increase in β-cell proliferation, despite no observed changes in neogenic potential or BCM [88]. Thus, although the effects of parenteral glucose on β-cell growth could be species-specific, more studies are needed to resolve these unanticipated disparities.

Glucose-mediated Irs2/PI3K/Akt signaling is a key determinant of enhanced β-cell growth and survival [136–139] and BCM expansion in response to insulin resistance [94]. Mice haplodeficient for glucokinase have a normal BCM under a regular chow diet, but fail to compensate for BCM in response to insulin resistance caused by a high fat diet [94]. This study demonstrated that normal BCM expansion to diet-induced insulin resistance requires CREB activation, in turn, to increase Irs2 and Pdx1 levels [94].

Whereas the coupling of glucose metabolism to β-cell function and growth is well established, the nature of how other nutrients such as amino acids impact β-cell growth is much less clear. The initial steps in insulin secretion and β-cell growth via the mTOR signaling pathway are driven by glucose-derived metabolic signals that involve K_{ATP} channel modulation and increased intracellular calcium concentrations [99]. Furthermore, increased intracellular calcium and amino acids are required for glucose-induced, mTOR-dependent DNA synthesis in cultured rat islets [100]. Hence, the mTOR pathway is a focal point for the integration of nutrient activation and increased cellular energy levels, as well for signals from growth factors and hormones. It exists as two distinct complexes, a rapamycin-sensitive complex (mTORC1) with the regulatory-associated protein raptor, and a rapamycin-resistant complex of mTOR and rictor (mTORC2) [140, 141]. The two downstream targets of mTORC1, the 70-kDa ribosomal protein S6 kinase (S6K1) and the eukaryotic initiation factor 4E-binding protein 1 (4EBP1), play key roles in regulating cell growth, DNA synthesis, proliferation, and survival [99]. Crosstalk between Irs2/PI3-kinase/Akt signaling and mTOR signaling modules has implications for fine-tuning BCM and preventing mTOR overactivity [142, 143].

The evolutionarily conserved Akt substrate GSK3β has recently been implicated in the pathophysiology of diabetes and appears to negatively regulate β-cell proliferation and BCM [93, 144]. Accordingly, it has been shown that (1) GSK3 activity is regulated by glucose in β-cell lines [144], (2) specific GSK3 inhibitors and RNA interference-mediated knockdown of GSK3 promoted β-cell replication and survival in β-cell lines and in islets [145] and, (3) transgenic mice overexpressing a constitutively active form of human GSK3β (S9A) driven by the rat insulin promoter exhibited impaired glucose tolerance, decreased BCM, and decreased β-cell proliferation [144]. Not surprisingly, Pdx1 levels were also decreased by 50% in these mice supporting an earlier study that reported that GSK3β targeted Pdx1 for degradation [92]. Thus GSK3 appears to be an excellent candidate for future diabetes intervention strategies.

Evidence is emerging for a regulatory axis between mTOR glucose/nutrient sensing and the ATP/energy sensor cAMP-activated protein kinase (AMPK) that may impact β-cell growth [143, 146], but not necessarily function [143]. This appears to be the essence of the β-cell's drive to balance ambient ATP levels with protein synthesis, growth, and proliferation in the milieu of dynamic changes in glucose and amino acid availability. AMPK activation antagonizes mTOR signaling and reduces S6K1 phosphorylation by a mechanism that involves TSC2 (tuberin) activation, leading to inhibition of mTOR activity [143]. Thus, β-cell growth mediated through the mTOR pathway may necessarily require AMPK inhibition, possibly through increased ATP production through the metabolism of branched chain amino acids and glutamine [143].

The tempering of β-cell growth through the insulin-signaling pathway may be provided by adipokines [146, 147]. For instance, whereas leptin signaling in β-cell lines inhibits the key phosphatase PTEN, effectively increasing PIP3 levels and enhancing downstream Akt signaling in a positive growth mode [147], β-cell leptin receptor deficiency has the opposite effect in mice [45]. Sustained mTOR activation can lead to Irs2 degradation [142, 148] that can be countered by adiponectin-stimulated AMPK activation [146]. Therapeutic strategies manipulating the mTOR module must consider the complicated nature of mTOR signaling in β-cell.

3.5.3 Neurally Derived Growth Factors

Despite being derived from two different embryonic fates, pancreatic β-cells and neurons share common gene regulatory mechanisms as well as the expression of a large number of proteins including the neurotrophins (NTs) nerve growth factor (NGF), brain-derived neurotrophic growth factor (BDNF), neurotrophin-3 (NT3), and NT4/5 that play roles in growth and survival of neuronal cells and to some extent in β-cells [149]. NTs elicit their effects through tyrosine-kinase (Trk) family of transmembrane receptors with Trk-A, Trk-B, and Trk-C binding with high affinity to NGF, BDNF (and NT4/5), and NT3, respectively [150].

Of the four NTs, NGF and its receptors has been the most studied. NGF binds to the high-affinity Trk-A and the low-affinity p75 neurotrophin receptors (p75NTR). Both receptors are expressed in β-cell lines, in islets and the exocrine tissue [151–154]. NGF receptors are also expressed in cultured fetal β-cells, in the ductal epithelium during early development, and in islets and peri-islet Schwann cells of STZ-treated rodents, and in NOD mice, suggesting potential roles in islet development and regeneration [8, 153, 165, 166]. Signaling via the NGF receptors has been shown to promote insulin secretion and survival in adult islets, transplanted islets, and in β-cell lines [155–158]. In this respect, islet apoptosis induced by NGF withdrawal was mediated by PI3-K/Akt signaling [159]. By contrast, although the transcripts for Trk-B and C receptors and their ligands, BDNF and NT3, are expressed in islets and in β-cell lines, the encoded proteins have been identified only in α-cells [160–163]. Nevertheless, in vivo administration of BDNF was shown to improve insulin sensitivity in the diabetic *db/db* mice that correlated with increased insulin signaling [164]. Importantly, BDNF ameliorated diabetes in these mice by increasing BCM and improving β-cell function [164]. Thus the NTs, such as BDNF, have pleiotropic actions on islets; however, precisely how they impact β-cell growth remains unclear.

3.6   CONCLUDING REMARKS

Although the nature of the control mechanisms for BCM homeostasis that impinge on the processes of proliferation, neogenesis, cellular hypertrophy, and survival is fragmentary, a consensus has emerged with the Irs2/Akt module playing key roles in each of these. Inputs from nutrient sensing pathways, hormone and growth factor cascades, and possibly neural influences converge on the β-cell's insulin signaling pathway to elicit an appropriate secretory response and BCM that reflects the drive to balance the body's current energy stores and plasma glucose levels with the prevailing insulin requirements. Unfortunately, many of these same growth and survival promoting molecules are also active in tumor progression. Future studies will resolve how closely the β-cell growth mechanisms characterized in rodents reflect those in humans through continued state-of-the-art research efforts involving gene manipulation, pharmacologic agents, cell lineage tracing, high resolution imaging, and developmental/regeneration biology. Despite the fact that we have much to learn about how these signaling pathways are integrated to specify β-cell function and mass under a set of physiological conditions and pathophysiological circumstances, it is imperative over the short term to extract and exploit the most promising approaches from these recent studies for translation to eventual therapies for insulin-dependent patients.

REFERENCES

1. Bonner-Weir S (2000) Islet growth and development in the adult. J Mol Endocrinol 24:297–302
2. Teta M, Long SY, Wartschow LM, Rankin MM, Kushner JA (2005) Very slow turnover of beta-cells in aged adult mice. Diabetes 54:2557–2567
3. Teta M, Rankin MM, Long SY, Stein GM, Kushner JA (2007) Growth and regeneration of adult beta cells does not involve specialized progenitors. Dev Cell 12:817–826
4. Deltour L, Leduque P, Paldi A, Ripoche MA, Dubois P, Jami J (1991) Polyclonal origin of pancreatic islets in aggregation mouse chimaeras. Development 112:1115–1121
5. Bonner-Weir S (2000) Life and death of the pancreatic beta cells. Trends Endocrinol Metab 11:375–378
6. Butler AE, Janson J, Bonner-Weir S, Ritzel R, Rizza RA, Butler PC (2003) Beta-cell deficit and increased beta-cell apoptosis in humans with type 2 diabetes. Diabetes 52:102–110
7. Butler PC, Meier JJ, Butler AE, Bhushan A (2007) The replication of beta cells in normal physiology, in disease and for therapy. Nat Clin Pract Endocrinol Metab 3:758–768
8. Weibel ER (1981) Stereological methods in cell biology: where are we-where are we going? J Histochem Cytochem 29:1043–1052
9. Bonner-Weir S, Deery D, Leahy JL, Weir GC (1989) Compensatory growth of pancreatic beta-cells in adult rats after short-term glucose infusion. Diabetes 38:49–53
10. Skau M, Pakkenberg B, Buschard K, Bock T (2001) Linear correlation between the total islet mass and the volume-weighted mean islet volume. Diabetes 50:1763–1770
11. Jetton TL, Lausier J, LaRock K, Trotman WE, Larmie B, Habibovic A, Peshavaria M, Leahy JL (2005) Mechanisms of compensatory β-cell growth in insulin resistant rats: roles of Akt kinase. Diabetes 54:2294–2304
12. Georgia S, Bhushan A (2004) Beta cell replication is the primary mechanism for maintaining postnatal beta cell mass. J Clin Invest 114:963–968
13. Dor Y (2006) β-cell proliferation is the major source of new pancreatic beta cells. Nat Clin Pract Endocrinol Metab 2:242–243
14. Bonner-Weir S, Toschi E, Inada A, Reitz P, Fonseca SY, Aye T, Sharma A (2004) The pancreatic ductal epithelium serves as a potential pool of progenitor cells. Pediatr Diabetes 5(Suppl 2):16–22
15. Bouwens L (2006) Beta cell regeneration. Curr Diabetes Rev 2:3–9
16. Dor Y, Brown J, Martinez OI, Melton DA (2004) Adult pancreatic beta-cells are formed by self-duplication rather than stem-cell differentiation. Nature 429:41–46
17. Okamoto H, Hribal ML, Lin HV, Bennett WR, Ward A, Accili D (2006) Role of the forkhead protein FoxO1 in beta cell compensation to insulin resistance. J Clin Invest 116:775–782
18. Bonner-Weir S, Baxter LA, Schuppin GT, Smith FE (1993) A second pathway for regeneration of adult exocrine and endocrine pancreas. Diabetes 42:1715–1720
19. Wang RN, Kloppel G, Bouwens L (1995) Duct to islet differentiation and islet growth in the pancreas of duct-ligated adult rats. Diabetologia 38:1405–1411
20. Jetton TL, Everill B, Lausier J, Roskens V, Habibovic A, LaRock K, Gokin A, Peshavaria M, Leahy JL (2008) Enhanced β-cell mass without increased proliferation following chronic mild glucose infusion. Am J Physiol Endocrinol Metab 294:E679–E687
21. Larsen MO, Rolin B, Raun K, Bjerre Knudsen L, Gotfredsen CF, Bock T (2007) Evaluation of β-cell mass and function in the Göttingen minipig. Diabetes Obes Metab 9(Suppl 2):170–179

22. Bouwens L, Pipeleers DG (1998) Extra-insular beta cells associated with ductules are frequent in adult human pancreas. Diabetologia 41:629–633

23. Finegood DT, Scaglia L, Bonner-Weir S (1995) Dynamics of beta-cell mass in the growing rat pancreas. Estimation with a simple mathematical model. Diabetes 44:249–256

24. Lipsett M, Finegood DT (2002) Beta-cell neogenesis during prolonged hyperglycemia in rats. Diabetes 51:1834–1841

25. Peshavaria M, Larmie BL, Lausier J, Satish B, Habibovic A, Roskens V, Larock K, Everill B, Leahy JL, Jetton TL (2006) Regulation of pancreatic beta-cell regeneration in the normoglycemic 60% partial-pancreatectomy mouse. Diabetes 55:3289–3298

26. Fernandez LA, Hatch EW, Armann B, Odorico JS, Hullett DA, Sollinger HW, Hanson MS (2005) Validation of large particle flow cytometry for the analysis and sorting of intact pancreatic islets. Transplantation 80:729–737

27. Scaglia L, Smith FE, Bonner-Weir S (1995) Apoptosis contributes to the involution of beta cell mass in the post partum rat pancreas. Endocrinology 136:5461–5468

28. Montanya E, Nacher V, Biarnés M, Soler J (2000) Linear correlation between beta-cell mass and body weight throughout the lifespan in Lewis rats: role of beta-cell hyperplasia and hypertrophy. Diabetes 49:1341–1346

29. Meier JJ, Bhushan A, Butler AE, Rizza RA, Butler PC (2005) Sustained beta cell apoptosis in patients with long-standing type 1 diabetes: indirect evidence for islet regeneration? Diabetologia 48:2221–2228

30. Meier JJ, Lin JC, Butler AE, Galasso R, Martinez DS, Butler PC (2006) Direct evidence of attempted beta cell regeneration in an 89-year-old patient with recent-onset type 1 diabetes. Diabetologia 49:1838–1844

31. Bernard C, Berthault M-F, Saulnier C, Ktorza A (1999) Neogenesis vs. apoptosis as main components of pancreatic β cells mass changes in glucose-infused normal and mildly diabetic adult rats. FASEB J 13:1195–1205

32. Simmons RA (2007) Role of metabolic programming in the pathogenesis of β-cell failure in postnatal life. Rev Endocr Metab Disord 8:95–104

33. Fernández E, Martín MA, Fajardo S, Escrivá F, Álvarez C (2007) Increased IRS-2 content and activation of IGF-I pathway contribute to enhance β-cell mass in fetuses from undernourished pregnant rats. Am J Physiol Endocrinol Metab 292:187–195

34. Zhang W, Feng D, Li Y, Iida K, McGrath B, Cavener DR (2006) PERK EIF2AK3 control of pancreatic β cell differentiation and proliferation is required for postnatal glucose homeostasis. Cell Metab 4:491–497

35. Portha B (2005) Programmed disorders of β-cell development and function as one cause for type 2 diabetes? The GK rat paradigm. Diabetes Metab Res Rev 21:495–504

36. Slack JM (1995) Developmental biology of the pancreas. Development 121:1569–1580

37. Murtaugh LC (2007) Pancreas and beta-cell development: from the actual to the possible. Development 134:427–438

38. Ackermann AM, Gannon M (2007) Molecular regulation of pancreatic β-cell mass development, maintenance, and expansion. J Mol Endocrinol 38:193–206

39. Sharma A, Zangen DH, Reitz P, Taneja M, Lissauer ME, Miller CP, Weir GC, Habener JF, Bonner-Weir S (1999) The homeodomain protein IDX-1 increases after an early burst of proliferation during pancreatic regeneration. Diabetes 48:507–513

40. Xu X, D'Hoker J, Stangé G, Bonné S, De Leu N, Xiao X, Van De Casteele M, Mellitzer G, Ling Z, Pipeleers D, Bouwens L, Scharfmann R, Gradwohl G, Heimberg H (2008) β cells can be generated from endogenous progenitors in injured adult mouse pancreas. Cell 132:197–207

41. Gradwohl G, Dierich A, LeMeur M, Guillemot F (2000) Neurogenin3 is required for the development of the four endocrine cell lineages of the pancreas. Proc Natl Acad Sci USA 97:1607–1611
42. Lee CS, De Leon DD, Kaestner KH, Stoffers DA (2006) Regeneration of pancreatic islets after partial pancreatectomy in mice does not involve the reactivation of neurogenin-3. Diabetes 55:269–272
43. Holland AM, Gonez LJ, Naselli G, Macdonald RJ, Harrison LC (2005) Conditional expression demonstrates the role of the homeodomain transcription factor Pdx1 in maintenance and regeneration of beta-cells in the adult pancreas. Diabetes 54:2586–2595
44. Bernal-Mizrachi E, Wen W, Stahlhut S, Welling CM, Permutt MA (2001) Islet beta cell expression of constitutively active Akt1/PKB alpha induces striking hypertrophy, hyperplasia, and hyperinsulinemia. J Clin Invest 108.1631–1638
45. Morioka T, Asilmaz E, Hu J, Dishinger JF, Kurpad AJ, Elias CF, Li H, Elmquist JK, Kennedy RT, Kulkarni RN (2007) Disruption of leptin receptor expression in the pancreas directly affects β cell growth and function in mice. J Clin Invest 117:2860–2868
46. Pende M, Kozma SC, Jaquet M, Oorschot V, Burcelin R, Le Marchand-Brustel Y, Klumperman J, Thorens B, Thomas G (2000) Hypoinsulinaemia, glucose intolerance and diminished beta-cell size in S6K1-deficient mice. Nature 408:994–997
47. Ruvinsky I, Sharon N, Lerer T, Cohen H, Stolovich-Rain M, Nir T, Dor Y, Zisman P, Meyuhas O (2005) Ribosomal protein S6 phosphorylation is a determinant of cell size and glucose homeostasis. Genes Dev 19:2199–2211
48. Velloso LA, Carneiro EM, Crepaldi SC, Boschero AC, Saad MJ (1995) Glucose- and insulin-induced phosphorylation of the insulin receptor and its primary substrates IRS-1 and IRS-2 in rat pancreatic islets. FEBS Lett 377:353–357
49. Rothenberg PL, Willison LD, Simon J, Wolf BA (1995) Glucose-induced insulin receptor tyrosine phosphorylation in insulin-secreting beta-cells. Diabetes 44:802–809
50. Harbeck MC, Louie DC, Howland J, Wolf BA, Rothenberg PL (1996) Expression of insulin receptor mRNA and insulin receptor substrate 1 in pancreatic islet beta-cells. Diabetes 45:711–717
51. Xu GG, Rothenberg PL (1998) Insulin receptor signaling in the beta-cell influences insulin gene expression and insulin content: evidence for autocrine beta-cell regulation. Diabetes 47:1243–1252
52. Hirayama I, Tamemoto H, Yokota H, Kubo SK, Wang J, Kuwano H, Nagamachi Y, Takeuchi T, Izumi T (1999) Insulin receptor-related receptor is expressed in pancreatic beta-cells and stimulates tyrosine phosphorylation of insulin receptor substrate-1 and -2. Diabetes 48:1237–1244
53. Fehmann H-C, Jehle P, Markus U, Goke B (1996) Functional active receptors for insulin-like growth factors-I (IGF-I) and IGF-II on insulin-, glucagon-, and somatostatin-producing cells. Metabolism 45:759–766
54. Kulkarni RN, Holzenberger M, Shih DQ, Ozcan U, Stoffel M, Magnuson MA, Kahn CR (2002) Beta-cell-specific deletion of the Igf1 receptor leads to hyperinsulinemia and glucose intolerance but does not alter beta-cell mass. Nat Genet 31:111–115
55. Withers DJ, Burks DJ, Towery HH, Altamuro SL, Flint CL, White MF (1999) Irs-2 coordinates Igf-1 receptor-mediated β-cell development and peripheral insulin signaling. Nat Genet 23:32–40
56. Withers DJ, Gutierrez JS, Towery H, Burks DJ, Ren JM, Previs S, Zhang Y, Bernal D, Pons S, Schulman GI, Bonner-Weir S, White MF (1998) Disruption of the IRS-2 gene causes type 2 diabetes in mice. Nature 391:900–904

64 Jetton et al.

57. Jhala US, Canettieri G, Screaton RA, Kulkarni RN, Krajewski S, Reed J, Walker J, Lin X, White M, Montminy M (2003) cAMP promotes pancreatic beta-cell survival via CREB-mediated induction of IRS2. Genes Dev 17:1575–1580
58. Lingohr MK, Briaud I, Dickson LM, McCuaig JF, Alárcon C, Wicksteed BL, Rhodes CJ (2006) Specific regulation of IRS-2 expression by glucose in rat primary pancreatic islet beta-cells. J Biol Chem 281:15884–15892
59. Park S, Dong X, Fisher TL, Dunn S, Omer AK, Weir G, White MF (2006) Exendin-4 uses Irs2 signaling to mediate pancreatic beta cell growth and function. J Biol Chem 281:1159–1168
60. Drucker DJ (2006) The biology of incretin hormones. Cell Metab 3:153–165
61. Kushner JA, Ye J, Schubert M, Burks DJ, Dow MA, Flint CL, Dutta S, Wright CV, Montminy MR, White MF (2002) Pdx1 restores beta cell function in Irs2 knockout mice. J Clin Invest 109:1193–1201
62. Kitamura T, Nakae J, Kitamura Y, Kido Y, Biggs WH, Wright CV, White MF, Arden KC, Accili D (2002) The forkhead transcription factor Foxo1 links insulin signaling to Pdx1 regulation of pancreatic beta cell growth. J Clin Invest 110:1839–1847
63. Hugl SR, White MF, Rhodes CJ (1998) Insulin-like growth factor I (IGF-I)-stimulated pancreatic β-cell growth is glucose-dependent. J Biol Chem 273:17771–17779
64. Buteau J, Roduit R, Susini S, Prentki M (1999) Glucagon-like peptide-1 promotes DNA synthesis, activates phosphatidylinositol 3-kinase and increases transcription factor pancreatic and duodenal homeobox 1 (PDX-1) DNA binding activity in beta (INS-1)-cells. Diabetologia 42:856–864
65. Holst LS, Mulder H, Manganiello V, Sundler F, Ahren B, Holm C, Degermanm E (1998) Protein kinase B is expressed in pancreatic β cells and activated upon stimulation with insulin-like growth factor I. Biochem Biophys Res Commun 250:181–186
66. Tuttle RL, Gill NS, Pugh W, Lee JP, Koeberlein B, Furth EE, Polonsky KS, Naji A, Birnbaum MJ (2001) Regulation of pancreatic beta-cell growth and survival by the serine/threonine protein kinase Akt1/PKBalpha. Nat Med 7:1133–1137
67. Garofalo RS, Orena SJ, Rafidi K, Torchia AJ, Stock JL, Hildebrandt AL, Coskran T, Black SC, Brees DJ, Wicks JR, McNeish JD, Coleman KG (2003) Severe diabetes, age-dependent loss of adipose tissue, and mild growth deficiency in mice lacking Akt2/PKB beta. J Clin Invest 112:197–208
68. Rane SG, Reddy EP (2000) Cell cycle control of pancreatic beta cell proliferation. Front Biosci 5:D1–D19
69. Cozar-Castellano I, Fiaschi-Taesch N, Bigatel TA, Takane KK, Garcia-Ocaña A, Vasavada R, Stewart AF (2006) Molecular control of cell cycle progression in the pancreatic beta-cell. Endocr Rev 27:356–370
70. Kushner JA, Ciemerych MA, Sicinska E, Wartschow LM, Teta M, Long SY, Sicinski P, White MF (2005) Cyclins D2 and D1 are essential for postnatal pancreatic beta-cell growth. Mol Cell Biol 25:3752–3762
71. Martín J, Hunt SL, Dubus P, Sotillo R, Néhmé-Pélluard F, Magnuson MA, Parlow AF, Malumbres M, Ortega S, Barbacid M (2003) Genetic rescue of Cdk4 null mice restores pancreatic beta-cell proliferation but not homeostatic cell number. Oncogene 22:5261–5269
72. Fatrai S, Elghazi L, Balcazar N, Cras-Méneur C, Krits I, Kiyokawa H, Bernal-Mizrachi E (2006) Akt induces beta-cell proliferation by regulating cyclin D1, cyclin D2, and p21 levels and cyclin-dependent kinase-4 activity. Diabetes 55:318–325
73. Kushner JA (2006) Beta-cell growth: an unusual paradigm of organogenesis that is cyclin D2/Cdk4 dependent. Cell Cycle 5:234–237

74. Cozar-Castellano I, Takane KK, Bottino R, Balamurugan AN, Stewart AF (2004) Induction of beta-cell proliferation and retinoblastoma protein phosphorylation in rat and human islets using adenovirus-mediated transfer of cyclin-dependent kinase-4 and cyclin D1. Diabetes 53:149–159

75. Vasavada RC, Cozar-Castellano I, Sipula D, Stewart AF (2007) Tissue-specific deletion of the retinoblastoma protein in the pancreatic beta-cell has limited effects on beta-cell replication, mass, and function. Diabetes 56:57–64

76. Cozar-Castellano I, Weinstock M, Haught M, Velázquez-Garcia S, Sipula D, Stewart AF (2006) Evaluation of beta-cell replication in mice transgenic for hepatocyte growth factor and placental lactogen: comprehensive characterization of the G1/S regulatory proteins reveals unique involvement of p21cip. Diabetes 55:70–77

77. Cozar-Castellano I, Haught M, Stewart AF (2006) The cell cycle inhibitory protein p21cip is not essential for maintaining beta-cell cycle arrest or beta-cell function in vivo. Diabetes 55:3271–3278

78. Uchida T, Nakamura T, Hashimoto N, Matsuda T, Kotani K, Sakaue H, Kido Y, Hayashi Y, Nakayama KI, White MF, Kasuga M (2005) Deletion of Cdkn1b ameliorates hyperglycemia by maintaining compensatory hyperinsulinemia in diabetic mice. Nat Med 11:175–182

79. Fontanière S, Casse H, Bertolino P, Zhang CX (2006) Analysis of p27(Kip1) expression in insulinomas developed in pancreatic beta-cell specific Men1 mutant mice. Fam Cancer 5:49–54

80. Georgia S, Bhushan A (2006) p27 regulates the transition of beta-cells from quiescence to proliferation. Diabetes 55:2950–2956

81. Rachdi L, Balcazar N, Elghazi L, Barker DJ, Krits I, Kiyokawa H, Bernal-Mizrachi E (2006) Differential effects of p27 in regulation of beta-cell mass during development, neonatal period, and adult life. Diabetes 55:3520–3528

82. Zhong L, Georgia S, Tschen SI, Nakayama K, Nakayama K, Bhushan A (2007) Essential role of Skp2-mediated p27 degradation in growth and adaptive expansion of pancreatic beta cells. J Clin Invest 117:2869–2876

83. Kushner JA, Simpson L, Wartschow LM, Guo S, Rankin MM, Parsons R, White MF (2005) Phosphatase and tensin homolog regulation of islet growth and glucose homeostasis. J Biol Chem 280:39388–39393

84. Stiles BL, Kuralwalla-Martinez C, Guo W, Gregorian C, Wang Y, Tian J, Magnuson MA, Wu H (2006) Selective deletion of Pten in pancreatic beta cells leads to increased islet mass and resistance to STZ-induced diabetes. Mol Cell Biol 26:2772–2781

85. Liang J, Slingerland JM (2003) Multiple roles of the PI3K/PKB (Akt) pathway in cell cycle progression. Cell Cycle 2:339–345

86. Nakamura N, Ramaswamy S, Vazquez F, Signoretti S, Loda M, Sellers WR (2000) Forkhead transcription factors are critical effectors of cell death and cell cycle arrest downstream of PTEN. Mol Cell Biol 20:8969–8982

87. Karnik SK, Chen H, McLean GW, Heit JJ, Gu X, Zhang AY, Fontaine M, Yen MH, Kim SK (2007) Menin controls growth of pancreatic beta-cells in pregnant mice and promotes gestational diabetes mellitus. Science 318:806–809

88. Alonso LC, Yokoe T, Zhang P, Scott DK, Kim SK, O'Donnell CP, Garcia-Ocaña A (2007) Glucose infusion in mice: a new model to induce beta-cell replication. Diabetes 56:1792–1801

89. Paris M, Bernard-Kargar C, Berthault MF, Bouwens L, Ktorza A (2003) Specific and combined effects of insulin and glucose on functional pancreatic beta-cell mass in vivo in adult rats. Endocrinology 144:2717–2727

90. Topp BG, McArthur MD, Finegood DT (2004) Metabolic adaptations to chronic glucose infusion in rats. Diabetologia 47:1602–1610

91. Jetton TL, Liu YQ, Trotman WE, Nevin PW, Sun XJ, Leahy JL (2001) Enhanced expression of insulin receptor substrate-2 and activation of protein kinase B/Akt in regenerating pancreatic duct epithelium of 60%-partial pancreatectomy rats. Diabetologia 44:2056–2065

92. Boucher MJ, Selander L, Carlsson L, Edlund H (2006) Phosphorylation marks IPF1/PDX1 protein for degradation by glycogen synthase kinase 3-dependent mechanisms. J Biol Chem 281:6395–6403

93. Tanabe K, Liu Z, Patel S, Doble BW, Li L, Cras-Méneur C, Martinez SC, Welling CM, White MF, Bernal-Mizrachi E, Woodgett JR, Permutt MA (2008) Genetic deficiency of glycogen synthase kinase-3beta corrects diabetes in mouse models of insulin resistance. PLoS Biol 6:e37

94. Terauchi Y, Takamoto I, Kubota N, Matsui J, Suzuki R, Komeda K, Hara A, Toyoda Y, Miwa I, Aizawa S, Tsutsumi S, Tsubamoto Y, Hashimoto S, Eto K, Nakamura A, Noda M, Tobe K, Aburatani H, Nagai R, Kadowaki T (2007) Glucokinase and IRS-2 are required for compensatory beta cell hyperplasia in response to high-fat diet-induced insulin resistance. J Clin Invest 117:246–257

95. Jetton TL, Liang Y, Pettepher CC, Zimmerman EC, Cox FG, Horvath K, Matschinsky FM, Magnuson MA (1994) Analysis of upstream glucokinase promoter activity in transgenic mice and identification of glucokinase in rare neuroendocrine cells in the brain and gut. J Biol Chem 269:3641–3654

96. Jetton TL, Moates JM, Lindner J, Wright CV, Magnuson MA (1998) Targeted oncogenesis of hormone-negative pancreatic islet progenitor cells. Proc Natl Acad Sci USA 95:8654–8659

97. Jetton TL, Postic C, Niswender KN, Moates JM, Magnuson MA (1994) Glucokinase gene expression in extrapancreatic neural and neuroendocrine cells. In: Baba S, Kaneko T (eds) Proceedings of the 15th International Diabetes Federation. Elsevier, Amsterdam, pp 193–197

98. McDaniel ML, Marshall CA, Pappan KL, Kwon G (2002) Metabolic and autocrine regulation of the mammalian target of rapamycin by pancreatic beta-cells. Diabetes 51:2877–2885

99. Kwon G, Marshall CA, Pappan KL, Remedi MS, McDaniel ML (2004) Signaling elements involved in the metabolic regulation of mTOR by nutrients, incretins, and growth factors in islets. Diabetes 53(Suppl 3):S225–S232

100. Kwon G, Marshall CA, Liu H, Pappan KL, Remedi MS, McDaniel ML (2006) Glucose-stimulated DNA synthesis through mammalian target of rapamycin (mTOR) is regulated by KATP channels: effects on cell cycle progression in rodent islets. J Biol Chem 281:3261–3267

101. Federici M, Hribal M, Perego L, Ranalli M, Caradonna Z, Perego C, Usellini L, Nano R, Bonini P, Bertuzzi F, Marlier LN, Davalli AM, Carandente O, Pontiroli AE, Melino G, Marchetti P, Lauro R, Sesti G, Folli F (2001) High glucose causes apoptosis in cultured human pancreatic islets of Langerhans: a potential role for regulation of specific Bcl family genes toward an apoptotic cell death program. Diabetes 50:1290–1301

102. Datta SR, Brunet A, Greenberg ME (1999) Cellular survival: a play in three Akts. Genes Dev 13:2905–2927

103. Danial NN, Walensky LD, Zhang CY, Choi CS, Fisher JK, Molina AJ, Datta SR, Pitter KL, Bird GH, Wikstrom JD, Deeney JT, Robertson K, Morash J, Kulkarni A, Neschen S, Kim S, Greenberg ME, Corkey BE, Shirihai OS, Shulman GI, Lowell BB, Korsmeyer SJ (2008) Dual role of proapoptotic BAD in insulin secretion and beta cell survival. Nat Med 14:144–153

104. Kim SJ, Nian C, Widenmaier S, McIntosh CH (2008) Glucose-dependent insulino-tropic polypeptide-mediated up-regulation of beta-cell antiapoptotic Bcl-2 gene expression is coordinated by cyclic AMP (cAMP) response element binding protein (CREB) and cAMP-responsive CREB coactivator 2. Mol Cell Biol 28: 1644–1656

105. Kim SJ, Winter K, Nian C, Tsuneoka M, Koda Y, McIntosh CH (2005) Glucose-dependent insulinotropic polypeptide (GIP) stimulation of pancreatic beta-cell survival is dependent upon phosphatidylinositol 3-kinase (PI3K)/protein kinase B (PKB) signaling, inactivation of the forkhead transcription factor Foxo1, and down-regulation of bax expression. J Biol Chem 280:22297–22307

106. Liadis N, Salmena L, Kwan E, Tajmir P, Schroer SA, Radziszewska A, Li X, Sheu L, Eweida M, Xu S, Gaisano HY, Hakem R, Woo M (2007) Distinct in vivo roles of caspase-8 in beta-cells in physiological and diabetes models. Diabetes 56:2302–2311

107. Johnson JD, Ahmed NT, Luciani DS, Han Z, Tran H, Fujita J, Misler S, Edlund H, Polonsky KS (2003) Increased islet apoptosis in Pdx1+/– mice. J Clin Invest 111:1147–1160

108. Rachman J, Gribble FM, Barrow BA, Levy JC, Buchanan KD, Turner RC (1996) Normalization of insulin responses to glucose by overnight infusion of glucagon-like peptide 1 (7–36) amide in patients with NIDDM. Diabetes 45:1524–1530

109. Nauck MA, Kleine N, Orskov C, Holst JJ, Willms B, Creutzfeldt W (1993) Normalization of fasting hyperglycaemia by exogenous glucagon-like peptide 1 (7–36 amide) in type 2 (non-insulin-dependent) diabetic patients. Diabetologia 36:741–744

110. Toft-Nielsen MB, Madsbad S, Holst JJ (1999) Continuous subcutaneous infusion of glucagon-like peptide 1 lowers plasma glucose and reduces appetite in type 2 diabetic patients. Diabetes Care 22:1137–1143

111. Willms B, Werner J, Holst JJ, Orskov C, Creutzfeldt W, Nauck MA (1996) Gastric emptying, glucose responses, and insulin secretion after a liquid test meal: effects of exogenous glucagon-like peptide-1 (GLP-1)-(7–36) amide in type 2 (noninsulin-dependent) diabetic patients. J Clin Endocrinol Metab 81:327–332

112. Zander M, Madsbad S, Madsen JL, Holst JJ (2002) Effect of 6-week course of glucagon-like peptide 1 on glycaemic control, insulin sensitivity, and beta-cell function in type 2 diabetes: a parallel-group study. Lancet 359:824–830

113. Scrocchi LA, Brown TJ, MaClusky N, Brubaker PL, Auerbach AB, Joyner AL, Drucker DJ (1996) Glucose intolerance but normal satiety in mice with a null mutation in the glucagon-like peptide 1 receptor gene. Nat Med 2:1254–1258

114. Pederson RA, Satkunarajah M, McIntosh CH, Scrocchi LA, Flamez D, Schuit F, Drucker DJ, Wheeler MB (1998) Enhanced glucose-dependent insulinotropic polypeptide secretion and insulinotropic action in glucagon-like peptide 1 receptor –/– mice. Diabetes 47:1046–1052

115. Hansotia T, Drucker DJ (2005) GIP and GLP-1 as incretin hormones: lessons from single and double incretin receptor knockout mice. Regul Pept 128:125–134

116. De León DD, Crutchlow MF, Ham JY, Stoffers DA (2006) Role of glucagon-like peptide-1 in the pathogenesis and treatment of diabetes mellitus. Int J Biochem Cell Biol 38:845–859

117. Li L, El-Kholy W, Rhodes CJ, Brubaker PL (2005) Glucagon-like peptide-1 protects beta cells from cytokine-induced apoptosis and necrosis: role of protein kinase B. Diabetologia 48:1339–1349

118. Holz GG, Chepurny OG (2005) Diabetes outfoxed by GLP-1? Sci STKE 268:2

119. Buteau J, Spatz ML, Accili D (2006) Transcription factor FoxO1 mediates glucagon-like peptide-1 effects on pancreatic beta-cell mass. Diabetes 55:1190–1196

120. Buteau J, Foisy S, Joly E, Prentki M (2003) Glucagon-like peptide 1 induces pancreatic beta-cell proliferation via transactivation of the epidermal growth factor receptor. Diabetes 52:124–132

121. Farilla L, Hui H, Bertolotto C, Kang E, Bulotta A, Di Mario U, Perfetti R (2002) glucagon-like peptide-1 promotes islet cell growth and inhibits apoptosis in Zucker diabetic rats. Endocrinology 143:4397–4408

122. Mu J, Woods J, Zhou Y-P, Roy RS, Li Z, Zycband E, Feng Y, Zhu L, Li C, Howard AD, Moller DE, Thornberry NA, Zhang BB (2006) Chronic inhibition of DPPIV with a sitagliptin analog preserves pancreatic β-cell mass and function in a rodent model of type 2 diabetes. Diabetes 55:1695–1704

123. Tourrel C, Bailbe D, Lacorne M, Meile MJ, Kergoat M, Portha B (2002) Persistent improvement of type 2 diabetes in the Goto-Kakizaki rat model by expansion of the beta-cell mass during the prediabetic period with glucagon-like peptide-1 or exendin-4. Diabetes 51:1443–1452

124. Xu G, Stoffers DA, Habener JF, Bonneir-Weir S (1999) Exendin-4 stimulates both beta-cell replication and neogenesis resulting in increased beta-cell mass and improved glucose tolerance in diabetic rats. Diabetes 48:2270–2276

125. Tourrel C, Balbe D, Lacorne M, Meile MJ, Kergoat M, Portha B (2001) GLP-1 and exendin-4 stimulate beta-cell mass neogenesis in STZ-treated newborn rats resulting in persistently improved glucose homeostasis at adult age. Diabetes 50:1562–1570

126. De Leon DD, Deng S, Madani R, Ahima RA, Drucker DJ, Stoffers DA (2003) Role of endogenous glucagon-like peptide-1 in islet regeneration after partial pancreatectomy. Diabetes 52:365–371

127. Lynn FC, Pamir N, Ng EH, McIntosh CH, Kieffer TJ, Pederson RA (2001) Defective glucose-dependent insulinotropic polypeptide receptor expression in diabetic fatty Zucker rats. Diabetes 50:1004–1011

128. Buteau J, Foisy S, Rhodes CJ, Carpenter L, Biden TJ, Prentki M (2001) Protein kinase C-zeta activation mediates glucagon-like peptide-1-induced pancreatic beta-cell proliferation. Diabetes 50:2237–2243

129. Wang X, Cahill CM, Pineyro MA, Zhou J, Doyle ME, Egan JM (1999) Glucagon-like peptide-1 regulates the β cell transcription factor, PDX-1, in insulinoma cells. Endocrinology 140:4904–4907

130. Stoffers DA, Kieffer TJ, Hussain MA, Drucker DJ, Bonner-Weir S, Habener JF, Egan JM (2000) Insulinotropic glucagon-like peptide 1 agonists stimulate expression of homeodomain protein IDX-1 and increase islet size in mouse pancreas. Diabetes 49:741–748

131. Perfetti R, Zhou J, Doyle ME, Egan JM (2000) Glucagon-like peptide-1 induces cell proliferation and pancreatic-duodenum homeobox-1 expression and increases endocrine cell mass in the pancreas of old, glucose-intolerant rats. Endocrinology 141:4600–4605

132. Wang X, Zhou J, Doyle ME, Egan JM (2001) Glucagon-like peptide-1 causes pancreatic duodenal homeobox-1 protein translocation from the cytoplasm to the nucleus of pancreatic β-cells by a cyclic adenosine monophosphate/protein kinase A-dependent mechanism. Endocrinology 142:1820–1827

133. Li Y, Cao X, Li LX, Brubaker PL, Edlund H, Drucker DJ (2005) Beta-cell Pdx1 expression is essential for the glucoregulatory, proliferative, and cytoprotective actions of glucagon-like peptide-1. Diabetes 54:482–491

134. Yusta B, Baggio LL, Estall JL, Koehler JA, Holland DP, Li H, Pipeleers D, Ling Z, Drucker DJ (2006) GLP-1 receptor activation improves beta cell function and survival following induction of endoplasmic reticulum stress. Cell Metab 4:391–406

135. Baggio LL, Drucker DJ (2007) Biology of incretins: GLP-1 and GIP. Gastroenterology 132:2131–2157

136. Srinivasan S, Bernal-Mizrachi E, Ohsugi M, Permutt MA (2002) Glucose promotes pancreatic islet beta-cell survival through a PI 3-kinase/Akt-signaling pathway. Am J Physiol Endocrinol Metab 283:E784–E793

137. Paris M, Bernard-Kargar C, Vilar J, Kassis N, Ktorza A (2004) Role of glucose in IRS signaling in rat pancreatic islets: specific effects and interplay with insulin. Exp Diabesity Res 5:257–263

138. Lingohr MK, Briaud I, Dickson LM, McCuaig JF, Alarcon C, Wicksteed BL, Rhodes CJ (2006) Specific regulation of IRS-2 expression by glucose in rat primary pancreatic islet beta-cells. J Biol Chem 281:15884–15892

139. Martinez SC, Cras-Meneur C, Bernal-Mizrachi E, Permutt MA (2006) Glucose regulates Foxo1 through insulin receptor signaling in the pancreatic islet β-cell. Diabetes 55:1581–1591

140. Loewith R, Jacinto E, Wullschleger S, Lorberg A, Crespo JL, Bonenfant D, Oppliger W, Jenoe P, Hall MN (2002) Two TOR complexes, only one of which is rapamycin sensitive, have distinct roles in cell growth control. Mol Cell 10:457–468

141. Abraham RT (2002) Identification of TOR signaling complexes: more TORC for the cell growth engine. Cell 111:9–12

142. Briaud I, Dickson LM, Lingohr MK, McCuaig JF, Lawrence JC, Rhodes CJ (2005) Insulin receptor substrate-2 proteasomal degradation mediated by a mammalian target of Rapamycin (mTOR)-induced negative feedback down-regulates protein kinase B-mediated signaling pathway in β-cells. J Biol Chem 280:2282–2293

143. Gleason CE, Lu D, Witters LA, Newgard CB, Birnbaum MJ (2007) The role of AMPK and mTOR in nutrient sensing in pancreatic β-cells. J Biol Chem 282:10341–10351

144. Liu Z, Tanabe K, Bernal-Mizrachi E, Permutt MA (2008) Mice with beta cell overexpression of glycogen synthase kinase-3β have reduced beta cell mass and proliferation. Diabetologia 51:623–631

145. Mussmann R, Geese M, Harder F, Kegel S, Andag U, Lomow A, Burk U, Onichtchouk D, Dohrmann C, Austen M (2007) Inhibition of GSK3 promotes replication and survival of pancreatic beta cells. J Biol Chem 282:12030–12037

146. Huypens PR (2007) Leptin and adiponectin regulate compensatory beta cell growth in accordance to overweight. Med Hypotheses 68:1134–1137

147. Ning K, Miller LC, Laidlaw HA, Burgess LA, Perera NM, Downes CP, Leslie NR, Ashford ML (2006) A novel leptin signalling pathway via PTEN inhibition in hypothalamic cell lines and pancreatic beta-cells. EMBO J 25:2377–2387

148. Guo S, Dunn SL, White MF (2006) The reciprocal stability of FOXO1 and IRS2 creates a regulatory circuit that controls insulin signaling. Mol Endocrinol 20:3389–3399

149. Atouf F, Czernichow P, Scharfmann R (1997) Expression of neuronal traits in pancreatic beta cells: implication of neuron-restrictive silencing factor/repressor element silencing transcription factor, a neuron-restrictive silencer. J Biol Chem 272:1929–1934

150. Lindsay RM (1996) Role of neurotrophins and trk receptors in the development and maintenance of sensory neurons: an overview. Philos Trans R Soc Lond B Biol Sci 351:365–373

151. Polak M, Scharfmann R, Seiheimer B, Eisenbarth G, Dressler D, Verma IM, Potter H (1993) Nerve growth factor induces neuron-like differentiation of an insulin-secreting pancreatic beta cell line. Proc Natl Acad Sci U S A 90:5781–5785

152. Rosenbaum T, Vidaltamayo R, Sanchez-Soto MC, Zentella A, Hiriart M (1998) Pancreatic beta cells synthesize and secrete nerve growth factor. Proc Natl Acad Sci USA 95:7784–7788

153. Scharfmann R, Tazi A, Polak M, Kanaka C, Czernichow P (1993) Expression of functional nerve growth factor receptors in pancreatic beta-cell lines and fetal rat islets in primary culture. Diabetes 42:1829–1836

154. Vidaltamayo R, Mery CM, Angeles-Angeles A, Robles-Diaz G, Hiriart M (2003) Expression of nerve growth factor in human pancreatic beta cells. Growth Factors 21:103–107

155. Rosenbaum T, Sanchez-Soto MC, Hiriart M (2001) Nerve growth factor increases insulin secretion and barium current in pancreatic beta-cells. Diabetes 50:1755–1762

156. Navarro-Tableros V, Sánchez-Soto MC, García S, Hiriart M (2004) Autocrine regulation of single pancreatic β-cell survival. Diabetes 53:2018–2023

157. Miao G, Mace J, Kirby M, Hopper A, Peverini R, Chinnock R, Shapiro J, Hathout E (2005) Beneficial effects of nerve growth factor on islet transplantation. Transplant Proc 37:3490–3492

158. Miao G, Mace J, Kirby M, Hopper A, Peverini R, Chinnock R, Shapiro J, Hathout E (2006) *In vitro* and *in vivo* improvement of islet survival following treatment with nerve growth factor. Transplantation 81:519–524

159. Pierucci D, Cicconi S, Bonini P, Ferrelli F, Pastore D, Matteucci C, Marselli L, Marchetti P, Ris F, Halban P, Oberholzer J, Federici M, Cozzolino F, Lauro R, Borboni P, Marlier LN (2001) NGF-withdrawal induces apoptosis in pancreatic beta cells *in vitro*. Diabetologia 44:1281–1295

160. Raile K, Klammt J, Garten A, Laue S, Blüher M, Kralisch S, Klöting N, Kiess W (2006) Glucose regulates expression of the nerve growth factor (NGF) receptors TrkA and p75NTR in rat islets and INS-1E beta-cells. Regul Pept 135:30–38

161. Bonini P, Pierucci D, Cicconi S, Porzio O, Lauro R, Marlier LN, Borboni P (2001) Neurotrophins and neurotrophin receptors mRNAs expression in pancreatic islets and insulinoma cell lines. J Pancreas 2:105–111

162. Lucini C, Costagliola C, Borzacchiello G, Castaldo L (2003) Neurotrophin 3 and its receptor TrkC immunoreactivity in glucagon cells of buffalo pancreas. Anat Histol Embryol 32:253–256

163. Lucini C, Maruccio L, De Girolamo P, Castaldo L (2003) Brain-derived neurotrophic factor in higher vertebrate pancreas: immunolocalization in glucagon cells. Anat Embryol (Berl) 206:311–318

164. Yamanaka M, Itakura Y, Inoue T, Tsuchida A, Nakagawa T, Noguchi H, Taiji M (2006) Protective effect of brain-derived neurotrophic factor on pancreatic islets in obese diabetic mice. Metabolism 55:1286–1292

165. Kanaka-Gantenbein C, Tazi A, Chernichow P, Scharfmann R (1995) *In vivo* presence of the high affinity nerve growth factor receptor Trk-A in the rat pancreas: differential localization during pancreatic development. Endocrinology 136:761–769

166. Teitelman G, Guz Y, Ivkovic S, Ehrlich M (1998) Islet injury induces neurotrophin expression in pancreatic cells and reactive gliosis of peri-islet Schwann cells. J Neurobiol 34:304–318

4

Race/Ethnic and Socioeconomic Disparities in Body Mass Index (BMI) and the Resulting Spread of Obesity and "Adult-Onset" Diabetes Epidemics Among Adolescents

Katherine E. Neubecker

Key Points

- Obesity among adolescents and young adults is a growing public health concern and disproportionately affects certain race/ethnic groups more than others. This chapter discusses how socioeconomic status, eating behavior, and exercise behavior as adolescents can help explain disparities in obesity rates among race/ethnic groups as young adults.

Keywords: Body mass index, BMI, Adolescent obesity, Race/ethnic, Socioeconomic, Healthcare disparity

4.1 INTRODUCTION

4.1.1 The Escalating Obesity Problem in the United States

Obesity is a growing health concern in the United States. According to the National Institutes of Health (NIH), the prevalence of overweight and obese individuals has increased dramatically over the past 30 years. Obesity

From: *Nutrition and Health: Management of Pediatric Obesity and Diabetes*,
Edited by: R.J. Ferry, Jr., DOI 10.1007/978-1-60327-256-8_4,
© Springer Science+Business Media, LLC 2011

rates had been relatively stable from 1960 to 1980 [1, 2] but have been increasing in subsequent years. According to the National Health and Nutrition Examination Survey (NHANES), a nationally representative sample of the U.S population, the prevalence of obesity among adults in 2007–2008 was 33.8%, and the prevalence of overweight and obese combined was 68.0%. Over the past 10 years, obesity rates for men increased significantly (adjusted odds ratio for 2007–2008 versus 1999–2008 was 1.32 (confidence interval 1.12–1.58). Fortunately, according to recent NHANES dates, obesity rates for women did not increase significantly over the past 10 years [3].

For *adults*, the term *overweight* is defined by body mass index (BMI) of 25–29.9 kg/m², and *obese* is defined by BMI >30 kg/m². High BMI is associated with increases in all-cause mortality and many diseases, including progression to Type 2 diabetes mellitus (T2DM), coronary artery disease, stroke, hypertension, sleep apnea, and certain cancers (such as breast, uterine, colorectal, and prostate cancers) [4]. Moreover, the comorbidities associated with high BMI contribute to the challenging problem of rising healthcare costs in the US Medical expenditures related to high BMI accounted for 9.1% of total US expenditures in 1998 and may have reached as high as $78.5 billion [5].

High BMI is a strong risk factor for T2DM in particular. As BMI increases in the adult population, so does the prevalence of T2DM. From 1980 through 2007, the incidence of diabetes in the United States almost tripled from 493,000 in 1980 to at least 1.5 million in 2007. In the 1990s, incidence increased in adults among all age groups. In the early 2000s, incidence appeared to have slowed in those above 45 years of age but continued to increase for 18–44 year olds [6].

4.1.2   Obesity and T2DM Epidemics Among Children and Adolescents

Unfortunately, obesity is not restricted to the adult population; it has recently become a major pediatric disease. Since 1980, the prevalence of obesity has tripled for school-aged children and adolescents [7]. In the pediatric population, overweight is defined as BMI between 85–95 percentiles, and obesity is defined as a BMI ≥95 percentile for children of the same age and gender [8]. For the age group of 2–19 years in 2007–2008, the prevalence of obesity was 17%, and the prevalence of overweight and obese combined was 31.7%. After more than a decade of publicity about this public health issue, some optimism derives from observations that the rate of increase of pediatric obesity might be slowing. Prevalence of obese and overweight children and adolescents did not change significantly from 1999 to 2006 [9]. However, the significant medical and financial burdens of obesity maintain concern and focus on obese children. Obese children often become obese adults [10], placing them at risk of increased mortality and morbidity. Some adverse effects of high BMI, such as hypertension and hyperlipidemia, can even become evident during childhood [11].

As with adults, as the prevalence of high BMI rises in the pediatric population, so does the prevalence of T2DM [12]. Prior to the past 20 years, T2DM usually struck adults, who were much more likely to be overweight or obese than those younger than 21. Thus, T2DM was often referred to as "adult-onset diabetes." However, T2DM is not just a problem among adults anymore. According to the NIH, no national, population-based study had been conducted on T2DM occurrence in children. Still, studies at San Antonio, Cincinnati, Charleston, Los Angeles, and other cities showed that the percentage of children and adolescents with newly diagnosed diabetes who were classified as having T2DM increased from less than 5% before 1994 to 30–50% in recent years [13].

Although rates of high BMI are rising among all race/ethnic groups in the United States, they are increasing most rapidly for specific minority populations, particularly African-Americans, Hispanics, and Native Americans [14]. As a result, weight-related diseases, including T2DM and hypertension, are found at higher rates for these minority groups than non-Hispanic Whites. Race/ethnic disparities in high BMI and T2DM are observable very early in life, even among children [15].

4.2   CONCEPTUAL FRAMEWORK: SOCIODEMOGRAPHIC AND BEHAVIORAL PATHWAYS TO HIGH BMI AND T2DM

The higher incidence of high BMI and T2DM in certain minority populations is partially due to genetics. African-Americans, compared to non-Hispanic Whites, experience higher rates of insulin-resistance, obesity, and other precursors to T2DM [3]. However, as depicted in the conceptual framework below, the author offers the hypothesis that sociodemographic and behavioral factors can also increase the risks of becoming overweight or obese, which can trigger T2DM. Low socioeconomic status is proposed to contribute to unhealthy behaviors, such as consumption of fattening foods and infrequent exercise, which can lead to high BMI and T2DM. Since African-Americans, Hispanics, and Native Americans constitute disproportionately large percentages of low-income groups, they are more likely to become overweight or obese and develop T2DM.

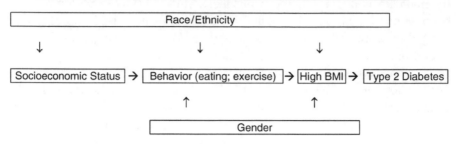

Conceptual Framework:

Sociodemographic and Behavioral Pathways to High BMI and Type 2 Diabetes

4.2.1   The Effects of Gender on Eating and Exercise Behavior and on BMI

Demographic characteristics, such as age and gender, impact eating and exercise behaviors. In general, men eat more than women in order to support their higher body mass. Also, for adolescents and young adults, males tend to exercise more frequently than do females, perhaps because active sports are sometimes emphasized more for males than females by schools and by society in general. Buckworth and Nigg found that college men exercise more than college women [16]. Salles-Costa *et al.* reported that relative to women, men participate more in group sports and physical activities that require more strength, such as tennis, soccer, volleyball, martial arts, jogging, and weight lifting. Women tend to engage in individual exercises and physical activities requiring less strength, such as walking and dancing [17]. Moreover, in many African-American communities, women walk significantly less than men do [18]. Also, because muscle weighs more than fat and males tend to have higher muscle mass than females, males often exhibit higher BMI [19].

4.2.2   The Impacts of Socioeconomic Status on Nutritional and Exercise Behavior

Clearly, behavioral factors, such as eating unhealthily or exercising infrequently, can contribute to being overweight and obese. Low socioeconomic status may make these unhealthy behaviors more likely and in effect raise the likelihood of high BMI and T2DM. First, a lack of financial resources can contribute to infrequent exercise because individuals with low income are less likely to afford memberships to exercise facilities, and low-income neighborhoods sometimes have high crime rates and are unsafe for outdoor exercise, such as walking or biking [20].

In addition, low socioeconomic status can increase tendencies toward unhealthy eating, because less money is available to spend on food, and cheap food in the United States is often unhealthy. At fast food establishments, a person can purchase several thousand calories for a few dollars. Fast food consumption by children has risen greatly over the years, which helps explain the increasing numbers of overweight and obese children. The proportion of food that children ate from restaurants and fast food establishments increased by almost 300% from 1977 to 1996 [21]. Since children are now eating more fast food, they are consuming more portions of high-calorie foods and fewer portions of vegetables, fruit, and milk. About 30% of children eat fast food on any given day. On days that children eat fast food, they consume an additional 187 kcal, which translates to about 6 lbs of calories per year [22]. Fast food consumption has risen not only for children but for adolescents as well. In one study, most adolescents overconsumed fast food, and overweight participants were especially likely to do so. Moreover, overweight adolescents were less likely to reduce food intake for the rest of the day after eating fast food meals than their nonoverweight counterparts [23].

4.2.3 The Impacts of Race/Ethnicity on Behavior Through Socioeconomic Status

As previously mentioned, certain race/ethnic groups might be genetically predisposed to having higher BMI. However, the socioeconomic status of race/ethnic groups likely influence BMI as well by affecting behavior. African-Americans, Hispanics, and Native Americans constitute disproportionately large percentages of low-income groups. Low income can contribute to behaviors such as unhealthy eating and infrequent exercise, which increases risk for high BMI and T2DM. Thus, race/ethnicity can impact behavior through socioeconomic status.

In some minority populations, those above normal body weight outnumber those with normal body weight, making overweight/obese the community norm. Minority neighborhoods often have numerous fast food restaurants that sell fattening foods, few supermarkets that provide fresh produce, and high neighborhood crime rates that discourage outdoor activities and limit safe places for walking and bicycling, including school routes [21]. Moreover, with regard to exercise, another study showed that many African-Americans with T2DM do not engage in regular activity, and their weight loss efforts often do not include physical activity [19].

4.2.4   Social Influences in Economically Disadvantaged
           Neighborhoods

The social influences within economically disadvantaged communities can perpetuate body weight problems. If many individuals in economically disadvantaged regions eat cheap ("fast") food, this enhances the "fast food culture" that can influence other community members to consume unhealthy, inexpensive food too. Social influences and commercial advertising within low-income neighborhoods can contribute to a norm of infrequent exercise. If many people in low-income neighborhoods do not exercise because they lack affordable access to fitness facilities or simply do not feel safe playing or exercising outside, this can reinforce the community norm of a sedentary lifestyle.

4.3   RESEARCH QUESTIONS AND HYPOTHESES

While the fact that certain race/ethnic groups suffer from higher prevalence of obesity and T2DM is well-known, the impact of specific sociodemographic and behavioral factors on high BMI and T2DM has not been well-defined in pediatrics. This issue is particularly vague for US adolescents, despite abundant data from adults. By analyzing the National Longitudinal Study of Adolescent Health, this review advances the literature on race/ethnic disparities among obesity and T2DM occurrence in adolescents by identifying the respective influences of race/ethnicity, income, eating behavior, and physical activity on high BMI rates among adolescents. Specifically, this chapter will address the following questions:

- How does socioeconomic status relate to eating and exercise behavior?
  Hypothesis #1: Low socioeconomic status is related to consumption of unhealthy foods and infrequent exercise.
- How does socioeconomic status relate to BMI and T2DM?
  Hypothesis #2: Low socioeconomic status is related to high BMI and T2DM.
- How does race/ethnicity relate to socioeconomic status, and through socioeconomic status, to behavior, BMI, and T2DM?
  Hypothesis #3: The race/ethnic groups of African-Americans, Hispanics, and Native Americans are associated with low socioeconomic status and thereby to unhealthy eating and exercise behaviors, high BMI, and T2DM.

Due to the fairly small sample size of the Adolescent Health Survey, relatively few cases of T2DM were available. However, many cases of overweight and obese adolescents were accessible for analysis, so sociodemographic and behavioral factors were analyzed with respect to their influences on BMI. These factors' influences on high BMI can be extended to T2DM, which often results from being overweight or obese.

4.4   METHODS

4.4.1   Data

The current research examines data from the public-use version of the National Longitudinal Study of Adolescent Health ("Add Health"), the largest, most comprehensive survey of adolescents ever completed. Add Health is a nationally representative study that examines health-related behaviors of adolescents in grades 7–12 and the effects manifested in young adulthood. Respondents were interviewed for the first two waves between 1994 and 1996 and reinterviewed for the third wave between 2001 and 2002 when they were 18–26 years old [24].

This review investigates the influences of demographic and behavioral factors during adolescence (Wave 1) on BMI during early adulthood (Wave 3). Out of the total 4,882 individuals with data available from Waves 1 and 3, only 3,844 were interviewed during both waves. Therefore, the number of cases (*N*) for each variable shown in Table 4.1 is out of a possible 3,844 cases.

4.4.2   Measures

Table 4.1 displays the variables used in this research and discussed in this section.

4.4.2.1   OUTCOME VARIABLES

BMI, the key outcome variable, is a generally accepted measure of body fat. In *adults*, BMI is calculated as weight (kg)/height (m)^2, and normal body composition is defined as BMI <25 kg/m^2, overweight as BMI 25–29.9 kg/m^2, and obese as BMI ≥30 kg/m^2. In the *pediatric* population, overweight is defined as BMI between 85–95 percentiles, and obesity is defined as BMI ≥95 percentile for children of the same age and gender. This study examines BMI of participants during early adulthood, so BMI calculations are based on the adult formula.

The Add Health survey asked participants whether or not they have diabetes, but did not distinguish between T1DM and T2DM. However, individuals who are diagnosed with diabetes at or above the age of 15 years tend to have T2DM rather than T1DM. Thus, the "Type 2 diabetes" variable that appears in Table 4.1 refers to individuals diagnosed with diabetes at age 15 or after. Since the data contains only 41 cases of T2DM, this study examines BMI as the outcome variable because substantially more cases of high BMI were available for analysis. However, results for high BMI can be extrapolated to T2DM because high BMI greatly predisposes to T2DM. Table 4.2 expresses the relationship between BMI and T2DM. As expected, fewer

Table 4.1 Distribution of the variables

	% (weighted)	% Missing (weighted)	N (unweighted)
Outcome variables			
Body mass index (kg/m^2)			
Normal weight (BMI <25)	46.5		
Overweight (25 ≤ BMI <30)	26.4		
Obese (BMI ≥30)	22.4		
Sum	95.3	4.7	3,648
Type 2 diabetes[b]			
Yes	0.7		
No	99.3		
Sum	99.9	0.1	3,668
Independent variables			
Case weight variable	100.0	0.0	3,844
Age at Wave 1[c]	100.0	0.0	3,844
Median: 15.4			
Mean: 15.5			
Gender			
Male	50.6		
Female	49.4		
Sum	100.0	0.0	3,844
Race/ethnicity variables[d]			
Non-Hispanic Whites	60.6		
African-Americans	12.1		
Hispanics	8.9		
Asians/Pacific Islanders	2.1		
Native Americans	0.8		
Other	0.3		
Multiple	1.7		
Sum	86.4	13.6	3,294
Mediating variables			
SOCIOECONOMIC STATUS VARIABLES			
Total household income per year	80.6	19.4	3,046
Median (thousands, $): 40.00			
Mean (thousands, $): 46.83			
Income categories			
$0–$9,999	6.1		
$10,000–$19,999	10.5		
$20,000–$29,999	11.9		
$30,000–$39,999	11.7		
>$40,000	40.5		
Sum	80.6	19.4	3,046
Receiving public assistance, such as welfare			
Yes	8.2		
No	81.7		
Sum	89.9	10.1	3,427

(continued)

Table 4.1 (continued)

	% (weighted)	% Missing (weighted)	N (unweighted)
BEHAVIOR VARIABLES			
Eating behavior variables (self-reports)			
# Times that consumed desserts (cookies/doughnuts/pies/cakes) yesterday			
None	44.7		
1 time	32.9		
2 or more times	22.4		
Sum	100.0	0.1	3,842
# Times that consumed starch (bread/cereal/rice/pasta) yesterday			
None	8.1		
1 time	29.0		
2 or more times	62.9		
Sum	100.0	0.1	3,842
# Times that consumed fruit or fruit juice yesterday			
None	22.56		
1 time	32.07		
2 or more times	45.32		
Sum	99.95	0.05	3,842
# Times that consumed vegetables yesterday			
None	31.75		
1 time	40.09		
2 or more times	28.11		
Sum	99.95	0.05	3,842
Exercise behavior variables (self-reports)			
# Times exercised in past week			
None	15.8		
1 or 2 times	31.9		
3 or 4 times	25.4		
5 or more times	26.8		
Sum	100.0	0.0	3,843
# Times played active sport in past week			
None	25.7		
1 or 2 times	27.3		
3 or 4 times	20.5		
5 or more times	26.5		
Sum	100.0	0.0	3,843

Source: National Longitudinal Study of Adolescent Health (http://www.cpc.unc.edu/projects/addhealth)
Note: Table frequencies are weighted. Refused/don't know responses are included in missing count.
[a]BMI=(weight in kilograms)/(height in meters^2). Out-of-range responses (height in feet=8+ or number of inches above last foot=12+) recorded as missing.
[b]The type 2 diabetes variable refers to people diagnosed with diabetes at >15 years of age because type 2 diabetes is usually the type of diabetes that strikes individuals >15 years of age.
[c] Age at Wave 1 was calculated using the following formula: (interview year – birth year) + (interview month – birth month). Age reported by student was not used because it had many missing responses.
[d]Taking the parent as the individual who completed the "Parent Questionnaire," the Parent's race, as opposed to Student's race, was used because the former has fewer missing responses. If the person who completed the "Parent Questionnaire" was not related to the student, the race variable was coded as missing. Thus, the race values presented on this table correspond with the Students' races.

Table 4.2 The relationship of income with behavior, the relationship of body mass index (BMI) with behavior, the relationship of body mass index (BMI) with race/ethnicity, income, and behavior, the relationship of race/ethnicity with income and behavior

Table 2a: The relationship of income with behavior

	Income Median $	Mean $
All cases	40,000	46,830
Type 2 diabetes		
Yes	24,000	29,790
No	40,000	46,950
Background variables		
Gender		
Male	39,000	46,000
Female	40,000	47,700
Race/ethnicity variables		
Non-Hispanic Whites	See Table 2c	
African-Americans	"	
Hispanics	"	
Asians/Pacific Islanders	"	
Native Americans	"	

Table 2b: The relationship of body mass index (BMI) with race/ethnicity, income, and behavior

	Body Mass Index Normal[a]	Overweight[b]	Obese[c]	Sum
All cases	48.8	27.7	23.5	100.0
Type 2 diabetes				
Yes	48.3	22.5	29.2	100.0
No	48.8	27.8	23.5	100.0
				(p<0.01)
Gender				
Male	46.2	31.0	22.8	100.0
Female	51.4	24.3	24.3	100.0
Non-Hispanic Whites	52.4	26.3	21.3	100.0
African-Americans	43.4	27.7	28.9	100.0
Hispanics	44.2	34.5	21.3	100.0
Asians/Pacific Islanders	60.6	23.6	15.9	100.0
Native Americans	34.0	22.8	43.2	100.0

Table 2c: The relationship of race/ethnicity with income and behavior

Race/Ethnicity**	All cases	NH White	AfAm	Hispanics	Asian/Pl	Native Amer	Other	Multiple races
All cases	100.0	70.2	14.0	10.3	2.5	0.9	0.3	1.9
Type 2 diabetes								
Yes	0.7	0.7	0.7	0.2	0.0	1.4	0.0	0.0
No	99.3	99.3	99.3	99.8	100.0	98.6	100.0	100.0
Sum	100.0	100.0	100.0	100.0	100.0	100.0	100.0	100.0
								(p<0.08)
Gender								
Male	50.6	50.5	49.9	52.8	53.6	50.4	48.1	45.9
Female	49.4	49.5	50.1	47.2	46.4	49.6	51.9	54.1
Sum	100.0	100.0	100.0	100.0	100.0	100.0	100.0	100.0
Non-Hispanic Whites	–	–	–	–	–	–	–	–
African-Americans	–	–	–	–	–	–	–	–
Hispanics	–	–	–	–	–	–	–	–
Asians/Pacific Islanders	–	–	–	–	–	–	–	–
Native Americans	–	–	–	–	–	–	–	–

						Sum									Sum	
Other "			61.6	20.4	17.9	100.0	–	–	–	–	–	–	–	–		
Multiple "			42.1	29.5	28.4	100.0	–	–	–	–	–	–	–	–		$p<0.01$
Mediating variables																
SOCIOECONOMIC STATUS VARIABLES																
Total household income per year																
Median (in thousands)	–		40.0	40.0	35.0		40.0	45.0	22.0	27.0	40.0	16.0	20.0	28.0		
Mean (in thousands)	–		49.4	45.3	42.5		46.8	52.4	29.6	33.6	46.6	20.9	27.3	29.7		
Income categories																
$0–$9,999			49.5	27.0	23.6	100.0	7.6	4.9	19.9	10.4	7.1	26.5	0.0	2.4		
$10,000–$19,999			41.6	30.9	27.5	100.0	13.0	9.2	22.8	25.7	5.9	31.3	11.3	23.9		
$20,000–$29,999			53.5	24.3	22.3	100.0	14.7	12.6	20.4	16.0	22.5	12.9	65.7	27.5		
$30,000–$39,999			48.1	25.1	26.8	100.0	14.5	14.7	11.6	17.8	13.5	12.6	0.0	9.6		
>$40,000			51.6	27.9	20.5	100.0	50.2	58.6	25.2	30.1	51.0	16.8	23.1	36.8		
Sum							Sum 100.0	100.0	100.0	100.0	100.0	100.0	100.0	100.0		$p<0.01$
Receiving public assistance, such as welfare																
Yes	11,000	15,030	44.5	32.3	23.2	100.0	9.1	5.5	22.4	14.3	2.7	24.3	20.1	11.9		
No	40,000	49,970	50.5	26.8	22.7	100.0	90.9	94.5	77.6	85.7	97.4	75.8	80.0	88.1		
Sum							Sum 100.0	100.0	100.0	100.0	100.0	100.0	100.0	100.0		$p<0.04$
BEHAVIOR VARIABLES																
Eating behavior variables (self-reports)																
# Times that consumed desserts (cookies/doughnuts/pies/cakes) yesterday																
None	36,000	46,300	43.5	28.7	27.8	100.0	44.7	43.2	44.0	43.2	41.9	17.8	14.7	58.9		
1 time	40,000	49,990	50.2	28.2	21.6	100.0	33.0	34.3	28.6	31.9	34.2	68.9	62.4	35.7		
2 or more times	40,000	43,310	57.0	25.2	17.9	100.0	22.4	22.4	27.4	20.0	23.9	13.4	22.9	5.5		

(continued)

Table 4.2 (continued)

	Table 2a: The relationship of income with behavior		Table 2b: The relationship of body mass index (BMI) with race/ethnicity, income, and behavior				Table 2c: The relationship of race/ethnicity with income and behavior							
	Income		Body Mass Index				Race/Ethnicity**							
	Median $	Mean $	Normal[a]	Overweight[b]	Obese[c]	Sum	All cases	NH White	AfAm	Hispanics	Asian/PI	Native Amer	Other	Multiple races
Sum		$p<0.01$				$p<0.01$	**Sum** 100.0	100.0	100.0	100.0	100.0	100.0	100.0	100.0
														$p<0.01$
# Times that consumed starches (bread/cereal/rice/pasta) yesterday														
None	29,000	36,520	44.3	28.3	27.4	100.0	8.1	6.0	13.1	9.1	7.1	4.4	8.0	13.2
1 time	36,000	44,610	43.8	29.8	26.5	100.0	29.0	27.4	31.4	35.5	27.0	20.6	16.1	29.5
2 or more times	40,000	49,120	51.6	26.7	21.7	100.0	62.9	66.5	55.5	55.4	65.9	75.0	75.9	57.3
Sum		$p<0.01$				$p<0.01$	**Sum** 100.0	100.0	100.0	100.0	100.0	100.0	100.0	100.0
														$p<0.01$
# Times that consumed fruit or fruit juice yesterday														
None	35,000	38,360	42.3	28.9	28.8	100.0	22.6	22.4	20.5	21.1	10.7	21.8	18.8	36.8
1 time	39,000	48,220	48.4	29.2	22.4	100.0	32.1	32.7	34.0	29.9	29.4	30.5	19.6	34.0
2 or more times	40,000	50,180	52.2	26.1	21.7	100.0	45.3	44.9	45.5	49.0	59.9	47.7	61.6	29.2
Sum		$p<0.01$					**Sum** 100.0	100.0	100.0	100.0	100.0	100.0	100.0	100.0
														$p<0.03$
# Times that consumed vegetables yesterday														
None	32,000	39,270	45.7	28.0	26.3	100.0	31.8	27.7	42.7	39.6	16.1	50.5	27.0	39.2
1 time	41,000	50,330	50.2	28.1	21.7	100.0	40.1	41.7	34.5	40.5	43.3	20.1	46.9	34.3

Table (continued)

	N	N	Normal BMI[a]	Overweight[b]	Obese[c]	Sum	p									p
2 or more times	40,000	50,230	50.3	26.9	22.9	100.0	p<0.02	28.1	30.6	22.8	19.9	40.6	29.5	26.1	26.6	p<0.01
Sum								100.0	100.0	100.0	100.0	100.0	100.0	100.0	100.0	
Exercise behavior variables (self-reports)																
# Times exercised in past week																
None	37,000	47,560	47.5	28.2	24.3	100.0		15.8	15.4	14.9	17.0	12.4	4.9	8.1	21.4	
1 or 2 times	40,000	46,830	49.5	26.3	24.3	100.0		31.9	31.9	31.9	33.1	28.1	41.7	32.1	30.1	
3 or 4 times	38,000	44,950	46.8	28.3	24.9	100.0		25.4	25.8	24.9	25.7	36.2	23.4	7.3	19.7	
5 or more times	40,000	48,260	50.7	28.6	20.8	100.0	p<0.03	26.8	26.9	28.4	24.3	23.3	30.0	52.6	28.8	p<0.03
Sum								100.0	100.0	100.0	100.0	100.0	100.0	100.0	100.0	
# Times played active sport in past week																
None	35,000	45,060	50.4	26.3	23.3	100.0		25.7	23.4	28.5	29.1	27.1	18.3	35.2	27.4	
1 or 2 times	37,000	43,470	46.7	27.7	25.6	100.0		27.3	27.4	25.9	28.8	22.1	27.3	9.4	35.8	
3 or 4 times	40,000	46,880	48.0	27.6	24.4	100.0		20.5	21.1	17.1	22.0	23.3	19.1	27.5	20.4	
5 or more times	45,000	51,710	50.0	29.2	20.8	100.0	p<0.01	26.5	28.2	28.6	20.1	27.6	35.3	28.0	16.4	p<0.02
Sum								100.0	100.0	100.0	100.0	100.0	100.0	100.0	100.0	

Source: National Longitudinal Study of Adolescent Health (http://www.cpc.unc.edu/projects/addhealth)

Note: Table frequencies are weighted. Chi-squares are based on unweighted frequencies.

**Race/Ethnicity Abbreviations: *NH White* non-Hispanic White; *AfAm* African-American; *Asian/PI* Asian/Pacific Islander; *Native Amer* Native American

[a]Normal BMI corresponds to BMI <25; [b]Overweight corresponds to 25 ≤BMI ≤30; [c]Obese corresponds to BMI >30

individuals with T2DM (48.3%) had normal BMI than individuals without T2DM (48.8%), and the obesity rate for people with T2DM (29.2%) exceeded the obesity rate for those without T2DM (23.5%), although these results were not statistically significant.

4.4.2.2 BACKGROUND VARIABLES

The first category under "background variables" in Table 4.1 is gender. Due to the very narrow age range (age at Wave 1 ranged from 12 to 17 years, with the median and mean ages both around 15.5 years), age was not included in the analysis. Race/ethnicity was divided into non-Hispanic Whites, African-Americans, Hispanics, Asians/Pacific Islanders, Native Americans, other, and multiple races.

4.4.2.3 MEDIATING VARIABLES

The Socioeconomic Status variables include receipt of public assistance (*e.g.*, welfare) and total household income per year, divided into $5,000 increments from $0 to $40,000. Above $40,000, cases are simply grouped into a "≥$40,000" category. This section devotes more detail to income groups below $40,000 because the current study is concerned with the impacts of low income on eating and exercise behavior and thus BMI and T2DM occurrence.

Behavior Variables include eating behavior (including consumption of fast food, desserts, starches, fruits or fruit juice, and vegetables) and exercise variables (including frequencies of exercise and playing active sports).

4.5 STATISTICS

The data have been weighted to ensure the accuracy of the means and medians of the "age at Wave 1" and "total household income per year" variables. However, the weights inflate the number of cases to population size. Thus, the standard deviations, if reported, would have been inaccurately small and therefore are not shown.

Table 4.2 performs cross-tabulations, accompanied by *p*-values where appropriate, of income with behavior, of BMI with race/ethnicity, income, and behavior, and of race/ethnicity with income and behavior. Table 4.3 displays the four multinomial logistic regression models that were generated to determine predictors of BMI.

Table 4.3 (multinomial logistic regression models) presents odds ratios for four multinomial logistic regression models that regress BMI on several predictor variables. For each model, the table first displays odds ratios for being obese relative to normal and then displays odds ratios for being overweight relative to normal. The term "normal" refers to having a BMI in the

Table 4.3
Multinominal logistic regression models

	Obesity							
Parameter	Model 1		Model 2		Model 3		Model 4	
*Odds ratios for obese relative to normal BMI	*Odds ratio	P	*Odds ratio	P	*Odds ratio	P	*Odds ratio	P
Likelihood		0.0496		0.033		<0.001		0.002
Intercept	0.384	<0.001	0.345	<0.001	0.616	0.003	0.569	0.005
Background variables								
Male (reference = female)	1.063	0.531	1.057	0.573	1.087	0.401	1.085	0.424
Race/ethnicity (reference = non-Hispanic White)								
African American	1.579	0.000	1.492	0.001	1.534	0.001	1.547	0.001
Hispanic	1.125	0.523	1.024	0.900	0.998	0.991	0.993	0.972
Asian/Pacific Islander	0.654	0.166	0.655	0.167	0.674	0.202	0.664	0.187
Native American	13.566	<0.001	12.022	<0.001	13.099	<0.001	13.025	<0.001
Other and multiple races	1.269	0.474	1.227	0.542	1.075	0.831	1.092	0.795
Mediating variables								
SOCIOECONOMIC STATUS VARIABLES								
Total household income/year (reference = above $40,000)								
$0–$9,999			1.277	0.198	1.190	0.369	1.176	0.402
$10,000–$19,999			1.494	0.011	1.359	0.055	1.363	0.054
$20,000–$29,999			1.083	0.585	1.006	0.966	1.008	0.956
$30,000–$39,999			1.392	0.020	1.329	0.048	1.312	0.060
BEHAVIOR VARIABLES								
Eating behavior variables (self-reports)								
One dessert consumed yesterday	(reference = none)				0.792	0.040	0.785	0.033
Two or more desserts consumed yesterday	(reference = none)				0.517	<0.001	0.511	<0.001
One starch consumed yesterday	(reference = two or more)				1.146	0.228	1.140	0.246
No starches consumed yesterday	(reference = two or more)				1.214	0.285	1.204	0.308
Fruit consumed yesterday	(reference = none)				0.681	0.001	0.676	0.001
One vegetable consumed yesterday	(reference = none)				0.786	0.045	0.785	0.045
Two or more vegetables consumed yesterday	(reference = none)				0.985	0.903	0.991	0.946
Exercise behavior variables (self-reports)								
Exercised 1–4 times in past week	(reference = none)						1.106	0.476
Exercised 5+ times in past week	(reference = none)						0.854	0.327
Played active sports in past week	(reference = none)						1.109	0.371
†Odds ratios for overweight relative to normal BMI	†Odds ratio	P	†Odds ratio	P	†Odds ratio	P	†Odds ratio	P
Likelihood (as mentioned earlier)		0.0496		0.033		<0.001		0.002
Intercept	0.417	<0.001	0.414	<0.001	0.458	<0.001	0.325	<0.001
Background variables								
Male (reference = female)	1.445	<0.001	1.447	<0.001	1.481	<0.001	1.445	0.000
Race/ethnicity (reference = non-Hispanic White)								
African American	1.089	0.481	1.059	0.648	1.073	0.578	1.075	0.569
Hispanic	1.700	0.001	1.619	0.002	1.571	0.004	1.579	0.004
Asian/Pacific Islander	0.799	0.389	0.816	0.436	0.804	0.407	0.817	0.444
Native American	4.116	0.046	3.804	0.061	4.017	0.052	3.934	0.056
Other and multiple races	1.307	0.386	1.318	0.375	1.226	0.515	1.240	0.493
Mediating variables								
SOCIOECONOMIC STATUS VARIABLES								
Total household income/year (reference = above $40,000)								
$0–$9,999			1.154	0.427	1.154	0.432	1.164	0.408
$10,000–$19,999			1.323	0.058	1.275	0.104	1.314	0.068
$20,000–$29,999			0.826	0.176	0.800	0.117	0.812	0.143
$30,000–$39,999			0.980	0.886	0.958	0.762	0.960	0.771

(continued)

86 Neubecker

Table 4.3
(continued)

	Obesity			
Parameter	Model 1	Model 2	Model 3	Model 4
BEHAVIOR VARIABLES				
Eating behavior variables (self-reports)				
One dessert consumed yesterday	(reference = none)		0.915 0.400	0.903 0.335
Two or more desserts consumed yesterday	(reference = none)		0.673 0.001	0.661 0.001
One starch consumed yesterday	(reference = two or more)		1.326 0.007	1.335 0.006
No starches consumed yesterday	(reference = two or more)		1.095 0.618	1.112 0.561
Fruit consumed yesterday	(reference = none)		0.931 0.546	0.896 0.353
One vegetable consumed yesterday	(reference = none)		0.986 0.898	0.963 0.736
Two or more vegetables consumed yesterday	(reference = none)		1.000 0.997	0.962 0.753
Exercise behavior variables (self-reports)				
Exercised 1–4 times in past week	(reference = none)			1.288 0.068
Exercised 5+ times in past week	(reference = none)			1.300 0.084
Played active sports in past week	(reference = none)			1.281 0.029

Model 1 regresses BMI only on the background variables of gender and race/ethnicity.
Model 2 adds the socioeconomic status variable of yearly household income to the analysis.
Model 3 adds eating behavior variables.
Model 4 adds the exercise behavior variables.

normal range (less than 25 kg/m^2). Also, the values in Table 4.3 are based on unweighted data because weighted data would produce unrealistically low p-values. To decrease the number of parameters in order to increase the p-value of the entire model, certain groups were combined in the multinomial regression models if they showed similar significance and directionality. The simplified groups are the race/ethnicity categories of "other and multiple," consumption of "one" and "two or more" fruits, involvement in exercise activities for "one or two" and "three or four" times in the past week, and participation in active sports for "one or two," "three or four," and "five or more" times in the past week.

4.6 RESULTS

4.6.1 Distribution of the Variables

Table 4.1 displays the weighted percentages, weighted percentages of missing responses, and unweighted N for all the variables. Most of the variables had low percentages of missing responses; BMI, T2DM, age at Wave 1, gender, and eating and exercise variables had fewer than 5% of responses missing. Race/ethnicity had a slightly higher percentage of missing responses (13.6%), as did total household income per year (19.4%) and receipt of public assistance (10.1%).

Across all individuals, nearly half were overweight (26.4%) or obese (22.4%). Thus, a minority of the sample (46.5%) had BMI in the "normal" range (<25 kg/m^2). Only 0.7% of the sample had T2DM ($n=41$). For the race/ethnicity variables, non-Hispanic Whites constituted the largest group at 60.6%, followed by African-Americans at 12.1%, Hispanics at 8.9%, Asians/Pacific Islanders at 2.1%, multiple races at 1.7%, and others at 0.3%. For the eating behavior variables, a fairly high percentage (44.7%) did not consume desserts the previous day. Also, the majority of the population (62.9%) consumed two or more starches the previous day, and few (8.1%) consumed no starches.

4.6.2 Relation of Socioeconomic Status with Eating and Exercise Behavior

Hypothesis #1: Low socioeconomic status is strongly related to consumption of unhealthy foods and infrequent exercise.

Table 4.2 (the relationship of income with behavior) partially supports Hypothesis #1. Individuals who consumed only one dessert the previous day exhibited the highest socioeconomic status: a mean income of \$49,990 and a median income of \$40,000. Individuals who consumed two or more desserts had the lowest mean income (\$43,310), and individuals who consumed no desserts had the lowest median income (\$36,000). Apparently, adolescents from households with the most money have a greater likelihood of consuming desserts in moderation (*e.g.*, once daily). Regarding consumption of starches, the greater the individuals' income levels, the more starch they consumed. This finding makes sense because the highest number of starches per day people could report in the study was "two or more," which is very low compared to the recommendation of five to six servings of starch per day by the US Department of Agriculture [25]. Most people with sufficient income would consume two or more starch servings per day, and individuals could be expected to consume less starch as their income decreased. Moreover, individuals with lower incomes were less likely to consume healthier foods, like fruit and vegetables. A positive, linear relationship existed between income and the consumption of fruit or fruit juice, and individuals who consumed any vegetables in one day had higher median and mean incomes than those who did not. Next, income and participation in active sports demonstrated a positive, linear relationship. Although a positive, linear relationship did not exist between income and amount of exercise, those who exercised the most (five or more times per week) had the highest incomes.

4.6.3 Relation of Socioeconomic Status with BMI and T2DM

Hypothesis #2: Low socioeconomic status is strongly related to high BMI and T2DM.

4.6.3.1 Low Income and High BMI

The relationship between low income and high BMI is supported by data from Table 4.2 (the relationship of BMI with race/ethnicity, income, and behavior). Individuals with normal BMI had the highest income, followed by overweight individuals and, finally, obese individuals. The BMI distributions across income categories showed statistical significance ($p < 0.01$). One of the low-income groups ($10,000–19,999 household earnings) exhibited the lowest percentage of individuals with normal BMI (41.6%) and the highest rates of overweight (30.9%) and obese (27.5%) individuals. The lowest income group of $0–$9,999 had relatively low rates of high BMI, perhaps because these people did not have enough money to afford much food at all, whereas the $10,000–19,999 group had enough money to purchase cheap, unhealthy food. The highest income group (greater than $40,000 per year) exhibited the lowest rates of obesity (20.5%). Individuals receiving public assistance manifested lower percentages of normal BMI (44.5%) than those without public aid (50.5%). People with government assistance also had higher proportions of obese and overweight individuals, 23.2 and 32.3%, respectively, than those without government assistance, 22.7 and 26.8%, respectively ($p < 0.04$).

4.6.3.2 Low Income and T2DM

Individuals with T2DM had much lower incomes ($24,000 median, $29,790 mean) than those without T2DM ($40,000 median, $46,950 mean), as demonstrated in Table 4.2. Since most of the subjects with T2DM developed the disease only after their income data was collected, their low incomes may not result from the disease. However, younger participants had lower incomes than older groups.

4.6.4   Relation of Race/Ethnicity with Socioeconomic Status, Behavior, BMI, and T2DM

Hypothesis #3: The race/ethnic groups of African-Americans, Hispanics, and Native Americans are strongly associated with low socioeconomic status and thereby to unhealthy eating and exercise behaviors, high BMI, and incidence of T2DM.

4.6.4.1 Race/Ethnicity and Income

Indeed, the race/ethnic groups of African-Americans, Hispanics, and Native Americans were associated with low socioeconomic status. Non-Hispanic Whites had the highest incomes per year, followed by Asians/

Pacific Islanders, Hispanics, African-Americans, and Native Americans, in that order. Non-Hispanic Whites and Asians/Pacific Islanders also exhibited lower percentages of public assistance use than did African-Americans, Hispanics, and Native Americans.

4.6.4.2 RACE/ETHNICITY AND EATING BEHAVIORS

Native Americans and African-Americans showed tendencies toward unhealthy eating behavior. Native Americans had the lowest proportion of individuals who ate no desserts (17.8%) and the highest proportion of individuals who ate one dessert during the day (68.9%). African-Americans exhibited the greatest percentage (27.4%) of individuals who consumed two or more desserts in 1 day. In contrast, Hispanics showed the highest proportion of individuals who consumed no desserts. Next, the majority of all race/ethnic groups marked the response for the maximum number of starches (two or more starches per day) on the survey. Not all race/ethnic groups with low-income levels and high obesity rates exhibited the same directionality for consumption of starches. Although Native Americans had the greatest proportion of individuals who consumed the maximum number of starches (75.0%), Hispanics (55.4%) and African-Americans (55.5%) had the lowest proportions that did so. African-Americans, Hispanics, and Native Americans exhibited relatively low rates of eating healthy foods at least twice per day; these three groups had lower proportions of consumption of fruits or fruit juice than Asians/Pacific Islanders and lower proportions of consumption of vegetables than Asians/Pacific Islanders and non-Hispanic Whites. These findings not only support the prediction in Hypothesis #3 that African-Americans, Hispanics, and Native Americans have higher tendencies toward unhealthy eating, but also that they have lower tendencies toward healthy eating.

4.6.4.3 RACE/ETHNICITY AND EXERCISE BEHAVIORS

Of all the race/ethnic groups, Hispanics showed the highest tendency toward no exercise at all, the second highest tendency toward only exercising one or two times per week, the third highest tendency toward exercising three or four times per week, and the fourth highest (and next to lowest) tendency toward exercising five or more times per week. Also, Hispanics showed the highest rate for doing no active sports and lowest rate for playing an active sport five or more times per week. Thus, the data strongly suggest that Hispanics engage in relatively little exercise. Native Americans showed the lowest rates for doing no exercise and active sports and the highest rates for exercising and for playing sports five or more times per week; these results were surprising given the extremely high obesity levels for Native Americans. Compared to other race/ethnic groups, African-Americans exhibited moderate rates both for exercising and for playing active sports either 0, "one or two," or "three or four" times per week. However, African-Americans showed the second highest rates both for exercising and for playing active sports extremely often (five or more times per week). Therefore, the data did *not* show that African-Americans and Native Americans do little exercise. Thus, the prediction outlined in Hypothesis #3 appears to be the case for Hispanics, but not so for African-Americans and Native Americans. Additionally, Asians/Pacific Islanders exercised quite frequently; they showed the highest percentage (36.2%) for exercising three or four times per week, which was 10.5% greater than that of non-Hispanic Whites, who exhibited the second highest percentage for exercising three or four times per week.

4.6.4.4 RACE/ETHNICITY AND BMI

The BMI disparities across race/ethnicity were statistically significant ($p < 0.01$). Excluding "other" and "multiple race/ethnicities," Asians/Pacific Islanders exhibited the highest percentage of normal BMI (60.6%), followed by non-Hispanic Whites (52.4%), then Hispanics (44.2%), next African-Americans (43.3%), and finally Native Americans (34.0%). Compared to the percentage of individuals with normal BMI across all cases (48.8%), Asians/Pacific Islanders and non-Hispanic Whites exhibited greater percentages of individuals with normal BMI, while Native Americans, African-Americans, and Hispanics, manifested lower percentages of individuals with normal BMI. Native Americans experienced an astonishingly high rate of obesity (43.2%), and African-Americans exhibited the second highest rate of obesity (28.9%). The rate of obesity across all race/ethnic groups was 23.5%. Hispanics showed the highest percentage of overweight individuals (34.5%), followed by African-Americans (27.7%). These results support the prediction stated in Hypothesis #3 that Hispanics, African-Americans, and Native Americans would exhibit relatively high BMI.

4.6.4.5 RACE/ETHNICITY AND T2DM

Although the relationship between race/ethnicity and T2DM was not statistically significant ($p < 0.08$), some interesting data were noted. None of the Asians/Pacific Islanders in the sample had T2DM, probably due to the small number of Asians/Pacific Islanders in the sample. In contrast, despite the small sample size of Native Americans, this group exhibited the highest rate of T2DM (1.4%) of all the race/ethnic groups.

4.6.5   Other Findings

4.6.5.1   BMI AND GENDER

In addition, a statistically significant gender effect was observed. Fewer males than females had normal BMI (46.2% compared to 51.4%, respectively), mostly because more males fell into the overweight category (31.0%) compared to females (24.3%). However, more females were obese (24.3%) than males (22.8%).

4.6.5.2   BMI AND EATING VARIABLES

Surprisingly, groups that consumed more dessert had lower percentages of overweight and obese individuals. Perhaps this indicates that desserts in moderation are acceptable, or that overweight and obese individuals did not want to admit eating dessert due to social desirability bias. The group with the highest consumption of starches (two or more per day) showed the highest proportion of individuals with normal BMI (51.6%) and the lowest levels of overweight (26.7%) and obese (21.7%) individuals. One should recall, however, that the group that consumed two or more starches per day also constituted a majority of the population (62.9%); the groups that consumed one starch and zero starches per day accounted for only 29.0% and 8.1% of the population, respectively. Additionally, groups that consumed more fruit, fruit juice, and vegetables had lower percentages of overweight and obese individuals. Surprisingly, people who exercised more did not exhibit lower BMI, and groups that played active sports more tended to have higher rates of overweight individuals. The discussion of the regression models below will include possible explanations for these unexpected relationships regarding exercise behavior.

4.6.6   Regression Models of Demographic Factors, Health Behavior, and BMI

Model 1 regresses BMI only on the background variables of gender and race/ethnicity. Model 2 adds the socioeconomic status variable of yearly household income to the analysis. Model 3 adds eating behavior variables. Finally, Model 4 adds the exercise behavior variables.

Model 1 regresses BMI on gender and race/ethnicity and reveals that BMI statistically differs by race/ethnicity (overall $p<0.05$). Compared to non-Hispanic Whites, Native Americans exhibited the highest odds of having high BMI (either obese or overweight) relative to normal BMI, followed by African-Americans and Hispanics, and finally Asians/Pacific Islanders. Despite the small sample size of Native Americans, they were an astonishing

13.6 times more likely to be obese and 3.9 times more likely to be overweight, compared to non-Hispanic Whites. Moreover, relative to non-Hispanic Whites, African-Americans exhibited 1.58 times more risk of being obese, and Hispanics exhibited 1.60 times more risk of being overweight. Hispanics also showed higher risk of being obese than non-Hispanic Whites, although this result was not statistically significant. Asians/Pacific Islanders exhibited noticeably low odds of being obese or overweight relative to normal BMI, compared to non-Hispanic Whites; however, this was not statistically significant, possibly due to their small sample size. In addition, males were 1.45 times more likely to be overweight, compared to females. This gender effect might be because males tend to exhibit higher BMIs since they tend to have more muscle mass, which weighs more than fat, compared to females [11].

Model 2 adds total household income per year to the multinomial regression model with nominally higher significance ($p < 0.04$) than Model 1 ($p < 0.05$), indicating that socioeconomic status plays a role in explaining the differentials in BMI across the sample. Receipt of public assistance is not included as a parameter because its effect is already encapsulated in total household income per year. In a previous model (not shown here), receipt of welfare did not show significance when included in the model with total household income per year. Although the relationship between income and BMI is not completely linear, a definite correlation exists between low income and increased tendency toward having high BMI relative to normal BMI. Compared to individuals from households earning greater than $40,000 per year, those with total household income per year below $40,000 were more likely to be obese than normal. These effects were statistically significant for the $10,000–19,999 and $30,000–39,999 income groups. Moreover, compared to individuals with total household income per year above $40,000, people with total household income per year less than $20,000 exhibited higher risk for being overweight relative to normal. This trend was statistically significant for the $10,000–19,999 income group. When total household income per year was added in Model 2, the race/ethnicity effects previously discussed still existed, although the effects were slightly reduced, indicating that income helps explain part of the disparity due to race/ethnicity. The gender effect detailed above (that "overweight" BMIs are more common in males) perpetuated as well.

Model 3 adds eating behavior variables to the analysis and adds further significance ($p < 0.001$) compared to Model 2 ($p < 0.05$), suggesting that eating behavior helps explain BMI. Surprisingly, compared to individuals who did not eat dessert the previous day, those who ate dessert had lower odds of being obese relative to normal, and those who ate two or more desserts the previous day manifested lower odds of being overweight relative to normal. These unexpected results might be due to a social desirability bias, whereby obese and overweight individuals might have underreported their dessert consumption because they were embarrassed to admit their true eating behavior. Another possibility is that overweight and obese individuals are more likely to be dieting and thus are less likely to be currently consuming desserts. This would support that not only can eating behavior impact BMI, but also BMI can impact eating behavior.

In addition, compared to people who ate two or more starches the previous day, those who ate only one starch were 1.3 times more likely to be overweight rather than normal. This finding suggests that consuming only one starch per day does not necessarily cause weight loss. As previously mentioned, the US Department of Health and Human Services and the US Department of Agriculture recommend five to six servings of starch per day. Therefore, one serving might not be sufficient for good nutrition and for maintaining normal BMI. Perhaps eating very little starch can lead people to consume more fattening foods instead and consequently develop higher BMI.

Also, compared to individuals who consumed no fruit the previous day, those who did eat fruit were only 0.68 times as likely to be obese rather than normal. Compared to individuals who ate no vegetables the day before, the ratio of those who consumed one serving of vegetables were only 0.79 times as likely to be obese. These results suggest that a diet including fruit and vegetables can be helpful for preventing weight problems. Additionally, the race/ethnicity, gender, and socioeconomic effects previously discussed were still evident and statistically significant in this model. Compared to non-Hispanic Whites, the elevated risks for African-Americans and Native Americans of being obese increased in Model 3 with the addition of eating variables. Also, the higher risk of Native Americans of being overweight increased in Model 3. Thus, differential reports of eating behavior actually widened the baseline race/ethnic differences for African-Americans and Native Americans; these were unexpected results. In contrast, the higher risk for Hispanics of being overweight relative to normal decreased in Model 3, suggesting that the eating behavior parameters added in this model do help explain the effects of being Hispanic on being overweight.

Finally, Model 4 adds Exercise Behavior Variables to the regression. The overall p-value increased slightly from Model 3 ($p<0.001$) to Model 4 ($p=0.002$), suggesting that the exercise variables added in Model 4 were not more useful predictors of BMI. As mentioned in the discussion of Table 4.2, African-Americans and Native Americans experienced large percentages of high BMI, yet they exercised and played sports quite frequently, whereas Hispanics, who also experienced large percentages of high BMI, exercised relatively infrequently. Thus, the relation between exercise and BMI is not consistent across race/ethnic groups. Still, Model 4 has high statistical significance ($p = 0.002$), which implies that the model could explain the disparities of high BMI across individuals. Engaging in exercise and active sports did not show statistical significance for obese relative to normal individuals but did show significance for overweight relative to normal. Surprisingly, individuals who exercised and individuals who played active sports were more likely to have BMIs in the overweight range rather than in the normal range. This might be because people who exercise have more muscle, which weighs more than fat. This could increase their BMI and classify them as "overweight" even though they are in good physical condition, a recognized limitation of BMI alone as a surrogate marker of body composition. Another explanation is that BMI can influence people's exercise behavior; overweight and obese people might be exercising more in order to lose weight. The effects of race/ethnicity, gender, socioeconomic status, and eating behavior already discussed persevered into the fourth model. The elevated risk for Native Americans of being overweight relative to normal slightly decreased in Model 4, suggesting that the addition of exercise variables in this model helped explain the effects of being Native American on being overweight. The other effects of race/ethnicity on BMI were not influenced a great deal by the addition of exercise variables in Model 4.

In summary, socioeconomic status and eating behavior (but not exercise behavior) appear to explain some of the disparities of BMI across race/ethnicity. After controlling for socioeconomic status and eating behavior, race/ethnic effects still existed. Thus, other factors not included in the multinomial regression models, such as genetic variability, are influencing the effects of race/ethnicity on BMI.

4.7   DISCUSSION

The data partially support the three hypotheses outlined in the introduction. The data provide some justification for Hypothesis #1, that low socioeconomic status is related to unhealthy eating behavior and infrequent exercise. The group that consumed the most desserts (two or more per day) exhibited the lowest mean income ($43,310), and people with low incomes were less likely to eat healthy foods like fruits and vegetables. Also, the group that exercised the most had the highest incomes, and a positive, linear relationship existed for income and participation in active sports.

Furthermore, the current analysis supports Hypothesis #2 that low socioeconomic status is related to high BMI. The highest incomes were found in people with normal BMI, followed by overweight and, finally, obese individuals. Moreover, compared to households earning greater than $40,000 per year, those earning below $40,000 exhibited higher odds of being obese relative to normal, and those earning below $20,000 exhibited higher odds of being overweight relative to normal.

In addition, the findings offer some support of Hypothesis #3, that the race/ethnic groups of Hispanics, African-Americans, and Native Americans are associated with low socioeconomic status and thereby to unhealthy eating and exercise behavior and higher BMI. Hispanics, African-Americans, and Native Americans had the lowest incomes and greatest tendencies toward receiving public assistance. Also, Hispanics, African-Americans, and Native Americans exhibited tendencies toward eating fattening foods and refraining from healthy foods. The data indicated that Hispanics, but not African-Americans or Native Americans, had lower tendencies toward exercise compared to non-Hispanic Whites. Furthermore, Hispanics, African-Americans, and Native Americans showed the greatest odds of having high BMI relative to normal BMI.

The current research has many implications for physicians, families, schools, and society. All adolescents should be taught the importance of healthy eating and exercise behaviors in preventing high BMI levels and associated health problems. However, physicians, families, and schools should especially encourage African-American, Hispanic, and Native American adolescents to eat more healthy foods and fewer fattening foods because these race/ethnic groups appear to show relatively high tendencies toward these behaviors. Also, Hispanics should be encouraged to exercise more frequently because they show low levels of physical activity and high proportions of overweight individuals. Schools could discourage unhealthy eating by replacing snack vending machines with fruit and water options in the cafeteria line, as one study advocated [26]. Schools could encourage physical activity by increasing the frequency of physical education classes and by encouraging students to exercise in school gyms after classes end for the day. A previous study suggested that cities promote healthful eating and exercise behavior by influencing urban environments and transport systems to promote physical activity, developing community-wide exercise programs, increasing communication about healthy eating and physical activity, and improving health services to promote breastfeeding and help currently overweight or obese people to lose weight [27].

Limitations of the current study include the nature of the BMI variable itself; because BMI only takes into account height and weight, and not proportions of muscle or fat. Thus, a muscular person could have the same BMI as someone who is simply overweight. Indeed, this would help explain why those who exercised five or more times per week and those who played active sports five or more times per week had the highest proportions of "overweight" individuals. The development of an indicator that takes into account muscle and fat proportions would be ideal for determining health. Also, this study attempted to use characteristics in Wave 1 (race/ethnicity, socioeconomic status, eating and exercise behavior) to predict BMI at a later point in time. A complication is that BMI at a later point in time is influenced by the BMI earlier in life. Thus, these models would have been a better predictor of weight change as opposed to weight at a single point in time. However, this was not possible in this analysis because the body weights at Wave 1 were self-reported, whereas weights at Wave 3 were not self-reported, so the two weights could not be adequately compared to determine weight change. Another limitation of the current study is that all BMI values under 25 were considered "normal," including very low BMI levels such as 19 and below. Although BMI numbers of 19 and below constituted only about 4% of the sample and thus probably did not significantly skew results, future research could exclude very low BMI levels from the "normal" category.

For future research, a dataset that provides measured (as opposed to self-reported) body weights on individuals at two different points in time would allow for the investigation of how certain characteristics and behaviors impact weight change over time. Moreover, analysis could be performed on larger datasets with many more T2DM patients. The current sample was relatively small and only contained 41 participants with T2DM, so the variables had to be analyzed with respect to high BMI as a proxy for T2DM. Investigating how certain variables not only impact BMI, but also development of T2DM, is the compelling next step. In addition, a future study could analyze how eating fast food influences race/ethnic differentials on BMI. Fast food consumption was not included in the public-use version of Add Health examined in this study, but this information is available on the private-use version. A future study using the private-use version of Add Health could investigate the "fast food culture" hypothesis outlined in the introduction that proposes that if many individuals in low-income neighborhoods eat cheap fast food, this can influence others to consume fast food as well. Because Add Health can compare the behavior of students with the behavior of their friends, a study could investigate whether friends exhibit similar patterns of fast food consumption. Also, future research could address other "peer effects," including whether friends exhibit similar exercise patterns. Indeed, people often eat and exercise with friends, so these peer effects might be substantial. In conclusion, differentials in BMI due to race/ethnicity are partially explained by socioeconomic status and eating and exercise behavior, but more research is needed to better understand the components of race/ethnicity that are contributing to the spread of the obesity and T2DM epidemics among adolescents in the United States.

Acknowledgments The author wishes to acknowledge the individuals affiliated with the Research Experience for Undergraduates (REU) Program at the Population Research Center at University of Texas at Austin, who provided invaluable conceptual and empirical guidance, as well as financial support, for this research. In particular, the author thanks Dr. Robert Hummer for his help with designing the conceptual pathway of the research and analyzing the results. The author also wishes to recognize Starling Pullum and Ginger Gossman, who helped with developing programming code and interpreting the data.

REFERENCES

1. Flegal KM, Carroll MD, Kuczamarski RJ, Johnson CL (1998) Overweight and obesity in the United States; prevalence and trends, 1960–994. Int J Obes Relat Metab Disord 22:39–47
2. Kuczamarski RJ, Flegal KM, Campbell SM, Johnson CL (1994) Increasing prevalence of overweight among US adults; the National Health and Nutrition Examination Surveys, 1960 to 1991. JAMA 272:205–211
3. NIH Obesity Research Task Force. Strategic Plan for NIH Obesity Research. http://www.obesityresearch.nih.gov/News/background.htm. Accessed 4 September 2004.
4. National Heart Lung and Blood Institute, National Institutes of Health. Clinical Guidelines on the Identification, Evaluation, and Treatment of Overweight and Obesity in Adults. http://www.nhlbi.nih.gov/guidelines/obesity/ob_home.htm. Accessed 1 July 2010.
5. Finkelstein EA, Fiebelkorn IC, Wang G (2003) National medical spending attributable to overweight and obesity: How much, and who's paying? Health Affairs W3:219–226
6. Centers for Disease Control and Prevention. Diabetes data and trends: incidence and age at diagnosis. http://www.cdc.gov/diabetes/statistics/incidence_national.htm. Accessed 12 July 2010.
7. Ogden CL, Flegal KM, Carroll MD, Johnson CL (2002) Prevalence and trends in over-weight among US children and adolescents, 1999–2000. JAMA 288:1728–1732
8. Center for Disease Control and Prevention. Defining Childhood Overweight and Obesity. http://www.cdc.gov/obesity/childhood/defining.html. Accessed 1 July 2010.
9. Ogden CL, Carroll MD, Curtin LR, Lamb MM, Flegal KM (2010) Prevalence of high body mass index in US children and adolescents, 2007–2008. JAMA 300:242–249
10. Serdula MK, Ivery D, Coates RJ, Freedman DS, Williamson DF, Byers T (1993) Do obese children become obese adults? A review of the literature. Prev Med 22:167–177
11. Freedman DS, Mei Z, Srinivasan SR, Berenson GS, Dietz WH (2007) Cardiovascular risk factors and excess adiposity among overweight children and adolescents: the Bogalusa Heart Study. J Pediatr 150:12–17
12. Arslanian SA (2002) Metabolic differences between Caucasian and African-American children and the relationship to type 2 diabetes mellitus. J Pediatr Endocrinol 15(Suppl 1):509–517
13. Many obese youth have condition that precedes type 2 diabetes: studies to address obesity-linked diseases in children. http://www.nih.gov/news/pr/mar2002/nichd-13.htm. Accessed 1 July 2010.
14. Denney JT, Krueger PM, Rogers RG, Boardman JD (2004) Race/ethnic and sex differentials in body mass among U.S. adults. Ethn Dis 14:389–398
15. Cossrow N, Falkner B (2004) Race/ethnic issues in obesity and obesity-related comorbidities. J Clin Endocrinol Metab 89:2590–2594

16. Buckworth J, Nigg C (2004) Physical activity, exercise, and sedentary behavior in college students. J Am Coll Health 53:28–34
17. Salles-Costa R, Heilborn ML, Werneck GL, Faerstein E, Lopes CS (2003) Gender and leisure-time physical activity. Cad Saúde Pública 19 (Suppl 2):S325–S333 [Portuguese].
18. Pearte CA, Gary TL, Brancati FL (2004) Correlates of physical activity levels in a sample of urban African Americans with type 2 diabetes. Ethn Dis 14:198–205
19. BMI calculator. Memorial Care: The standard of excellence in health care website. http://www.memorialcare.org/health/BMIcalculator.cfm. Accessed 2 July 2010.
20. Fitzgibbon ML, Stolley MR (2004) Environmental changes may be needed for prevention of overweight in minority children. Pediatr Ann 33:45–49
21. St-Onge MP, Keller KL, Heymsfield SB (2003) Changes in childhood food consumption patterns: a cause for concern in light of increasing body weights. Am J Clin Nutr 78: 1068–1073
22. Bowman SA, Gortmaker SL, Ebbeling CB, Pereira MA, Ludwig DS (2004) Effects of fast-food consumption on energy intake and diet quality among children in a national household survey. Pediatrics 113:112–118
23. Ebbeling CB, Sinclair KB, Pereira MA, Garcia-Lago E, Feldman HA, Ludwig DS (2004) Compensation for energy intake from fast food among overweight and lean adolescents. JAMA 291:2828–2833
24. Carolina Population Center. The national longitudinal study of adolescent health. http://www.cpc.unc.edu/projects/addhealth. Accessed 15 July 2004.
25. U.S. Department of Agriculture Center for Nutrition Policy and Promotion. http://www.mypyramid.gov/pyramid/grains_amount.aspx#. Accessed 2 July 2010.
26. Bell AC, Swinburn BA (2004) What are the key food groups to target for preventing obesity and improving nutrition in schools? Eur J Clin Nutr 58:258–263
27. Swinburn BA, Caterson I, Seidell JC, James WP (2004) Diet, nutrition and the prevention of excess weight gain and obesity. Public Health Nutr 7:123–146

Part II
Obesity: Clinical Assessments

5

Assessment and Treatment of Cardiovascular Disease in Obese Children

Piers R. Blackett, Petar Alaupovic, Kevin Short, and Kenneth C. Copeland

Key Points

- Pediatric obesity predicts adult obesity, unfortunately.
- Pediatric obesity is linked to early development of elevated risk for subsequent cardiovascular disease.
- Obese children and adolescents deserve comprehensive, cardiovascular risk assessment.
- Interventions to promote healthier nutrition and increased physical activity remain the mainstays for prevention, treatment, and ultimate risk reduction.

Keywords: Obesity, Atherogenesis, Metabolic syndrome, Lifestyle, Dyslipidemia, Hypertension, Apolipoproteins, Inflammation, Cytokines, Treatment

5.1 INTRODUCTION

5.1.1 Overview

The increase in prevalence and severity of obesity in children [169] is concerning, as is progression to type 2 diabetes (T2DM) [138] and its known cardiovascular consequences. Obese children and adolescents

From: *Nutrition and Health: Management of Pediatric Obesity and Diabetes,*
Edited by: R.J. Ferry, Jr., DOI 10.1007/978-1-60327-256-8_5,
© Springer Science+Business Media, LLC 2011

tend to become obese as adults [60] and a high percentage have associated hypertension, dyslipidemia, and insulin resistance [57] which often persist and progress into adulthood [59]. Body mass index (BMI) during childhood significantly predicts adult risk factors [160], and strong persistence of weight status between childhood and adulthood [59] may contribute to adult risk. Childhood obesity, hypertension, dyslipidemia, and insulin resistance – individually and as a cluster – influence cardiovascular risk factors in adolescence and early adulthood [22]. These problems possess clinical significance, since it has been proposed that insulin resistance and compensatory hyperinsulinemia relate to the pathogenesis of both hypertension and dyslipidemia [142] and their deleterious effects lead to atherosclerosis well before the appearance of diabetes [179].

Adult obesity predicts cardiovascular disease (*e.g.*, myocardial infarction, stroke, cardiovascular deaths) [191], but these end-points do not generally occur at young ages. Consequentially, childhood studies have been restricted to showing associations with risk factors. However, it has been demonstrated with noninvasive measures that arterial intimal thickening and arterial stiffness are altered with obesity [14, 81], supporting claims that early, preventable and reversible cardiovascular changes are detectable and can be clinically defined in young patients with obesity.

Good evidence confirms that biochemical mediators of atherosclerosis which have been associated with obesity in adults are also increased in obese children. These observations support a role for obesity – particularly visceral fat – as an accelerator of atherosclerosis in both adults and children. The adverse effects of adipocytes, particularly when abdominally situated, are related to their secretion of cytokines, hormones, and free fatty acids into the portal circulation [167, 168]. Hepatic influx of portally derived fatty acids is a known mediator of increased triglyceride-rich lipoprotein production [65]. Adipocyte-derived cytokines and hormones are known to accelerate progression to both glucose intolerance and vascular disease. Puberty increases insulin resistance [4], and the increase is attributed to increases in sex steroids, growth hormone, and growth factors (such as insulin-like growth factor binding protein-3) associated with the normal adolescent growth spurt [35, 36]. Obesity during puberty further accentuates insulin resistance in both sexes [153]. Expression of obesity-related cardiovascular risk is also influenced by ethnic background [57]. For example, African American youth are most susceptible to hypertension [16], whereas Native Americans show greatest risk for progression to T2DM [136] particularly if obese [188].

5.1.2   Prediction of Adult Risk

The relationship of childhood and adolescent obesity to adult cardiovascular risk has been well documented. The Carnegie (Boyd Orr) cohort, first surveyed in Britain from 1937 to 1939, was evaluated for the effect of BMI on subsequent cardiovascular mortality after 57 years [71]. When the effect of childhood BMI >75%ile was compared with childhood BMI between 25 and 49%ile, the hazard ratio for ischemic heart disease was 2.0. In the Bogalusa heart study [157], adolescents overweight at ages 13–17 years tended to remain overweight into young adulthood (ages 27–31 years), an unhealthy habitus which was associated with clustering of risk factors including elevated total cholesterol:HDL-C ratio, insulin level, and systolic hypertension. Prevalence of hypertension was increased 8.5-fold in those adults who had been obese as adolescents, and dyslipidemia was 3.1–8.3-fold higher in the obese cohort compared to the lean controls. Subsequent Bogalusa studies of a cohort aged 8–17 years [160] showed a positive relationship between BMI and a cluster of four risk variables: BMI, fasting insulin, systolic or mean arterial blood pressure, and total cholesterol:HDL-C or triglyceride:HDL-C ratio. After a mean follow-up period of 11.6 years, the proportion of individuals who developed this clustering increased across BMI and insulin quartiles. The relationship to childhood BMI remained significant even after adjusting for childhood insulin, but the converse was not true. Thus, childhood BMI and insulin were significant predictors of childhood clustering with BMI being the strongest. In the Harvard Growth Study [125], adolescents who were evaluated between 1922 and 1935 were re-evaluated in 1988. Being overweight in adolescence was associated with higher risk for coronary heart disease and atherosclerosis in adulthood, and it was a more powerful predictor of adult risk than being overweight in adulthood. These findings support the influence of obesity and obesity-associated risk factors on the pathogenesis of atherosclerosis beginning in childhood and adolescence, then progressing to occlusive arterial disease in adulthood.

5.1.3   Early Atherogenesis

Obesity appears to enhance the development of atherosclerotic lesions [118], a process which begins early in life. It was initially suspected that atherosclerosis began in childhood, when investigators performing autopsies on young men killed in the Korean War found striking evidence of fatty streaks and atherosclerotic plaques in young adult males [52]. Subsequent studies on young soldiers killed during the Vietnam War revealed that 45% had evidence of coronary atherosclerosis [120]. More recently, both the Bogalusa and Pathobiological Determinants of Atherosclerosis in Youth (PDAY) studies have provided more detailed evidence that risk factors are proportionate to the area of vascular lesions [17, 105] and that obesity is a significant contributing factor, especially in males [118]. The PDAY research group examined topographic distributions of atherosclerosis in the right coronary arteries and abdominal aortas in more than 2,000 autopsied persons, ages 15–34 years. The images obtained from fatty streaks stained with Sudan IV were digitized, and the raised lesions were manually outlined for computerized mapping and quantitation of selected areas of each artery [117]. Fourteen percent of the cohort had a BMI >30 kg/m^2, and the extent of both fatty streaks and raised lesions was associated with high non-HDL-C, low HDL-C, hypertension, elevated glycohemoglobin, and presence of obesity – with the relationship between obesity and fatty streaks greater in males than females [119]. Multiple combinations of risk factors were found to be associated with accelerated progression to raised fatty streaks by mid-adolescence and possibly earlier [116]. The significance of these findings is particularly disturbing, in view of extensive epidemiological evidence of a secular increase in the prevalence of obesity in childhood and adolescence [169]. Since the age of onset for T2DM is decreasing [138], it follows that the associated cardiovascular risk – known to precede diabetes [179] – may also occur at a younger age than in previous generations.

Based on biochemical and physical evidence, it is reasonable to propose that obesity plays a significant central role in progression of early stages of atherogenesis, culminating in the formation of the fatty streak and subsequent plaque formation. The process begins with nonatherosclerotic thickening, consisting of increases in smooth muscle, elastin and proteoglycans, but with initial lesions devoid of lipid [126]. Consistent with the response to the retention hypothesis [190], which proposes that atherogenic lipoproteins are retained in the intima by binding to extracellular proteoglycans [30, 190], it is possible that obesity – particularly when co-existent with dyslipidemia or hypertension – is likely to accelerate progression of subendothelial lipid retention and subsequent plaque formation. Further insight on the effect of obesity on arterial change is provided by studies on calcium deposition in asymptomatic adults, by quantitation of arterial calcium deposition at two time points approximately 8 years apart. In this report, several indices of obesity predicted progression of calcium deposition, inferring lesion progression [29].

More recent evidence suggests that the increase in lipid within fatty streaks is associated with monocyte adhesion to the arterial endothelium, migration into the intima, and macrophage formation. The cumulative result is pathological intimal thickening and foam cell formation [126]. Components of the arterial wall (such as smooth muscle, elastin, collagen, and the endothelium [11]) constitute structural and functional layers, and potentially contribute to vascular distensibility and thickness. Endothelium-derived nitric oxide modulates basal vasodilatory tone under normal conditions [54], but the enzyme nitric oxide synthase (NOS), an insulin-dependent enzyme, becomes impaired with insulin resistance, resulting in decreased vascular tone. Changes in the endothelium are associated with and contribute to infiltration of monocytes and lipoproteins as secondary events [10, 75].

5.2   THE METABOLIC SYNDROME

5.2.1   Overview

Cardiovascular risk factors, initially described and characterized as an obesity-associated cluster in adults, also occur in children, forming what is now termed the metabolic syndrome [90, 142] (Fig. 5.1), which provides a framework for a clinical approach to screening and intervention. There is evidence that each component of the syndrome has genetic components [147, 162] and its development is primed by gestational factors such as obesity and diabetes during pregnancy [23]. Insulin resistance contributes to increased expression of the metabolic syndrome [142] and is enhanced by puberty [74], particularly when the adolescents become overweight or obese [40], leading to elevations in blood pressure, dyslipidemia, glucose intolerance, and elevated C-reactive protein (CRP) [27] (Fig. 5.1). De Ferranti demonstrated ethnic differences in prevalence of the syndrome, with a higher prevalence in Hispanic adolescents than Caucasians and African Americans [47]. These data support the likelihood that populations who are prone to insulin resistance and T2DM also tend to have greater cardiovascular risk, even in adolescence, suggesting that "the clock for cardiovascular disease starts ticking" before diabetes develops [179].

5.2.2   Defining Cut Points

Defining the metabolic syndrome as a disease cluster in pediatric populations has been more problematic than in adults because multiple definitions, with different age-appropriate cut points, have been proposed. Table 5.1 lists five examples. For example, the NHANES III adolescent population has been evaluated for prevalence of the metabolic syndrome using two different

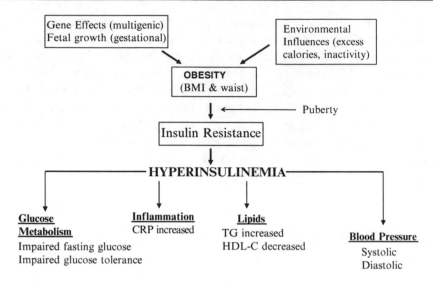

Fig. 5.1. The metabolic syndrome in childhood and adolescence.

definitions [34, 47], demonstrating that calculation of the prevalence is increased when less stringent criteria are used.

Weiss and colleagues evaluated obese children and adolescents attending the Yale pediatric clinic [187], defining obesity as a BMI above 2 standard deviations (Z score >2). They observed a high prevalence of the syndrome (Table 5.1) using more stringent criteria than in most studies, with 38.7% of the moderately obese (BMI Z score >2) and 49% of the severely obese (BMI Z score >2.5) meeting their definition of metabolic syndrome. It is possible that the expected referral bias for their clinic-based population resulted in a high prevalence of severely obese children and adolescents, not only with overt diabetes but also with cardiovascular risk. However, it might be argued that use of less stringent criteria would lead to more effective prevention strategy.

Since criteria such as waist circumference, triglyceride, HDL-C, and blood pressure are continuous variables, the cut points can be based on percentile-based values at points where the criteria are considered abnormal. Since percentiles change with age during adolescence, it has been possible to construct curves for the percentile cut points relative to equivalent adult values – as recommended by the Adult Treatment Panel III (ATP III) from the National Cholesterol Education Program (NCEP) Expert Panel on Detection, Evaluation, and Treatment of High Blood Cholesterol in Adults and the International Diabetes Foundation (IDF). For example, charts constructed

Table 5.1
Different criteria (actual values or percentiles for age) for the metabolic syndrome in adolescence

	de Ferranti	Jolliffe	Cruz	Goodman	Weiss
Waist circumference	>75th	Males: 92nd Females: 72nd	>90th	>102 cm (make) >88 cm (female)	BMI Z score >2.0
Triglyceride	>100 mg/dL	89th	>90th	>150 mg/dL	>95th
HDL-C	<50 mg/dL (male 12–14 years) <45 mg/dL (male 15–19 years) <50 mg/dL (female 12–19 years)	Males: 26th Females: 43rd	<10th	<40 mg/dL (male) <50 mg/dL (female)	<5th
Blood pressure	SBP >90th	Males SBP 92nd DBP 97th Females SBP 93rd DBP 99th	>90th	>85/130 mmHg	SBP and DBP >95th
Fasting glucose	>13.75 mM >110 mg/dL	5.6 mM (100 mg/dL)	>13.75 mM >110 mg/dL	>13.75 mM >110 mg/dL	Post glucose load (IGT): >7.8 mM (140 mg/dL) <11.1 mM (200 mg/dL)

by the United States Centers for Disease Control (CDC) can used for plotting the BMI and charts for each of the individual metabolic syndrome criteria offer an age-specific assessment of risk [88], except for fasting glucose, which remains stable across age [88]. Since the initial selection of adult NCEP ATP III cut points was arbitrary and based on a consensus approximation of the cut points to degree of long-term risk, there is variable approximation to percentiles among the individual criteria. Therefore, translating these values to equivalent percentiles for adolescents tends to be liberally inclusive for some of the criteria. This appears to be particularly so for the HDL-C cut point which was estimated to be at the 26–43%ile for male and female adolescents by Joliffe *et al.* [88] (Table 5.1), resulting in a high prevalence of abnormal HDL-C in adolescents.

With these inconsistencies in mind, there is good rationale for use of the 90%iles [40] to define risk factors in adolescents, since values >90%ile have been widely regarded as abnormal [41], although justification by long-term follow-up has not yet been achieved. In contrast, metabolic syndrome cut points were initially selected based on adult risk. However, the prevailing populations from which the data were derived may not necessarily represent the norm. Since the secular trend for the past three decades has been to increase body weight relative to height [169], it follows that adolescent percentiles above the median for BMI trend upwards and associated risk factors are likely to follow the same trend. Our own approach to evaluating Oklahoman Native Americans and Caucasian adolescents was to use a selection of recommended criteria. We selected a BMI Z score >2 [187], an HDL level <10%ile for age and gender, triglyceride level >90%ile for age and gender [41], fasting glucose >100 mg/dL (as recommended by the American Diabetes Association), and either a systolic or diastolic blood pressure >90%ile for age and gender [41].

The cut point for an impaired fasting glucose was initially set at 110 mg/dL by the American Diabetes Association committee. This cutoff was based on prevailing evidence for associated diabetic microvascular complications. However, subsequent assessment of outcomes warranted lowering it to 100 mg/dL, because glucose levels above this cut point potentially predict both microvascular and macrovascular disease. It follows that the lower value is a better cut point for the NCEP definition of the metabolic syndrome. Weiss *et al.* propose that a 2-h glucose tolerance test should be performed in children to determine whether impaired glucose tolerance is present, defined as the 2-h glucose >140 mg/dL (but not >200 mg/dL which would define diabetes). The same authors considered the 2-h glucose to be superior for detecting the presence of insulin resistance in adolescents when compared to use of a fasting glucose level.

5.2.3 Clinical Use

It has been debated whether identifying the metabolic syndrome is useful for clinical purposes [92]. The argument is based on insufficient evidence to justify calling the cluster a syndrome without a proven central cause. Additionally, limiting clinical assessment to the defined criteria provided by NCEP may obscure or miss significant risk in individuals whose cardiovascular risk factors are not criteria – such as an elevated LDL-cholesterol, a significant family history of cardiovascular events, or smoking. However, the concept and practical use of the syndrome has been defended based on data showing significant disease prediction and the usefulness of criteria for treatment according to recommended guidelines [70]. Since each of the components has a relationship to myocardial infarction [131, 196], detecting one or more of the NCEP components is clinically relevant and detection of three or more abnormal criteria together increases the risk for coronary heart disease or stroke in adults two- to threefold [5, 101].

The controversies raised for adults apply also to adolescents [90], but with the added problem of defining age-appropriate cut points and deciding which criteria are the most predictive and can be used cost-effectively in the clinical setting. The accumulating evidence suggests that a comprehensive risk appraisal should routinely be adopted for children and adolescents referred for obesity, and used as the basis for a problem-oriented approach to risk reversal. The triad of evaluation and treatment options (consisting of diet, exercise, and behavioral modification) is central to clinical management and should also include assessment of the innate or nonmodifiable, preventable, and treatable factors contributing to the current health status of the patient (Table 5.2). Evaluation also should include consideration of social factors determining food choices, commercial sources of foods, exercise choices, and access to safe playgrounds. Familial risk factors, overt disease, and family lifestyle will influence the child's choices and opportunities. Nonmodifiable factors – such as age, gender, ethnic background, and family history – should always be considered (Table 5.2), since these clearly influence outcomes.

It has been proposed that evaluation and treatment of metabolic syndrome criteria should be revised for clinical pediatric use by taking into account ten evidence-based items from which to quantify risk. Among these are family history of early cardiovascular risk, T2DM, or hypertension; abnormal birth weight (particularly those born small for gestational age, SGA); ethnic origin from a group at risk; specific clinical features (high BMI, waist circumference, or blood pressure; acanthosis nigricans); and metabolic abnormalities (impaired glucose tolerance or overt T2DM) [24]. Triglyceride and HDL-C, although established components of metabolic

Table 5.2
Obesity-associated factors influencing cardiovascular risk

Innate
Family history of premature CHD
Monogenic obesity
Multigenic etiologies
Age
Gender
Ethnic background
Preventable
Inactivity
Dietary excesses
Behavioral
Appetite
Depression
Low self-esteem
Lack of family support
Smoking (exacerbating)
Treatable
Excess body fat
BMI
Waist circumference
Dyslipidemia
Raised LDL-C
Low HDL-C
Raised triglyceride
Hypertension
Systolic BP
Diastolic BP
Insulin resistance
Impaired glucose tolerance
Diabetes mellitus

syndrome definitions for adults, were excluded for use in children based on insufficient evidence that these predict which children (or adolescents) will display high-risk lipoprotein levels as adults. However, accumulating evidence that lipid levels are associated with the occurrence of atherosclerotic lesions at a young age [17, 116] may warrant re-evaluation and inclusion. Also, it is considered appropriate to emphasize and modify dietary treatment to reverse the dyslipidemias if present [12].

Treatable risk factors – the subject of this chapter – can also be targeted, but as in adults, the use of pharmaceutical agents needs careful consideration (see Sects. 5.4, 5.5). A complete assessment requires going beyond the metabolic syndrome criteria and consideration of novel risk factors (such as Lp(a), homocysteine, adiponectin, and CRP) which can compound risk and could potentially influence response to therapeutic approaches. These novel risk measures should be assessed when individual or familial risk is excessive and traditional risk measures are normal.

The family history includes listing first- and second-degree relatives with T2DM, coronary artery disease and stroke (including hyperlipidemia if known), and hypertension. Ethnic background is often relevant, particularly if the patient's ethnicity is known to predispose to a disease or trait. For example, the Hispanic and American Indian populations, known to be at higher risk for developing T2DM, also display high rates of the metabolic syndrome in adolescence [2, 47]. African American women display a higher prevalence of the metabolic syndrome than men, and this difference is attributable to obesity and the disproportionate presence of hypertension and T2DM [33]. Hypertension is more prevalent in African American and Hispanic adolescents, particularly when they become overweight [121]. American Indian populations, similar to Pacific and Indian Ocean Islanders, have particularly higher risk of developing obesity beginning in childhood, subsequent T2DM and associated cardiovascular disease [78, 188].

5.3 PHYSICAL MEASURES OF CARDIOVASCULAR ASSESSMENT

5.3.1 Overview

The extent of the evaluation will depend on the clinical setting and whether the evaluation is to be recorded and analyzed in a research environment, with appropriate institutional research committee approval or in various clinical settings (which could be a university-based clinic, outreach clinics serving specific communities, private practices with specific prevention interests, or schools). Besides obtaining basic measurements such as the computed BMI and blood pressure, certain physical measurements have excellent potential for widespread clinical use in the assessment of vascular risk associated with obesity. Pulse wave analysis assesses loss of normal distensibility of the vascular wall. Intima-media thickness (IMT) by Doppler ultrasound provides a measure of thickening, which is shown to be predictive of cardiovascular risk in adults [110]. These techniques and data on their use in children and adolescents have been reviewed [150, 174], and the authors predict that they will become standardized and much more available for routine clinical use.

5.3.2 Physical Examination Measurements

5.3.2.1 Height, Weight, and Body Mass Index

It is important to determine height and weight measurements as accurately as possible, using a reputable and calibrated stadiometer for height and a scaled (or electronic) machine for weight. BMI, or computed BMI Z score, can be obtained readily from height and weight measurements. It has been argued that BMI is more accurate than a waist measurement. When compared to age- and sex-related normative data, BMI is better for comparing serial measurements [187]. Electronic medical recording (EMR) enables graphing the height, weight, and BMI, and EMR can be readily shown to the patient or client. All values should be plotted using established charts such as those made available by the United States' CDC and Prevention Web site (http://www.cdc.gov/nchs/about/major/nhanes/growthcharts/charts.htm).

5.3.2.2 Waist

Published waist measurement norms for children and adolescents in NHANES III are available [53]. The waist is measured using a tape measure at just above the uppermost lateral border of the right ilium, at the end of a normal expiration, and recorded to the nearest millimeter [53]. Studies on the topical distribution of fat in relation to cardiovascular disease have shown that visceral fat is more closely associated with cardiovascular risk in adults than other fat depots [98]. Elevations in blood pressure and triglycerides, low HDL-C, and insulin resistance have all been associated with increased waist circumference in children [104, 134, 148]. The waist-to-hip ratio, although favored for adults, appears less suited for children because of the changes in hip circumference influenced by puberty. Consequently, the waist-to-height ratio has been preferred, but does not appear to be superior to BMI for association with risk factors [58]. Nevertheless, children and adolescents aged 8–18 years with a waist circumference >90%ile were shown to be more likely to have an atherogenic lipoprotein profile and increased biomarkers of endothelial dysfunction such as intercellular adhesion molecule-1 and E-selectin [25].

5.3.2.3 Blood Pressure

Blood pressure is measured when the subject is relaxed and sedentary after selection of an appropriate sized cuff, which in length is two-thirds that of the upper arm (http://www.cdc.gov/nchs/data/nhanes/nhanes3/cdrom/NCHS/MANUALS/PRESSURE.PDF). Three readings are taken, and the mean of the latter two readings is computed. It is essential to follow guidelines on correct positioning: patient sitting with the back supported, both feet on the floor, and the tested arm supported at the heart level [69].

Ambulatory blood pressure monitoring has been gaining in popularity and has potential use for evaluation of children [69], particularly for identification of increased nocturnal blood pressure [111]. However, the method requires an oscillometric device, which is influenced by arterial stiffness [177]. Children with low arterial stiffness have poor reproducibility, suggesting that use is limited, although application for assessment of adolescents has been documented [184], and there is potential for clinical use in detecting diurnal fluctuations. Obese children and adolescents aged 7–18 years were studied to assess factors linking obesity to ambulatory blood pressure rises [63]. The risk of having increased systolic and diastolic hypertension increased, respectively, with the BMI Z score and waist circumference. In multivariate regression analysis, daytime systolic blood pressure was independently associated with urinary norepinephrine, suggesting activation of the sympatho-adrenal system in obesity.

Progress in blood pressure measurement and information on devices can be viewed online at http://www.dableducational.org.

5.3.3 Left Ventricular Mass

The left ventricle mass (LVM), determined by echocardiography, has been shown to be an independent determinant of increased cardiovascular morbidity in adults in the Framingham Heart Study [107]. Linear growth in childhood is a determinant of cardiac growth, but excess weight leads to an increase in LVM beyond that expected for normal growth [173]. The effect of obesity on LVM in adolescence has been confirmed, and the effect is greater in African Americans than European Americans, and also greater in boys than in girls [49].

LVM relates to components of the metabolic syndrome in childhood, and this association follows and strengthens into young adulthood [154]. The magnitude of increase in BMI between ages 13 and 27 years positively correlates to the increase in LVM, suggesting that curtailing weight gain in adolescence could help prevent excess growth of LVM [154]. It has been debated whether surrogate measures of body mass proportional to height (such as BMI and ponderal index) can be regarded as representing the effect of obesity on LVM independent of height [44]. However, the relationship between LVM and body fat mass, measured by dual X-ray absorptiometry (DEXA) and analyzed independently of height, was reported to be weak [44]. Nevertheless, the cumulative burden of adiposity estimated by the area under the curve for serial BMI measures from childhood (4–17 years) to adulthood (20–38 years) is a significant correlate and predictor of LVM [109].

Beside LVM, in adults, left ventricular dilatation (a measure of left ventricular end-diastolic diameter) is predicted better by childhood BMI than by systolic blood pressure [72]. It is possible that the elevated dilatation could result from excessive vascularity of the adipose tissue, resulting in increased blood volume and cardiac output. Adipocyte-generated cytokines could also have an effect on cardiac function, particularly when derived from abdominal fat, since left atrial enlargement was found to be present in childhood and related to abdominal obesity and insulin resistance [76].

5.3.4 Arterial Wall Stiffness

Structural changes in the arterial wall are associated with BMI and serum insulin levels [166] in adolescents, resulting in a loss of distensibility of the vessel measured by pulse wave analysis. Gender and age are significant determinants of pulse wave velocity in adolescents because the velocity is higher in boys, and increases with age and blood pressure are seen in both sexes [127]. Low plasma apoA-I, insulin resistance, visceral distribution of fat, and possibly elevated leptin levels [152] – all correlate with vessel distensibility, suggesting that these factors might influence changes in the arterial wall leading to stiffness, particularly when associated with obesity.

An association of serum cholesterol concentrations with arterial stiffness has been observed in children [106]; but in subsequent studies in adolescents, the same authors observed a stronger association between arterial stiffness and obesity than with serum cholesterol [189]. However, the association with cholesterol appeared to have a threshold effect at approximately 4.5 mmol/L (174 mg/dL). In these studies, the association with obesity was progressive, beginning with a BMI of approximately 20 kg/m^2, lower than the 85%ile defining overweight or obesity in the United States. The authors also observed an additive effect of diastolic blood pressure and associations with the number of risk factors for the metabolic syndrome [189].

More recently, pulse wave forms have been measured simultaneously for the brachial and ankle pulses by a volume plethysmographic method and heart sound recorder. The time duration between the two wave forms and the heart beat is calculated as the heart–ankle time duration minus the heart–brachial time duration [85] and is considered to be representative of the mechanical properties of the large-sized central elastic and medium-sized peripheral muscular arteries [195]. A relationship of insulin resistance to arterial stiffness determined by brachial-ankle pulse wave velocity was independent of obesity in 256 adolescent males [103]. The associated hyperinsulinemia and slight increase in blood glucose may exert effects on the vessel wall through promoting sodium absorption [161], stimulating the sympathetic nervous system [194] and increasing vascular smooth muscle growth [15]. Although glucose is not abnormally increased until glucose intolerance ensues, high ambient glucose concentration increases the likelihood of glycosylation of cell wall proteins and in altered glycosylated end-products. These products are likely to increase stiffness and thickening [171], when glucose intolerance has developed.

Nitric oxide formation and release (induced by NOS normally) occur in the endothelium and are reduced with insulin resistance, resulting in impaired vasodilation, susceptibility to injury, and subsequent stiffening of the vessel wall [123]. This mechanism is thought to play a major role in the endothelial dysfunction and associated stiffness of the common carotid artery in severely obese children [166]. Severe obesity in adolescence results in endothelial dysfunction and stiffness [81, 166] and in increased wall thickness by ultrasound [81]. Stiffness appears related to IMT determined by ultrasound, and the two arterial wall measures may represent similar structural changes with loss of distensibility preceding but overlapping with increased thickness.

5.3.5   Intima-Media Thickness

IMT determined by ultrasound has gained popularity as a technique to determine early vascular change. It has been established as a marker of atherosclerosis in adults [48]. Carotid IMT independently predicts vascular events in adults [110] at each of four age quartiles ranging from 19 to 90 years over a mean follow-up interval of 4.2 years. Also, there is evidence that risk factors during childhood (with the exception of CRP [91]) predict adult IMT [46, 141]. IMT is increased in obese children [14] and in children with hypercholesterolemia [99] and type 1 diabetes [99]. In obese children, IMT is also related to blood pressure and impaired insulin sensitivity [143]. Inversely associated with obesity in children [137], circulating adiponectin level was found to be independently associated with IMT [14], when controlled for gender, Tanner stage of puberty, and BMI. This suggests that the low adiponectin levels characteristic of obese children constitute an important, novel risk factor. In adults, hypoadiponectinemia has been shown to predict coronary artery disease [139] and has been found to have an independent negative association with common carotid IMT in middle-aged adults [82].

CRP and the cytokine interleukin-6 (IL-6) correlate positively with IMT in obese children [93], suggesting that the arterial thickening is partially mediated by inflammatory factors or establishes the setting for enhanced inflammatory activity. In addition, insulin resistance and oxidant status may also influence IMT changes in obese prepubertal children [62]. Postabsorptive insulin resistance measured by the surrogate marker QUICK-I has been shown to be independently related to IMT in a group of early pubescent children [8].

It is evident that IMT in obese children is influenced by more than one risk factor. In a comprehensive evaluation of risk factors, Reinuhr *et al.* found IMT of obese children to associate independently with systolic blood pressure, blood glucose, and CRP, suggesting a combined play of blood pressure, glucose intolerance, and inflammation [143]. Increased IMT has been observed in obese children aged 6–14 years compared to age-matched controls [81], although many obesity-associated risk factors (such as blood pressure, triglycerides, and insulin resistance) also differ between obese and nonobese children. In an attempt to identify the precise obesity-associated risk factors influencing IMT, Beauloye *et al.* examined the effects of glucose, insulin, CRP, adhesion molecules (ICAM, VCAM, E-selectin), lipid profile, resistin, and adiponectin [14]. They reported that – when controlled for gender, Tanner stage, and relative BMI – only adiponectin was associated with IMT, confirming findings published in adult men but not in women [128].

5.4   BIOCHEMICAL MEASUREMENTS OF CARDIOVASCULAR RISK

5.4.1   *Overview*

The link between obesity and changes in the arterial wall consist of several biochemical mediators. Dyslipidemia and insulin resistance have long been associated with cardiovascular and T2DM risk. More recently, the adipocyte has been found to contribute by secreting free fatty acids, cytokines, and hormones known to affect the arterial wall (Fig. 5.2).

5.4.2   *Insulin Resistance*

Insulin resistance precedes the onset of diabetes and enhances processes associated with cardiovascular risk, as evidenced by classic epidemiological studies [179]. Increased insulin levels (both absolute and relative to glucose levels) are associated with obesity at a young age [20, 21]. Derived from the molar product of glucose and insulin divided by 22.5, the homeostasis index is a convenient measure of insulin resistance in the fasting state [114]. This index correlates closely with insulin resistance determined by the glucose clamp technique, the recognized gold standard for defining insulin resistance. The homeostasis index is associated with the dyslipidemia of obesity, but lack of insulin assay standardization prohibits establishing norms and general use. Other widely used techniques – including the oral glucose tolerance test and the rapid sequence intravenous glucose tolerance test – provide equally reliable and valuable measurements of insulin resistance. Fasting insulin levels are generally increased in obese

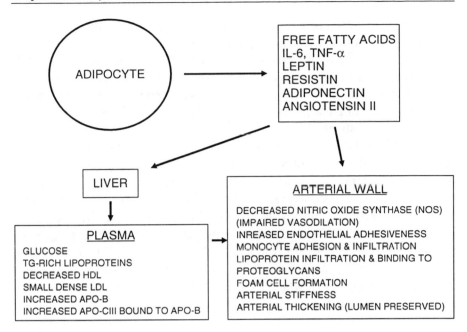

Fig. 5.2. Mediators of early atherosclerosis in obesity.

adolescents and can be used as a surrogate measure of insulin resistance, but evidence for use as a treatment target is lacking.

5.4.3   Obesity-Related Dyslipidemia

A standard recommendation for evaluation of children and adolescents with obesity includes a fasting lipid profile [12]. In recent years, standardization of lipid measurements between laboratories has become increasingly important, because target levels of blood cholesterol and triglyceride are part of evidenced-based approaches used to diagnose lipid abnormalities, assess cardiovascular disease risk, and monitor therapy. Accordingly, it is desirable to calibrate and match triglyceride and cholesterol values with a standard source, such as the CDC reference methods. Alternatively, dry chemistry methodology requiring small volume finger-stick samples can be used for screening programs. Availability at the point of care (POC) enables health care providers to confront the patient with results rapidly, an approach which facilitates instruction and has a behavioral advantage. The dyslipidemia typically associated with obesity is characterized by the fasting, first morning lipid profile. Dyslipidemia results from insulin resistance and is diagnosed by increased triglyceridemia and decreased circulating HDL-C. LDL-C is seldom increased, but molding of triglyceride-enriched LDL particles by increased hepatic lipase occurs, resulting in smaller and denser LDL (which facilitate transendothelial passage into the arterial intima) [9]. Similar particle size characteristics are present in childhood, and small LDL size is positively correlated with relative weight [56]. Elevated triglyceride is an independent risk factor for atherosclerosis, and triglyceride-rich particles play a role in pathogenesis. Hepatic VLDL production is increased in insulin resistant states [108] and results from the abundant supply of free fatty acids from fat cells (particularly visceral fat, which provides fatty acids for hepatic uptake via the portal veins). Visceral fat is first acquired in childhood and is proportionate to a general increase in body fat [68]. When present in adolescence, visceral adiposity is associated with postmortem evidence of coronary artery pathology [100], further suggesting its importance as a therapeutic target. The dyslipidemia associated with insulin-resistant states has been best characterized in adults [28, 64] and occurs in association with abdominal obesity [28]. Children and adolescents manifest the same derangements when they become obese and insulin resistant (Fig. 5.3) [7, 34, 187].

Adipocyte-derived free fatty acids are important substrates for hepatic synthesis of VLDL [64]. In insulin resistance, lipoprotein lipase activity is impaired, resulting in reduced clearance of triglyceride-rich particles. Cholesterol-ester transfer protein enhances triglyceride exchange for cholesterol ester contained in HDL. Consequently, HDL becomes triglyceride-rich, rendering it a good substrate for hepatic lipase. Subsequent formation of lipid-poor and smaller HDL results in degradation of the particle and renal uptake, leading to further reduction in HDL-C.

Particle size determined by nuclear magnetic resonance (NMR) can provide a complete size profile, including VLDL, LDL, and HDL size [56]. Obesity in adolescents has been associated positively with VLDL size and negatively with LDL size [56]. This same dyslipidemic profile has been associated with fatty liver in obese adolescents [26], a finding that supports measurements of aspartate and alanine transaminase levels as markers of liver function in a comprehensive biochemical assessment of obese adolescents. Using the same analysis techniques, increased small LDL particle number can be detected in obese children who have normal LDL-C, particularly when the metabolic syndrome or T2DM is present [38, 87].

5.4.4 Apolipoproteins

Information derived from a classic lipid profile can be enhanced by commercially available methods to assess apolipoproteins, which can serve to provide additional insight on deranged lipoprotein transport in cases with obesity and insulin resistance (Fig. 5.3). However, apolipoprotein measurements

LIPOPROTEIN TRANSPORT IN INSULIN RESISTANCE

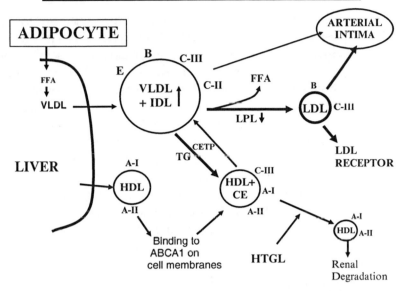

Fig. 5.3. Adipocytes, particularly those located in the viscera, provide fatty acids for hepatic uptake and incorporation into VLDL. Each VLDL particle containing one apoB molecule per particle acquires apoC-III, apoC-II, apoE, and some minor apolipoproteins. VLDL is progressively molded by lipoprotein lipase located in muscle and fat, resulting in formation of IDL and LDL with lowered triglyceride content. The molding process is impaired in insulin resistant states such as obesity. Smaller particles containing choles-terol, apoB, and apoC-III cross the vascular endothelium and become located subinti-mally. ApoC-III-mediated binding to proteoglycans and endothelial activation occurs. HDL lowering occurs in part as a result of exchange of triglyceride in VLDL with cho-lesterol ester in HDL resulting in formation of triglyceride-rich HDL, a good substrate for hepatic triglyceride lipase (HTGL). HTGL-induced lipolysis results in small HDL which is prone to degradation. The net effect is reduced and dysfunctional HDL with impaired reverse cholesterol transport, HDL degradation, and formation of atheroscle-rotic triglyceride-rich particles and small dense LDL with susceptibility to oxidation.

have not been widely recognized as clinically useful, possibly because of lack of standardization, as well as widespread reliance on lipid and lipopro-tein cholesterol values in clinical practice. Nevertheless, their evaluation in research studies continues to provide insight on mechanism and association with disease states (such as cardiovascular outcomes and obesity, particu-larly apoB, apoA-I [155, 179], and the B:A-I ratio [180]). It is also likely that apoB has use in children and may aid decisions on treatment with the availability of a normal range and laboratory standardization [102].

5.4.4.1 APOB:APOA-I RATIO

Apolipoprotein B (apoB) serves to form VLDL in the hepatocyte, transport lipids in the plasma, and modulate their uptake by LDL receptors. ApoB levels are proportionate to the number of apoB-containing particles, because each VLDL particle, IDL particle (intermediate density lipoprotein), and LDL particle contains one molecule of apoB. Hepatic influx of fatty acids increases plasma apoB and patients with obesity and insulin resistance tend to have a higher apoB [65]. In contrast to apoB, apoA-I is protective and functions to facilitate cholesterol efflux from cells by binding to the cholesterol transporter ATP-binding cassette transporter (ABCA1) on cell surfaces, and enhancing lecithin-cholesterol acyl transferase (LCAT), which esterifies the cell-derived free cholesterol to form cholesterol ester in the HDL core. Thus, the apoB:apoA-I ratio reflects the function of two apolipoproteins which work in opposing directions to enhance atherosclerosis and serve as atherosclerosis markers when alone or combined as the apoB:apoA-I ratio.

ApoB, apoA-I, and the apoB:apoA-I ratio have been validated as risk factors in prospective studies. The AMORIS [6], INTERHEART [196], and ULSAM [51] studies have shown apoB:apoA-I ratio to predict risk of both nonfatal and fatal myocardial infarction in adults. Furthermore, a recent meta-analysis supports clinical use of this ratio as a risk marker in adults [163]. ApoB:apoA-I has been associated with the metabolic syndrome and its individual components in a representative U.S. population (NHANES III), and the association with insulin resistance was independent of other components and inflammatory risk factors [124]. Measurement of the apoA-I:apoB ratio in childhood may be related to parental incidence of myocardial infarction [158], indicating that the ratio may reflect genetic risk.

The association of apoB with insulin resistance can be explained by insulin's regulatory role in lipoprotein transport. Insulin regulates lipoprotein lipase activity, controlling free fatty acid flux and availability for hepatic uptake. The triglyceride-to-HDL-C ratio represents similar biochemical processes and in adolescents is associated with insulin resistance measured by the insulin clamp [73].

5.4.4.2 APOC-III

Recent studies have strengthened the argument that changes in surface apolipoprotein distribution play a role in atherogenesis [64], particularly in high triglyceride states such as insulin resistance associated with obesity [146]. ApoC-III increases in hypertriglyceridemic states and modulates lipoprotein lipase activity [182] and particle uptake by LDL receptors [164]. Excess apoC-III (relative to apoB) enhances binding of apoB to proteoglycan in the arterial wall [129] and promotes monocyte binding to endothelial cells [95]. These pathophysiological studies provide rationale for observations in epidemiological studies, which demonstrate that apoC-III bound to apoB-containing particles enhances atherosclerosis in subjects undergoing arterial bypass grafts [79], in patients with diabetes [105], and in a subgroup of participants in the CARE study on atherosclerotic risk in adults [146]. ApoC-III levels in American Indian children were found to be proportionate to their insulin resistance as determined by the homeostasis index [19], suggesting that their tendency to become obese at an early age predisposes them to early risk for atherosclerosis.

Based on evidence that efficient lipolysis of triglycride-rich particles results in transfer of apoC-III to HDL particles [31], Alaupovic et al. have proposed that the C-III ratio (ratio of apoC-III in HDL to that in non-HDL) represents the efficiency of lipolysis and correlates with lipoprotein lipase activity [1]. To obtain the C-III ratio, after precipitation with heparin and manganese, apoC-III can be measured in both the supernate (associated with apoA-I-containing particles) and precipitate (associated with apoB-containing particles). ApoC-III in the heparin precipitate and the C-III ratio are associated with HOMA insulin resistance, BMI Z score, and waist circumference, particularly in boys [19]. This relationship with insulin appears partially influenced by the presence of an insulin response element in the apoC-III gene promoter, possibly accounting for association of apoC-III with the metabolic syndrome [130]. The promoter normally plays a role in downregulation of apoC-III synthesis; however, upregulation of apoC-III and VLDL production occurs in the insulin resistant state [3].

5.4.4.3 LP(A)

A plasminogen-like protein, apo(a), binds covalently to apoB to form Lp(a), which confers additive risk to individuals with classic risk factors. The status of Lp(a) as a clinically important risk factor in *adults* has remained controversial [89]; however, a meta-analysis has shown it to be an independent risk factor [43]. When increased, Lp(a) may predispose to both thrombosis and atherogenesis. A consensus reference method is recommended to avoid being affected by the known variation in isoform size [89, 112]. Lp(a) concentration is largely determined by the apo(a) gene which programs for a variable number of plasminogen-like ring structures called kringles. The number of kringles is inversely proportional to Lp(a) concentration [176]. Large isoforms associated with low concentrations are common in Caucasian populations [175]. In general, higher Lp(a) concentration is associated with higher cardiovascular risk and, when elevated, may warrant lowering the LDL-C target below 70 mg/dL and the addition of niacin (if tolerated).

Estrogens lower Lp(a) [13]. In the *young* obese patient, Lp(a) serves as a novel risk factor providing information on risk, when the family history indicates early cardiovascular disease, particularly if classic risk factors appear normal [185]. Association with risk factors appears to be determined by both gender and age [183].

Lp(a) is positively associated with BMI, waist-to-hip ratio, and percent body fat (determined by bioelectrical impedance) in young adult males [183]. Lp(a) assessment in children is indicated when clustering of risk is present or when high familial risk is unexplained by conventional testing. Detection of high levels may require lowering therapeutic targets for cholesterol in order to provide adequate risk reduction.

5.4.4.4 ApoE

ApoE, a polymorphic apolipoprotein, also may determine risk by modulating particle uptake by LDL receptors [164]. Population studies have revealed three isoforms, differing from one another by one amino acid. $ApoE_3$ is the most common allele occurring in about 77%, with $apoE_4$ in 15%, and $apoE_2$ in 8% of western Caucasian populations [45]. Individuals with one or more of the $apoE_4$ alleles tend to have about 10% higher circulating cholesterol. Those with $apoE_2$ or $apoE_4$ alleles tend to have a higher triglyceride [42]. Those with the E_2E_2 genotype have a low cholesterol, except in 1–2% who develop dyslipidemia in association with other genetic or environmental factors including obesity.

The apoE alleles have an interactive influence on the relationship of obesity [86, 113] and dietary intake [178] on plasma lipid profiles in adults. Since the apoE allele contributes to risk for atherosclerosis in young subjects studied following early death [77], apoE may contribute to the pathogenesis of early atherosclerosis in adolescence, particularly in the presence of obesity. $ApoE_2$ modulates triglyceride levels in obese children and its relative influence is followed by $apoE_4$ [159]. Thus, apoE polymorphisms appear to modulate the association between obesity and dyslipidemias beginning in childhood.

5.4.4.5 LpA-I and LpA-I:A-II

ApoA-I and apoA-II serve as the main apolipoproteins in HDL, and their presence defines the HDL particles as containing both (LpA-I:A-II) or apoA-I alone (LpA-I). LpA-I carries more cholesterol and has a greater protective role in reverse cholesterol transport. LpA-I and LpA-I:A-II, respectively, approximate the larger HDL_2 and smaller HDL_3 particles [83].

We recently investigated the influence of BMI on high density lipoproteins in Cherokee children and adolescents aged 5–19 years to determine the relationships between obesity and LpA-I and LpA-I:A-II [20]. Significant correlations between waist circumference (a surrogate measure of visceral fat) and HDL cholesterol, LpA-I, and LpA-I:A-II, supported a compounding influence of visceral fat on the tendency to decrease high density lipoproteins. We observed that the obesity-related lowering of HDL-C occurs as early as age 5 years. In general, the decline in HDL-C values with BMI Z score quartiles was significant for all age groups of Cherokee children and adolescents, but declines in LpA-I and LpA-I:A-II were less remarkable. The finding confirms a predominant decrease in the cholesterol "load" for the respective lipoprotein "transport vehicles" (mainly apoA-I and apoA-II), which remains relatively constant. Adiposity may therefore result in less transfer of cholesterol to the HDL particles either from a cellular source via the ABCA1 cassette located on cell surfaces or from lipolysis of VLDL. Multiple regression modeling supported a negative influence of adiposity on HDL-C and to a lesser extent on LpA-I and LpA-I:A-II. Homeostatic index (HOMA-IR) was negatively associated with LpA-I:A-II. Therefore, HDL's role in children as a cholesterol acceptor from lipoprotein and cellular sources appears compromised by insulin resistance.

The trend for HDL-C, LpA-I, and LpA-I:A-II to decrease with age in boys (more so than in girls) supports a gender-specific effect of puberty, and suggests that boys acquire a greater cardiovascular risk at puberty, particularly if the boy is obese. In the accompanying insulin-resistant state of puberty, triglyceride enrichment of HDL (mediated by cholesterol ester transport protein in exchange for cholesterol ester) [15] results in HDL degradation by hepatic lipase, an enzyme known to be androgen sensitive. Endogenous testosterone production in prepubertal males is associated with the enzyme activity [156] leading to lower HDL-C levels.

5.4.4.6 NMR LIPOPROTEIN PROFILE

Based on published data, it appears that the size and particle concentration determined by NMR is ideal for investigating dyslipidemia occurring in obese insulin-resistant adolescents, who often have variations from normal throughout the profile [25, 26, 56]. A single analysis provides information on all the density classes and appears superior to alternative methods for estimating density subclasses. The patient's plasma sample is subjected to a short pulse of energy within a magnetic field. The resonant sound that is broadcast by the lipid molecules is recorded and analyzed to determine the number and size of lipoproteins present. Lipids associated with larger lipoproteins broadcast a signal that is characteristically distinct from those of smaller lipoproteins providing a spectrum of particle sizes and total number for each density class. A computer algorithm separates the signals into groups and then quantifies the number of particles in that group.

Data obtained from the profiles – particularly LDL particle number – have been highly predictive of cardiovascular disease in adults [39] and have proven useful to choose treatment for obvious dyslipidemia by metabolic syndrome criteria, despite normal LDL-C. These patients are likely to display increased LDL particle concentration associated with small particle size; however, similar information and clinical judgment can be obtained by determining apoB [37, 155]. Adolescents tend to have an abnormal profile when their BMI is increased [56] or when they have an increased waist circumference [25]. The profile becomes even more atherogenic when they possess liver fat accumulation or evidence of nonalcoholic fatty liver disease (NAFLD) [26].

5.5   ADHESION MOLECULES AND INFLAMMATION

Obesity in children is associated with increased markers of early endothelial change. The adhesion molecules and inflammatory markers ICAM-1, VCAM-1, P-selectin, and CRP are found to be higher in obese compared to normal children [50] and adolescents [67]. Circulating endothelin 1 level is also higher in obese children (compared to normal peers) and correlates significantly with BMI, triglycerides, and cholesterol [66]. Since adhesion molecules function to promote recruitment of inflammatory cells and transendothelial migration, increases in children may serve to promote early pathological vascular changes [22]. The health of the arterial wall may be compromised further by thrombomodulin (a marker of endothelial cell damage), which is increased in obese adolescents [172].

Adipocytes, together with an inflammatory cell infiltrate, clearly propagate inflammatory changes in the obese state [167] (Fig. 5.2). Adipocytes secrete several proteins with inflammatory and endocrine properties termed adipokines. These include cytokines [e.g., tumor necrosis factor-α (TNF-α) and IL-6] and chemokines (e.g., monocyte chemoattractant protein-1 (MCP-1)). Other secretions from adipocytes include plasminogen activator inhibitor-1 (PAI-1), angiotensinogen, cholesterol ester transfer protein (CETP), vascular endothelial growth factor (VEGF), and adiponectin. With its extensive secretory functions, the adipocyte illustrates the complex interaction among several key systems involved in regulating cardiovascular health. Significant changes in adipocyte-derived proteins occur in the obese state, implicating these substances as likely cardiovascular risk factors.

An acute phase reactant produced primarily by the liver, CRP is an established independent risk factor for cardiovascular disease [144]. Obese adults display high circulating CRP levels, which can be lowered by weight loss [149]. TNF-α – which is known to modulate immune and inflammatory processes – exerts multiple effects on the adipocyte: inhibition of differentiation [165], stimulation of lipolysis [145], apoptosis [140], and adipocyte-specific insulin resistance [80]. In obesity, TNF-α expression is increased in adipocytes, muscle, and macrophages [97]. TNF-α regulates cytokine secretions by the adipocyte [186], including increased secretion of itself, IL-6, and MCP-1 [181]. TNF-α decreases gene expression of adiponectin within human preadipocytes, contributing to the increase in insulin resistance [94]. Therefore, TNF-α contributes to induction of insulin resistance and monocyte recruitment [181]. In addition to adipocyte-mediated cytokine secretion, expansion of the fat mass is associated with macrophage accumulation and enhanced cytokine production [186].

Obesity in children has been characterized as being associated with oxidative stress and an adverse adipokine profile. When children with the metabolic syndrome were divided into three groups of normal weight, overweight, and overweight with the metabolic syndrome, differences across groups were found for triglyceride, HDL-C, HOMA, adiponectin, leptin, CRP, IL-6, and 8-isoprotane (a measure of oxidative stress). Oxidative stress worsened throughout the continuum of obesity, especially when associated with the metabolic syndrome [96]. It has been proposed that the inflammatory process within adipose tissue is adipocyte driven, and that the process is enhanced by hypoxia. One reason is that pockets of expanding fat become distant from the blood supply and relatively low in oxygenation. The resulting hypoxia then results in stimulation of cytokines and angiogenic factors to improve the blood supply [168]. This postulated process may partly explain the increasing severity of the cytokine increase with the degree of obesity.

5.6   INTERVENTION

5.6.1   Overview

Based on both epidemiological and pathological evidence to date, it is logical to conclude that if obesity in childhood is prevented or reversed, much of the tracking and progressive worsening of cardiovascular risk would be held in check or reversed. However, we are only just beginning to obtain evidence on feasibility and efficacy of interventions that influence not only obesity-related outcomes, but also reverse physical cardiovascular risk measurements and biochemical risk markers, within a few months of the first observation. However, in resistant cases, achieving long-term goals requires longer time periods.

5.6.2   Lifestyle

It is well accepted that lifestyle forms the basis of weight management in childhood, while pharmacological therapies have had limited success [61]. Gastric bypass procedures may be effective in causing preferential loss of centrally located fat [84], suggesting feasibility for this approach to treat severe adolescent obesity (discussed further in Chap. 20). It is encouraging that moderate weight loss in overweight adolescents improves dyslipidemia and insulin resistance [18]. Insulin resistance is an important target of intervention, since it predicts cardiovascular risk from ages 13 to 19 years interactively with BMI [151].

5.6.3   IMT Reversal by Exercise

Despite difficulty in defining specific causes of the observed IMT thickening in obese children, it is encouraging that the changes can be reversed by exercise too. Woo *et al.* showed that the addition of an exercise program to dietary modification resulted in reduced IMT and increased flow-mediated dilation [192]. When obese adolescents participated in an exercise program for 6 months, both IMT and vascular function improved. These improvements correlated with favorable changes in obesity measures, blood pressure, lipid values (triglyceride and LDL/HDL ratio), and inflammation (CRP and fibrinogen) [122]. Wunch *et al.* managed to bring about substantial weight loss in 56 prepubertal children, defined by a reduction of BMI Z score by at least 0.5. The decrease in IMT occurring over the 12-month study period paralleled a decrease in blood pressure, triglycerides, insulin, and insulin resistance index, as well as increased HDL-C [193].

Interventions to increase physical activity in children can result in weight loss or slow the rate of weight gain, but both outcomes are difficult to attain and sustain in the clinical setting. However, it seems possible that exercise – even without much weight loss – exerts some favorable effects on vascular function. In adults, dietary measures and exercise contribute to improvements in endothelial function and IMT in patients on treatment with pharmaceutical agents [32].

5.6.4   Dyslipidemia Treatment

The characteristic increase in triglyceride and decrease in HDL-C seen in association with insulin resistance and co-existing obesity is responsive to lifestyle interventions [132, 170], which should always be a central component of the therapeutic plan for children and adolescents. If hypercholesterolemia co-exists, there are specific guidelines for targeting LDL-C.

Metformin is advocated by some clinicians for children with impaired glucose tolerance or obesity [61], along with insulin resistance and a family history of T2DM. Metformin has an added effect on triglyceride lowering. A fibrate (*e.g.*, fenofibrate) can be used for refractory cases of hypertriglyceridemia when the triglyceride remains above 200 mg/dL. However, fibrates have not yet been FDA approved for pediatric use.

Published guidelines for use of lipid-lowering drugs in children have been largely based on targeting a reduction in LDL-C. Pharmacologic therapy has been recommended after a trial of diet therapy has been ineffective for 6–12 months, and when either: (1) LDL-C is above 190 mg/dL (4.9 mmol/L) with no other risk factors for coronary artery disease; or (2) when LDL-C is above 160 mg/dL (4.1 mmol/L) with a family history of early coronary artery disease or if two or more risk factors are present. The treatment goal is to attain an LDL-C <130 mg/dL (3.35 mmol/L) or ideally <110 mg/dL (2.85 mmol/L). If these criteria for drug therapy are met, a statin is recommended as first-line treatment. Lowering the effective dose of the statin is desirable for children and can be done by adding 10 mg of ezetimibe (Zetia) daily. This combination also has a triglyceride lowering effect and lowers non-HDL [133]. The development of an extended release form of niacin has made it a possible agent of choice to elevate HDL-C; however, flushing, although reduced in severity, remains a significant compliance-limiting side effect. A selective antagonist of the prostaglandin D(2) receptor subtype 1 (Laropiprant®) has been developed [135], and trials incorporating its use combined with niacin show promise, suggesting that use in children and adolescents may be considered.

More recent American Heart Association guidelines published in 2007 have added recommendations for children if they have additional risk factors [115]. For children with high risk lipid abnormalities, the presence of additional risk factors or high risk conditions may allow lowering of the LDL-C cut points, targets, and treatment ages under 10 years. Additional risk factors include male gender, strong family history of cardiovascular disease or events, associated low HDL-C, high triglycerides, small dense LDL, overweight/obesity and the metabolic syndrome, other medical conditions with risk for cardiovascular disease [*e.g.*, diabetes mellitus, HIV, systemic lupus erythematosis, or organ transplantation], smoking and passive smoke exposure, and novel risk factors [*e.g.*, elevated Lp(a), homocysteine, or CRP]. Low HDL-C, high triglyceride, elevated CRP, and a family history positive for cardiovascular disease are frequent in young obese patients. In obese children who are refractory to lifestyle measures (the majority), the new modifications allow earlier pharmacologic intervention for cases with LDL-C values in the intermediate range (*i.e.*, 130–160 mg/dL) making a treatment target of <110 mg/dL more attainable in cases who fail to respond to lifestyle measures. Despite controversial argument for large-scale pharmacological intervention based on more liberal guidelines, data support more aggressive primary prevention strategies at earlier ages. However, since there is a paucity of trial data for pharmacological treatment of children less than 10 years of age, treatment according to protocol-based studies is advised.

Since triglyceride-rich lipoprotein particles are frequently encountered in association with elevations in apoB (reflecting hepatic influx of fatty acids) [64], it can be argued that non-HDL (a close correlate of apoB) should be regarded as an important target for therapy. Since determination of non-HDL is readily available from the standard lipid profile (by subtracting HDL-C from total cholesterol), it can be used as a marker of dyslipidemia as recommended by NCEP. The recommended targets for non-HDL are 30 mg/dL higher than for LDL-C.

5.6.5 Hypertension Treatment

Guidelines for management of hypertension associated with obesity have been published elsewhere [55]. The DASH diet for adults is thought to be effective in children and consists of fruits, vegetables, low fat dairy, whole grains, reduced saturated fat and refined sugar, and low salt. Increased physical activity should always be recommended, provided the blood pressure is mild or under satisfactory control. Estimating the plasma renin activity can be used as a basis for treatment selection. ACE inhibitors should be used for subjects with a high renin, provided renal blood flow is normal. If renin is low, a thiazide diuretic can be used. In general, ACE inhibitors remain the first choice, and the minimal effective dose is 0.08 mg/kg/day. Several ACE inhibitors have been studied in children, including enalapril, fosinopril, and lisinopril. Although their pediatric applications have been extensive, long-term safety and efficacy data remain limited.

For primary hypertension, the target is to lower the blood pressure <95%ile. For secondary hypertension, the therapeutic goal is <90%ile in order to prevent hypertensive organ damage. Evaluation of hypertension and estimation of targets requires use of blood pressure percentile charts for age, gender, and height. The Harriet Lane handbook and other widely available clinical references can be used. Use of the electronic medical record to incorporate calculated percentiles has been an advantage in many healthcare systems.

5.7 CONCLUSIONS

The current epidemic of obesity in children and adolescents has far-reaching public health implications, in no small part due to associated cardiovascular health risks in adult life. Risk evaluation is essential for effective management and serial follow-up of obese children and adolescents, especially those having the cluster of comorbidities known as the metabolic syndrome. Although there is substantial controversy as to the definition of the metabolic syndrome in childhood, it is clear that the same obesity-associated comorbidities exist in children and significantly resemble those described in adults. Those caring for obese children and adolescents should use a checklist of recognizable and diagnosable problems, including the use of recommended cut points, in order to provide a framework for characterizing cardiovascular risk and to develop reasonable treatment goals.

Knowledge of the causes and mechanisms underlying the metabolic syndrome in childhood has increased substantially over the past decade. Both newly described vascular markers (*e.g.*, ICAM-1 and VCAM-1) and classic markers of inflammation (*e.g.*, cytokines and CRP) are implicated in the pediatric metabolic syndrome, representing potential therapeutic targets. Possibly as a result of lipoprotein infiltration and inflammation, quantitative changes in arterial thickness and stiffness can now be documented by cutting edge technologies with potential to enhance assessment and treatment monitoring.

Direct measurement of the components of circulating lipids and lipoproteins (*e.g.*, apolipoproteins) is not only possible, but potentially provides a more detailed clinical assessment of cardiovascular risk and can facilitate decisions on choice of treatment. However, widespread clinical use has not yet emerged despite the moderate to high correlations between conventional lipid measurements and apolipoproteins. Furthermore, evidence that they are superior risk predictors in early adulthood and at older ages supports inclusion of apolipoprotein measures in the clinic. This paradigm shift in practice could be facilitated with more assay standardization and wider availability of age-related normative data for the apolipoproteins. There is strong support for evaluating adults and at risk adolescents by measuring the apoB:A-I ratio, apoB and apoC-III bound to apoB-containing lipoproteins, or heparin-precipitated apoC-III. Lp(a) is re-emerging as a potent risk factor, with recent improvements in assays including genotyping. The same applies for apoE. The lipoprotein particle size and number profile by NMR can provide adjunctive information to assist in clinical decision making, but similar information to the determination of LDL particle concentration can be obtained from plasma apoB assay. Since CRP has been established as a measure of cardiovascular risk in adult studies, it may be an additional component to the metabolic syndrome.

Evidence suggests that many of these factors are reversible with effective treatment. However, extensive evidence and optimal clinical practice indicate that the central component of obesity and cardiovascular risk management should always be lifestyle, but comprehensive lifestyle treatments are costly, poorly reimbursed, and rarely effective in the long term, particularly when obesity has become severe. Pharmaceutical treatments should be used when recommended dyslipidemia and hypertension cut points are exceeded or when risk is increased by the co-existence of additional risk factors.

REFERENCES

1. Alaupovic P (1981) David Rubinstein memorial lecture: the biochemical and clinical significance of the interrelationship between very low density and high density lipoproteins. Can J Biochem 59:565–579
2. Alaupovic P, Blackett P, Wang W, Lee E (2008) Characterization of the metabolic syndrome by apolipoproteins in the Oklahoma Cherokee. J Cardiometab Syndr 3:193–199
3. Altomonte J, Cong L, Harbaran S et al. (2004) Foxo1 mediates insulin action on apoC-III and triglyceride metabolism. J Clin Invest 114:1493–1503
4. Amiel SA, Sherwin RS, Simonson DC, Lauritano AA, Tamborlane WV (1986) Impaired insulin action in puberty. A contributing factor to poor glycemic control in adolescents with diabetes. N Engl J Med 315:215–219
5. Anuurad E, Chiem A, Pearson TA, Berglund L (2007) Metabolic syndrome components in African-Americans and European-American patients and its relation to coronary artery disease. Am J Cardiol 100:830–834
6. Aronson D (2008) Hyperglycemia and the pathobiology of diabetic complications. Adv Cardiol 45:1–16
7. Arslanian S, Suprasongsin C (1996) Insulin sensitivity, lipids, and body composition in childhood: is "syndrome X" present? J Clin Endocrinol Metab 81:1058–1062
8. Atabek ME, Pirgon O, Kivrak AS (2007) Evidence for association between insulin resistance and premature carotid atherosclerosis in childhood obesity. Pediatr Res 61:345–349
9. Austin MA (2000) Triglyceride, small, dense low-density lipoprotein, and the atherogenic lipoprotein phenotype. Curr Atheroscler Rep 2:200–207
10. Back MR, Carew TE, Schmid-Schoenbein GW (1995) Deposition pattern of monocytes and fatty streak development in hypercholesterolemic rabbits. Atherosclerosis 116:103–115
11. Bank AJ, Wang H, Holte JE, Mullen K, Shammas R, Kubo SH (1996) Contribution of collagen, elastin, and smooth muscle to in vivo human brachial artery wall stress and elastic modulus. Circulation 94:3263–3270
12. Barlow SE, Dietz WH (1998) Obesity evaluation and treatment: Expert Committee recommendations. The Maternal and Child Health Bureau, Health Resources and Services Administration and the Department of Health and Human Services. Pediatrics 102:E29
13. Bayrak A, Aldemir DA, Bayrak T, Corakci A, Dursun P (2006) The effect of hormone replacement therapy on the levels of serum lipids, apolipoprotein AI, apolipoprotein B and lipoprotein (a) in Turkish postmenopausal women. Arch Gynecol Obstet 274:289–296
14. Beauloye V, Zech F, Tran HT, Clapuyt P, Maes M, Brichard SM (2007) Determinants of early atherosclerosis in obese children and adolescents. J Clin Endocrinol Metab 92:3025–3032
15. Begum N, Song Y, Rienzie J, Ragolia L (1998) Vascular smooth muscle cell growth and insulin regulation of mitogen-activated protein kinase in hypertension. Am J Physiol 275:C42–C49

16. Berenson G, Srinivasan S, Chen W, Li S, Patel D (2006) Racial (black-white) contrasts of risk for hypertensive disease in youth have implications for preventive care: the Bogalusa Heart Study. Ethn Dis 16:S4-2-9
17. Berenson GS, Srinivasan SR, Bao W, Newman WP III, Tracy RE, Wattigney WA (1998) Association between multiple cardiovascular risk factors and atherosclerosis in children and young adults. The Bogalusa Heart Study. N Engl J Med 338:1650–1656
18. Berkowitz RI, Fujioka K, Daniels SR et al. (2006) Effects of sibutramine treatment in obese adolescents: a randomized trial. Ann Intern Med 145:81–90
19. Blackett PR, Blevins KS, Quintana E et al. (2005) ApoC-III bound to apoB-containing lipoproteins increase with insulin resistance in Cherokee Indian youth. Metabolism 54:180–187
20. Blackett PR, Blevins KS, Stoddart M et al. (2005) Body mass index and high-density lipoproteins in Cherokee Indian children and adolescents. Pediatr Res 58:472–477
21. Blackett PR, Taylor T, Russell D, Lu M, Fesmire J, Lee ET (1996) Lipoprotein changes in relation to body mass index in Native American adolescents. Pediatr Res 40:77–81
22. Blankenberg S, Barbaux S, Tiret L (2003) Adhesion molecules and atherosclerosis. Atherosclerosis 170:191–203
23. Boney CM, Verma A, Tucker R, Vohr BR (2005) Metabolic syndrome in childhood: association with birth weight, maternal obesity, and gestational diabetes mellitus. Pediatrics 115:e290–e296
24. Brambilla P, Lissau I, Flodmark CE et al. (2007) Metabolic risk-factor clustering estimation in children: to draw a line across pediatric metabolic syndrome. Int J Obes (Lond) 31:591–600
25. Burns SF, Arslanian SA (2009) Waist circumference, atherogenic lipoproteins, and vascular smooth muscle biomarkers in children. J Clin Endocrinol Metab 94:4914–4922
26. Cali AM, Zern TL, Taksali SE et al. (2007) Intrahepatic fat accumulation and alterations in lipoprotein composition in obese adolescents: a perfect pro-atherogenic state. Diab Care 30(12):3093–3098
27. Cardoso-Saldana G, Juarez-Rojas JG, Zamora-Gonzalez J et al. (2007) C-reactive protein levels and their relationship with metabolic syndrome and insulin resistance in Mexican adolescents. J Pediatr Endocrinol Metab 20:797–805
28. Carr MC, Brunzell JD (2004) Abdominal obesity and dyslipidemia in the metabolic syndrome: importance of type 2 diabetes and familial combined hyperlipidemia in coronary artery disease risk. J Clin Endocrinol Metab 89:2601–2607
29. Cassidy AE, Bielak LF, Zhou Y et al. (2005) Progression of subclinical coronary atherosclerosis: does obesity make a difference? Circulation 111:1877–1882
30. Chait A, Wight TN (2000) Interaction of native and modified low-density lipoproteins with extracellular matrix. Curr Opin Lipidol 11:457–463
31. Chajek T, Eisenberg S (1978) Very low density lipoprotein. Metabolism of phospholipids, cholesterol, and apolipoprotein C in the isolated perfused rat heart. J Clin Invest 61:1654–1665
32. Chan SY, Mancini GB, Burns S et al. (2006) Dietary measures and exercise training contribute to improvement of endothelial function and atherosclerosis even in patients given intensive pharmacologic therapy. J Cardiopulm Rehabil 26:288–293
33. Clark LT, El-Atat F (2007) Metabolic syndrome in African Americans: implications for preventing coronary heart disease. Clin Cardiol 30:161–164
34. Cook S, Weitzman M, Auinger P, Nguyen M, Dietz WH (2003) Prevalence of a metabolic syndrome phenotype in adolescents: findings from the third National Health and Nutrition Examination Survey, 1988–1994. Arch Pediatr Adolesc Med 157:821–827

35. Copeland KC, Eichberg JW, Parker CR Jr (1985) Bartke A: Puberty in the chimpanzee: somatomedin-C and its relationship to somatic growth and steroid hormone concentrations. J Clin Endocrinol Metab 60:1154–1160
36. Copeland KC, Kuehl TJ, Castracane VD (1982) Pubertal endocrinology of the baboon: elevated somatomedin-C/insulin-like growth factor I at puberty. J Clin Endocrinol Metab 55:1198–1201
37. Cromwell WC, Barringer TA (2009) Low-density lipoprotein and apolipoprotein B: clinical use in patients with coronary heart disease. Curr Cardiol Rep 11:468–475
38. Cromwell WC, Otvos JD (2006) Heterogeneity of low-density lipoprotein particle number in patients with type 2 diabetes mellitus and low-density lipoprotein cholesterol <100 mg/dl. Am J Cardiol 98:1599–1602
39. Cromwell WC, Otvos JD, Keyes MJ et al. (2007) LDL particle number and risk of future cardiovascular disease in the Framingham Offspring Study – implications for LDL management. J Clin Lipidol 1:583–592
40. Cruz ML, Goran MI (2004) The metabolic syndrome in children and adolescents. Curr Diab Rep 4:53–62
41. Cruz ML, Weigensberg MJ, Huang TT, Ball G, Shaibi GQ, Goran MI (2004) The metabolic syndrome in overweight Hispanic youth and the role of insulin sensitivity. J Clin Endocrinol Metab 89:108–113
42. Dallongeville J, Lussier-Cacan S, Davignon J (1992) Modulation of plasma triglyceride levels by apoE phenotype: a meta-analysis. J Lipid Res 33:447–454
43. Danesh J, Collins R, Peto R (2000) Lipoprotein(a) and coronary heart disease. Meta-analysis of prospective studies. Circulation 102:1082–1085
44. Daniels SR, Kimball TR, Morrison JA, Khoury P, Witt S, Meyer RA (1995) Effect of lean body mass, fat mass, blood pressure, and sexual maturation on left ventricular mass in children and adolescents. Statistical, biological, and clinical significance. Circulation 92:3249–3254
45. Davignon J, Gregg RE, Sing CF (1988) Apolipoprotein E polymorphism and atherosclerosis. Arteriosclerosis 8:1–21
46. Davis PH, Dawson JD, Riley WA, Lauer RM (2001) Carotid intimal-medial thickness is related to cardiovascular risk factors measured from childhood through middle age: the Muscatine Study. Circulation 104:2815–2819
47. de Ferranti SD, Gauvreau K, Ludwig DS, Neufeld EJ, Newburger JW, Rifai N (2004) Prevalence of the metabolic syndrome in American adolescents: findings from the Third National Health and Nutrition Examination Survey. Circulation 110: 2494–2497
48. de Groot E, Hovingh GK, Wiegman A et al. (2004) Measurement of arterial wall thickness as a surrogate marker for atherosclerosis. Circulation 109:III33–III38
49. Dekkers C, Treiber FA, Kapuku G, Van Den Oord EJ, Snieder H (2002) Growth of left ventricular mass in African American and European American youth. Hypertension 39:943–951
50. Desideri G, De Simone M, Iughetti L et al. (2005) Early activation of vascular endothelial cells and platelets in obese children. J Clin Endocrinol Metab 90:3145–3152
51. Dunder K, Lind L, Zethelius B, Berglund L, Lithell H (2004) Evaluation of a scoring scheme, including proinsulin and the apolipoprotein B/apolipoprotein A1 ratio, for the risk of acute coronary events in middle-aged men: Uppsala Longitudinal Study of Adult Men (ULSAM). Am Heart J 148:596–601
52. Enos WF, Holmes RH, Beyer J (1986) Landmark article, July 18, 1953: Coronary disease among United States soldiers killed in action in Korea. Preliminary report. By William F. Enos, Robert H. Holmes and James Beyer. JAMA 256:2859–2862

53. Fernandez JR, Redden DT, Pietrobelli A, Allison DB (2004) Waist circumference percentiles in nationally representative samples of African-American, European-American, and Mexican-American children and adolescents. J Pediatr 145:439–444

54. Fernandez N, Martinez MA, Climent B *et al.* (2003) *In vivo* coronary effects of endothelin-1 after ischemia-reperfusion. Role of nitric oxide and prostanoids. Eur J Pharmacol 481:109–117

55. Flynn JT, Daniels SR (2006) Pharmacologic treatment of hypertension in children and adolescents. J Pediatr 149:746–754

56. Freedman DS, Bowman BA, Otvos JD, Srinivasan SR, Berenson GS (2000) Levels and correlates of LDL and VLDL particle sizes among children: the Bogalusa heart study. Atherosclerosis 152:441–449

57. Freedman DS, Dietz WH, Srinivasan SR, Berenson GS (1999) The relation of over weight to cardiovascular risk factors among children and adolescents: the Bogalusa Heart Study. Pediatrics 103:1175–1182

58. Freedman DS, Kahn HS, Mei Z *et al.* (2007) Relation of body mass index and waist-to-height ratio to cardiovascular disease risk factors in children and adolescents: the Bogalusa Heart Study. Am J Clin Nutr 86:33–40

59. Freedman DS, Khan LK, Dietz WH, Srinivasan SR, Berenson GS (2001) Relationship of childhood obesity to coronary heart disease risk factors in adulthood: the Bogalusa Heart Study. Pediatrics 108:712–718

60. Freedman DS, Khan LK, Serdula MK, Dietz WH, Srinivasan SR, Berenson GS (2005) The relation of childhood BMI to adult adiposity: the Bogalusa Heart Study. Pediatrics 115:22–27

61. Freemark M (2007) Pharmacotherapy of childhood obesity: an evidence-based, conceptual approach. Diab Care 30:395–402

62. Giannini C, de Giorgis T, Scarinci A *et al.* (2007) Obese related effects of inflammatory markers and insulin resistance on increased carotid intima media thickness in prepubertal children. Atherosclerosis 200(2):446

63. Gilardini L, Parati G, Sartorio A, Mazzilli G (2007) Pontiggia B. Sympathoadrenergic and metabolic factors are involved in ambulatory blood pressure rise in childhood obesity. J Hum Hypertens, Invitti C

64. Ginsberg HN (2002) New perspectives on atherogenesis: role of abnormal triglyceride-rich lipoprotein metabolism. Circulation 106:2137–2142

65. Ginsberg HN, Zhang YL, Hernandez-Ono A (2005) Regulation of plasma triglycerides in insulin resistance and diabetes. Arch Med Res 36:232–240

66. Glowinska B, Urban M, Hryniewicz A, Peczynska J, Florys B, Al-Hwish M (2004) Endothelin-1 plasma concentration in children and adolescents with atherogenic risk factors. Kardiol Pol 61:329–338

67. Glowinska B, Urban M, Peczynska J, Florys B (2005) Soluble adhesion molecules (sICAM-1, sVCAM-1) and selectins (sE selectin, sP selectin, sL selectin) levels in children and adolescents with obesity, hypertension, and diabetes. Metabolism 54:1020–1026

68. Goran MI (1999) Visceral fat in prepubertal children: Influence of obesity, anthropometry, ethnicity, gender, diet, and growth. Am J Hum Biol 11:201–207

69. Graves JW, Althaf MM (2006) Utility of ambulatory blood pressure monitoring in children and adolescents. Pediatr Nephrol 21:1640–1652

70. Grundy SM (2007) Metabolic syndrome: a multiplex cardiovascular risk factor. J Clin Endocrinol Metab 92:399–404

71. Gunnell DJ, Frankel SJ, Nanchahal K, Peters TJ, Davey Smith G (1998) Childhood obesity and adult cardiovascular mortality: a 57-y follow-up study based on the Boyd Orr cohort. Am J Clin Nutr 67:1111–1118

72. Haji SA, Ulusoy RE, Patel DA et al. (2006) Predictors of left ventricular dilatation in young adults (from the Bogalusa Heart Study). Am J Cardiol 98:1234–1237

73. Hannon TS, Bacha F, Lee SJ, Janosky J, Arslanian SA (2006) Use of markers of dyslipidemia to identify overweight youth with insulin resistance. Pediatr Diabetes 7:260–266

74. Hannon TS, Janosky J, Arslanian SA (2006) Longitudinal study of physiologic insulin resistance and metabolic changes of puberty. Pediatr Res 60:759–763

75. Hironaka K, Yano M, Kohno M et al. (1997) In vivo aortic wall characteristics at the early stage of atherosclerosis in rabbits. Am J Physiol 273:H1142–H1147

76. Hirschler V, Acebo HL, Fernandez GB, de Lujan Calcagno M, Gonzalez C, Jadzinsky M (2006) Influence of obesity and insulin resistance on left atrial size in children. Pediatr Diabetes 7:39–44

77. Hixson JE (1991) Apolipoprotein E polymorphisms affect atherosclerosis in young males. Pathobiological determinants of atherosclerosis in youth (PDAY) research group. Arterioscler Thromb 11:1237–1244

78. Hodge AM, Dowse GK, Zimmet PZ, Collins VR (1995) Prevalence and secular trends in obesity in Pacific and Indian Ocean island populations. Obes Res 3(Suppl 2):77s–87s

79. Hodis HN, Mack WJ, Azen SP et al. (1994) Triglyceride- and cholesterol-rich lipoproteins have a differential effect on mild/moderate and severe lesion progression as assessed by quantitative coronary angiography in a controlled trial of lovastatin. Circulation 90:42–49

80. Hotamisligil GS (2003) Inflammatory pathways and insulin action. Int J Obes Relat Metab Disord 27(Suppl 3):S53–S55

81. Iannuzzi A, Licenziati MR, Acampora C et al. (2006) Carotid artery stiffness in obese children with the metabolic syndrome. Am J Cardiol 97:528–531

82. Iglseder B, Mackevics V, Stadlmayer A, Tasch G, Ladurner G, Paulweber B (2005) Plasma adiponectin levels and sonographic phenotypes of subclinical carotid artery atherosclerosis: data from the SAPHIR Study. Stroke 36:2577–2582

83. Ikewaki K, Zech LA, Kindt M, Brewer HB Jr, Rader DJ (1995) Apolipoprotein A-II production rate is a major factor regulating the distribution of apolipoprotein A-I among HDL subclasses LpA-I and LpA-I:A-II in normolipidemic humans. Arterioscler Thromb Vasc Biol 15:306–312

84. Inge T, Wilson KA, Gamm K, Kirk S, Garcia VF, Daniels SR (2007) Preferential loss of central (trunk) adiposity in adolescents and young adults after laparoscopic gastric bypass. Surg Obes Relat Dis 3:153–158

85. Ito N, Ohishi M, Takagi T et al. (2006) Clinical usefulness and limitations of brachial-ankle pulse wave velocity in the evaluation of cardiovascular complications in hypertensive patients. Hypertens Res 29:989–995

86. Jemaa R, Elasmi M, Naouali C et al. (2006) Apolipoprotein E polymorphism in the Tunisian population: frequency and effect on lipid parameters. Clin Biochem 39:816–820

87. Jeyarajah EJ, Cromwell WC, Otvos JD (2006) Lipoprotein particle analysis by nuclear magnetic resonance spectroscopy. Clin Lab Med 26:847–870

88. Jolliffe CJ, Janssen I (2007) Development of age-specific adolescent metabolic syndrome criteria that are linked to the Adult Treatment Panel III and International Diabetes Federation criteria. J Am Coll Cardiol 49:891–898

89. Jones GT, van Rij AM, Cole J et al. (2007) Plasma lipoprotein(a) indicates risk for 4 distinct forms of vascular disease. Clin Chem 53:679–685

90. Jones KL (2006) The dilemma of the metabolic syndrome in children and adolescents: disease or distraction? Pediatr Diabetes 7:311–321

91. Juonala M, Viikari JS, Ronnemaa T, Taittonen L, Marniemi J, Raitakari OT (2006) Childhood C-reactive protein in predicting CRP and carotid intima-media thickness in adulthood: the Cardiovascular Risk in Young Finns Study. Arterioscler Thromb Vasc Biol 26:1883–1888

92. Kahn R, Buse J, Ferrannini E, Stern M (2005) The metabolic syndrome: time for a critical appraisal: joint statement from the American Diabetes Association and the European Association for the Study of Diabetes. Diab Care 28:2289–2304

93. Kapiotis S, Holzer G, Schaller G et al. (2006) A proinflammatory state is detectable in obese children and is accompanied by functional and morphological vascular changes. Arterioscler Thromb Vasc Biol 26:2541–2546

94. Kappes A, Loffler G (2000) Influences of ionomycin, dibutyryl-cycloAMP and tumour necrosis factor-alpha on intracellular amount and secretion of apM1 in differentiating primary human preadipocytes. Horm Metab Res 32:548–554

95. Kawakami A, Aikawa M, Libby P, Alcaide P, Luscinskas FW, Sacks FM (2006) Apolipoprotein CIII in apolipoprotein B lipoproteins enhances the adhesion of human monocytic cells to endothelial cells. Circulation 113:691–700

96. Kelly AS, Steinberger J, Kaiser DR, Olson TP, Bank AJ, Dengel DR (2006) Oxidative stress and adverse adipokine profile characterize the metabolic syndrome in children. J Cardiometab Syndr 1:248–252

97. Kern PA, Ranganathan S, Li C, Wood L, Ranganathan G (2001) Adipose tissue tumor necrosis factor and interleukin-6 expression in human obesity and insulin resistance. Am J Physiol Endocrinol Metab 280:E745–E751

98. Kissebah AH, Vydelingum N, Murray R et al. (1982) Relation of body fat distribution to metabolic complications of obesity. J Clin Endocrinol Metab 54:254–260

99. Koeijvoets KC, Rodenburg J, Hutten BA, Wiegman A, Kastelein JJ, Sijbrands EJ (2005) Low-density lipoprotein receptor genotype and response to pravastatin in children with familial hypercholesterolemia: substudy of an intima-media thickness trial. Circulation 112:3168–3173

100. Kortelainen ML, Sarkioja T (2001) Visceral fat and coronary pathology in male adolescents. Int J Obes Relat Metab Disord 25:228–232

101. Kurl S, Laukkanen JA, Niskanen L et al. (2006) Metabolic syndrome and the risk of stroke in middle-aged men. Stroke 37:806–811

102. Kwiterovich PO Jr (2008) Recognition and management of dyslipidemia in children and adolescents. J Clin Endocrinol Metab 93:4200–4209

103. Lee JW, Lee DC, Im JA, Shim JY, Kim SM, Lee HR (2007) Insulin resistance is associated with arterial stiffness independent of obesity in male adolescents. Hypertens Res 30:5–11

104. Lee S, Bacha F, Arslanian SA (2006) Waist circumference, blood pressure, and lipid components of the metabolic syndrome. J Pediatr 149:809–816

105. Lee SJ, Campos H, Moye LA, Sacks FM (2003) LDL containing apolipoprotein CIII is an independent risk factor for coronary events in diabetic patients. Arterioscler Thromb Vasc Biol 23:853–858

106. Leeson CP, Whincup PH, Cook DG et al. (2000) Cholesterol and arterial distensibility in the first decade of life: a population-based study. Circulation 101:1533–1538

107. Levy D, Garrison RJ, Savage DD, Kannel WB, Castelli WP (1990) Prognostic implications of echocardiographically determined left ventricular mass in the Framingham Heart Study. N Engl J Med 322:1561–1566

108. Lewis GF (1997) Fatty acid regulation of very low density lipoprotein production. Curr Opin Lipidol 8:146–153

109. Li X, Li S, Ulusoy E, Chen W, Srinivasan SR, Berenson GS (2004) Childhood adiposity as a predictor of cardiac mass in adulthood: the Bogalusa Heart Study. Circulation 110:3488–3492

110. Lorenz MW, von Kegler S, Steinmetz H, Markus HS, Sitzer M (2006) Carotid intima-media thickening indicates a higher vascular risk across a wide age range: prospective data from the Carotid Atherosclerosis Progression Study (CAPS). Stroke 37:87–92

111. Lurbe E, Torro I, Aguilar F *et al.* (2008) Added impact of obesity and insulin resistance in nocturnal blood pressure elevation in children and adolescents. Hypertension 51:635–641

112. Marcovina SM, Koschinsky ML, Albers JJ, Skarlatos S (2003) Report of the National Heart, Lung, and Blood Institute Workshop on Lipoprotein(a) and Cardiovascular Disease: recent advances and future directions. Clin Chem 49:1785–1796

113. Marques-Vidal P, Bongard V, Ruidavets JB *et al.* (2003) Obesity and alcohol modulate the effect of apolipoprotein E polymorphism on lipids and insulin. Obes Res 11:1200–1206

114. Matthews DR, Hosker JP, Rudenski AS, Naylor BA, Treacher DF, Turner RC (1985) Homeostasis model assessment: insulin resistance and beta-cell function from fasting plasma glucose and insulin concentrations in man. Diabetologia 28:412–419

115. McCrindle BW, Urbina EM, Dennison BA *et al.* (2007) Drug therapy of high-risk lipid abnormalities in children and adolescents: a scientific statement from the American Heart Association Atherosclerosis, Hypertension, and Obesity in Youth Committee, Council of Cardiovascular Disease in the Young, with the Council on Cardiovascular Nursing. Circulation 115:1948–1967

116. McGill HC Jr, McMahan CA, Herderick EE, Malcom GT, Tracy RE, Strong JP (2000) Origin of atherosclerosis in childhood and adolescence. Am J Clin Nutr 72:1307S–1315S

117. McGill HC Jr, McMahan CA, Herderick EE *et al.* (2000) Effects of coronary heart disease risk factors on atherosclerosis of selected regions of the aorta and right coronary artery. PDAY Research Group. Pathobiological Determinants of Atherosclerosis in Youth. Arterioscler Thromb Vasc Biol 20:836–845

118. McGill HC Jr, McMahan CA, Herderick EE *et al.* (2002) Obesity accelerates the progression of coronary atherosclerosis in young men. Circulation 105:2712–2718

119. McGill HC Jr, McMahan CA, Zieske AW *et al.* (2000) Associations of coronary heart disease risk factors with the intermediate lesion of atherosclerosis in youth. The Pathobiological Determinants of Atherosclerosis in Youth (PDAY) Research Group. Arterioscler Thromb Vasc Biol 20:1998–2004

120. McNamara JJ, Molot MA, Stremple JF, Cutting RT (1971) Coronary artery disease in combat casualties in Vietnam. JAMA 216:1185–1187

121. McNiece KL, Poffenbarger TS, Turner JL, Franco KD, Sorof JM, Portman RJ (2007) Prevalence of hypertension and pre-hypertension among adolescents. J Pediatr 150:640–644, 644.e1

122. Meyer AA, Kundt G, Lenschow U, Schuff-Werner P, Kienast W (2006) Improvement of early vascular changes and cardiovascular risk factors in obese children after a six-month exercise program. J Am Coll Cardiol 48:1865–1870

123. Montagnani M, Quon MJ (2000) Insulin action in vascular endothelium: potential mechanisms linking insulin resistance with hypertension. Diabetes Obes Metab 2:285–292

124. Moran A, Jacobs DR Jr, Steinberger J *et al.* (2008) Changes in insulin resistance and cardiovascular risk during adolescence: establishment of differential risk in males and females. Circulation 117:2361–2368

125. Must A, Jacques PF, Dallal GE, Bajema CJ, Dietz WH (1992) Long-term morbidity and mortality of overweight adolescents. A follow-up of the Harvard Growth Study of 1922 to 1935. N Engl J Med 327:1350–1355

126. Nakashima Y, Fujii H, Sumiyoshi S, Wight TN, Sueishi K (2007) Early human atherosclerosis: accumulation of lipid and proteoglycans in intimal thickenings followed by macrophage infiltration. Arterioscler Thromb Vasc Biol 27:1159–1165

127. Niboshi A, Hamaoka K, Sakata K, Inoue F (2006) Characteristics of brachial-ankle pulse wave velocity in Japanese children. Eur J Pediatr 165:625–629

128. Nilsson PM, Engstrom G, Hedblad B et al. (2006) Plasma adiponectin levels in relation to carotid intima media thickness and markers of insulin resistance. Arterioscler Thromb Vasc Biol 26:2758–2762

129. Olin-Lewis K, Krauss RM, La Belle M et al. (2002) ApoC-III content of apoB-containing lipoproteins is associated with binding to the vascular proteoglycan biglycan. J Lipid Res 43:1969–1977

130. Olivieri O, Bassi A, Stranieri C et al. (2003) Apolipoprotein C-III, metabolic syndrome, and risk of coronary artery disease. J Lipid Res 44:2374–2381

131. Opie LH (2007) Metabolic syndrome. Circulation 115:e32–e35

132. Orchard TJ, Temprosa M, Goldberg R et al. (2005) The effect of metformin and intensive lifestyle intervention on the metabolic syndrome: the Diabetes Prevention Program randomized trial. Ann Intern Med 142:611–619

133. Ose L, Shah A, Davies MJ et al. (2006) Consistency of lipid-altering effects of ezetimibe/simvastatin across gender, race, age, baseline low density lipoprotein cholesterol levels, and coronary heart disease status: results of a pooled retrospective analysis. Curr Med Res Opin 22:823–835

134. Ouyang F, Christoffel KK, Brickman WJ et al. (2010) Adiposity is inversely related to insulin sensitivity in relatively lean Chinese adolescents: a population-based twin study. Am J Clin Nutr 91(3):662–671

135. Paolini JF, Bays HE, Ballantyne CM et al. (2008) Extended-release niacin/laropiprant: reducing niacin-induced flushing to better realize the benefit of niacin in improving cardiovascular risk factors. Cardiol Clin 26:547–560

136. Pavkov ME, Hanson RL, Knowler WC, Bennett PH, Krakoff J, Nelson RG (2007) Changing patterns of type 2 diabetes incidence among Pima Indians. Diab Care 30:1758–1763

137. Pilz S, Horejsi R, Moller R et al. (2005) Early atherosclerosis in obese juveniles is associated with low serum levels of adiponectin. J Clin Endocrinol Metab 90:4792–4796

138. Pinhas-Hamiel O, Dolan LM, Daniels SR, Standiford D, Khoury PR, Zeitler P (1996) Increased incidence of non-insulin-dependent diabetes mellitus among adolescents. J Pediatr 128:608–615

139. Pischon T, Girman CJ, Hotamisligil GS, Rifai N, Hu FB, Rimm EB (2004) Plasma adiponectin levels and risk of myocardial infarction in men. JAMA 291:1730–1737

140. Prins JB, Niesler CU, Winterford CM et al. (1997) Tumor necrosis factor-alpha induces apoptosis of human adipose cells. Diabetes 46:1939–1944

141. Raitakari OT, Juonala M, Kahonen M et al. (2003) Cardiovascular risk factors in childhood and carotid artery intima-media thickness in adulthood: the Cardiovascular Risk in Young Finns Study. JAMA 290:2277–2283

142. Reaven GM (1988) Banting lecture 1988. Role of insulin resistance in human disease. Diabetes 37:1595–1607

143. Reinehr T, Kiess W, de Sousa G, Stoffel-Wagner B, Wunsch R (2006) Intima media thickness in childhood obesity: relations to inflammatory marker, glucose metabolism, and blood pressure. Metabolism 55:113–118

138 Blackett et al.

_144. Ridker PM, Rifai N, Rose L, Buring JE, Cook NR (2002) Comparison of C-reactive protein and low-density lipoprotein cholesterol levels in the prediction of first cardiovascular events. N Engl J Med 347:1557–1565
145. Ryden M, Arvidsson E, Blomqvist L, Perbeck L, Dicker A, Arner P (2004) Targets for TNF-alpha-induced lipolysis in human adipocytes. Biochem Biophys Res Commun 318:168–175
146. Sacks FM, Alaupovic P, Moye LA et al. (2000) VLDL, apolipoproteins B, CIII, and E, and risk of recurrent coronary events in the cholesterol and recurrent events (CARE) trial. Circulation 102:1886–1892
147. Sale MM, Woods J, Freedman BI (2006) Genetic determinants of the metabolic syndrome. Curr Hypertens Rep 8:16–22
148. Savva SC, Tornaritis M, Savva ME et al. (2000) Waist circumference and waist-to-height ratio are better predictors of cardiovascular disease risk factors in children than body mass index. Int J Obes Relat Metab Disord 24:1453–1458
149. Selvin E, Paynter NP, Erlinger TP (2007) The effect of weight loss on C-reactive protein: a systematic review. Arch Intern Med 167:31–39
150. Short KR, Blackett PR, Gardner AW, Copeland KC (2009) Vascular health in children and adolescents: effects of obesity and diabetes. Vasc Health Risk Manag 5:973–990
151. Sinaiko AR, Steinberger J, Moran A et al. (2005) Relation of body mass index and insulin resistance to cardiovascular risk factors, inflammatory factors, and oxidative stress during adolescence. Circulation 111:1985–1991
152. Singhal A, Farooqi IS, Cole TJ et al. (2002) Influence of leptin on arterial distensibility: a novel link between obesity and cardiovascular disease? Circulation 106:1919–1924
153. Sinha R, Fisch G, Teague B et al. (2002) Prevalence of impaired glucose tolerance among children and adolescents with marked obesity. N Engl J Med 346:802–810
154. Sivanandam S, Sinaiko AR, Jacobs DR Jr, Steffen L, Moran A, Steinberger J (2006) Relation of increase in adiposity to increase in left ventricular mass from childhood to young adulthood. Am J Cardiol 98:411–415
155. Sniderman AD, Faraj M (2007) Apolipoprotein B, apolipoprotein A-I, insulin resistance and the metabolic syndrome. Curr Opin Lipidol 18:633–637
156. Sorva R, Kuusi T, Dunkel L, Taskinen MR (1988) Effects of endogenous sex steroids on serum lipoproteins and postheparin plasma lipolytic enzymes. J Clin Endocrinol Metab 66:408–413
157. Srinivasan SR, Bao W, Wattigney WA, Berenson GS (1996) Adolescent overweight is associated with adult overweight and related multiple cardiovascular risk factors: the Bogalusa Heart Study. Metabolism 45:235–240
158. Srinivasan SR, Berenson GS (1995) Serum apolipoproteins A-I and B as markers of coronary artery disease risk in early life: the Bogalusa Heart Study. Clin Chem 41:159–164
159. Srinivasan SR, Ehnholm C, Elkasabany A, Berenson GS (2001) Apolipoprotein E polymorphism modulates the association between obesity and dyslipidemias during young adulthood: The Bogalusa Heart Study. Metabolism 50:696–702
160. Srinivasan SR, Myers L, Berenson GS (2002) Predictability of childhood adiposity and insulin for developing insulin resistance syndrome (syndrome X) in young adulthood: the Bogalusa Heart Study. Diabetes 51:204–209
161. ter Maaten JC, Voordouw JJ, Bakker SJ, Donker AJ, Gans RO (1999) Salt sensitivity correlates positively with insulin sensitivity in healthy volunteers. Eur J Clin Invest 29:189–195
162. Teran-Garcia M, Bouchard C (2007) Genetics of the metabolic syndrome. Appl Physiol Nutr Metab 32:89–114

163. Thompson A, Danesh J (2006) Associations between apolipoprotein B, apolipoprotein AI, the apolipoprotein B/AI ratio and coronary heart disease: a literature-based meta-analysis of prospective studies. J Intern Med 259:481–492
164. Tomiyasu K, Walsh BW, Ikewaki K, Judge H, Sacks FM (2001) Differential metabolism of human VLDL according to content of ApoE and ApoC-III. Arterioscler Thromb Vasc Biol 21:1494–1500
165. Torti FM, Torti SV, Larrick JW, Ringold GM (1989) Modulation of adipocyte differentiation by tumor necrosis factor and transforming growth factor beta. J Cell Biol 108:1105–1113
166. Tounian P, Aggoun Y, Dubern B et al. (2001) Presence of increased stiffness of the common carotid artery and endothelial dysfunction in severely obese children: a prospective study. Lancet 358:1400–1404
167. Trayhurn P (2005) Endocrine and signalling role of adipose tissue: new perspectives on fat. Acta Physiol Scand 184:285–293
168. Trayhurn P, Wood IS (2004) Adipokines: inflammation and the pleiotropic role of white adipose tissue. Br J Nutr 92:347–355
169. Troiano RP, Flegal KM, Kuczmarski RJ, Campbell SM, Johnson CL (1995) Overweight prevalence and trends for children and adolescents. The National Health and Nutrition Examination Surveys, 1963 to 1991. Arch Pediatr Adolesc Med 149:1085–1091
170. Tuomilehto J, Lindstrom J, Eriksson JG et al. (2001) Prevention of type 2 diabetes mellitus by changes in lifestyle among subjects with impaired glucose tolerance. N Engl J Med 344:1343–1350
171. Ulrich P, Cerami A (2001) Protein glycation, diabetes, and aging. Recent Prog Horm Res 56:1–21
172. Urban M, Wojtkielewicz K, Glowinska B, Peczynska J (2005) Soluble thrombomodulin – a molecular marker of endothelial cell injury in children and adolescents with obesity. Endokrynol Diabetol Chor Przemiany Materii Wieku Rozw 11:73–77
173. Urbina EM, Gidding SS, Bao W, Pickoff AS, Berdusis K, Berenson GS (1995) Effect of body size, ponderosity, and blood pressure on left ventricular growth in children and young adults in the Bogalusa Heart Study. Circulation 91:2400–2406
174. Urbina EM, Williams RV, Alpert BS et al. (2009) Noninvasive assessment of subclinical atherosclerosis in children and adolescents: recommendations for standard assessment for clinical research: a scientific statement from the American Heart Association. Hypertension 54:919–950
175. Utermann G, Duba C, Menzel HJ (1988) Genetics of the quantitative Lp(a) lipoprotein trait. II. Inheritance of Lp(a) glycoprotein phenotypes. Hum Genet 78:47–50
176. Utermann G, Menzel HJ, Kraft HG, Duba HC, Kemmler HG, Seitz C (1987) Lp(a) glycoprotein phenotypes. Inheritance and relation to Lp(a)-lipoprotein concentrations in plasma. J Clin Invest 80:458–465
177. van Popele NM, Bos WJ, de Beer NA et al. (2000) Arterial stiffness as underlying mechanism of disagreement between an oscillometric blood pressure monitor and a sphygmomanometer. Hypertension 36:484–488
178. Vincent S, Planells R, Defoort C et al. (2002) Genetic polymorphisms and lipoprotein responses to diets. Proc Nutr Soc 61:427–434
179. Walldius G, Jungner I (2004) Apolipoprotein B and apolipoprotein A-I: risk indicators of coronary heart disease and targets for lipid-modifying therapy. J Intern Med 255:188–205
180. Walldius G, Jungner I, Holme I, Aastveit AH, Kolar W, Steiner E (2001) High apolipoprotein B, low apolipoprotein A-I, and improvement in the prediction of fatal myocardial infarction (AMORIS study): a prospective study. Lancet 358:2026–2033

181. Wang B, Jenkins JR, Trayhurn P (2005) Expression and secretion of inflammation-related adipokines by human adipocytes differentiated in culture: integrated response to TNF-alpha. Am J Physiol Endocrinol Metab 288:E731–E740

182. Wang CS, McConathy WJ, Kloer HU, Alaupovic P (1985) Modulation of lipoprotein lipase activity by apolipoproteins. Effect of apolipoprotein C-III. J Clin Invest 75:384–390

183. Wang W, Lee ET, Alaupovic P, Blackett P, Blevins KS (2005) Correlation between lipoprotein(a) and other risk factors for cardiovascular disease and diabetes in Cherokee Indians: the Cherokee Diabetes Study. Ann Epidemiol 15:390–397

184. Wang X, Poole JC, Treiber FA, Harshfield GA, Hanevold CD, Snieder H (2006) Ethnic and gender differences in ambulatory blood pressure trajectories: results from a 15-year longitudinal study in youth and young adults. Circulation 114:2780–2787

185. Wang XL, Wang J (2003) Lipoprotein(a) in children and adolescence. Pediatr Endocrinol Rev 1:109–119

186. Weisberg SP, McCann D, Desai M, Rosenbaum M, Leibel RL, Ferrante AW Jr (2003) Obesity is associated with macrophage accumulation in adipose tissue. J Clin Invest 112:1796–1808

187. Weiss R, Dufour S, Groszmann A et al. (2003) Low adiponectin levels in adolescent obesity: a marker of increased intramyocellular lipid accumulation. J Clin Endocrinol Metab 88:2014–2018

188. West KM (1974) Diabetes in American Indians and other native populations of the New World. Diabetes 23:841–855

189. Whincup PH, Gilg JA, Donald AE et al. (2005) Arterial distensibility in adolescents: the influence of adiposity, the metabolic syndrome, and classic risk factors. Circulation 112:1789–1797

190. Williams KJ, Tabas I (1995) The response-to-retention hypothesis of early atherogenesis. Arterioscler Thromb Vasc Biol 15:551–561

191. Wilson PW, D'Agostino RB, Sullivan L, Parise H, Kannel WB (2002) Overweight and obesity as determinants of cardiovascular risk: the Framingham experience. Arch Intern Med 162:1867–1872

192. Woo KS, Chook P, Yu CW et al. (2004) Overweight in children is associated with arterial endothelial dysfunction and intima-media thickening. Int J Obes Relat Metab Disord 28:852–857

193. Wunsch R, de Sousa G, Toschke AM, Reinehr T (2006) Intima-media thickness in obese children before and after weight loss. Pediatrics 118:2334–2340

194. Young JB (1988) Effect of experimental hyperinsulinemia on sympathetic nervous system activity in the rat. Life Sci 43:193–200

195. Yu WC, Chuang SY (2007) Lin YP. Brachial-ankle vs carotid-femoral pulse wave velocity as a determinant of cardiovascular structure and function. J Hum Hypertens, Chen CH

196. Yusuf S, Hawken S, Ounpuu S et al. (2004) Effect of potentially modifiable risk factors associated with myocardial infarction in 52 countries (the INTERHEART study): case-control study. Lancet 364:937–952

6 Community-Based Approaches to Reduce Pediatric Obesity

Keith L. Perkins and
Dawn M. McNamee

Key Points

- Community-based approaches must be tailored to local needs and resources, engage key stakeholders, and become self-sustaining.
- Community-based approaches comprise the most cost effective interventions to address the public health aspects of pediatric obesity and T2DM.

Keywords: Community, Pediatric obesity, Prevention

6.1 USA-BASED PROGRAMS

Childhood obesity has become a worldwide problem that requires community solutions and interventions to help prevent the long-term consequences of this major medical problem. Fortunately, the obesity epidemic in children has inspired many individuals, foundations, and communities to implement change and to encourage participation in programs which prevent and reverse childhood obesity. This chapter highlights various programs around the world working to change a generation (Table 6.1).

6.1.1 Seed to Table Program (Maplewood, Missouri)

"Quick and fast" are the words we want to hear when it comes to our food. One school district, however, is taking strides to add more patience to food preparation from the soil to the mouth. In Maplewood, Missouri,

From: *Nutrition and Health: Management of Pediatric Obesity and Diabetes*,
Edited by: R.J. Ferry, Jr., DOI 10.1007/978-1-60327-256-8_6,
© Springer Science+Business Media, LLC 2011

Table 6.1

Community-based programs aimed at reducing and preventing pediatric obesity

Program	Base	Champion	Community	Website	Support
Seed to Table	School	Debi Gibson	Maplewood MO	http://www.mrhsd.org/gardens/index.html	Missouri Foundation for Health
America Scores	Community	Fredrick Popp, CEO	United States	www.americascores.org	AmeriCorps
Healthy Kids, Healthy Communities	Community		United States	http://www.healthykidshealthy-communities.org/	Robert Wood Foundation
Healthy Schools Initiative	School	South Carolina Dept. of Health	South Carolina	http://www.scdhec.gov/health/chcdp/schools/healthy_schools.htm	CDC
Healthy 100 Kids	Clinic	Florida Hospital for Children	Florida	http://www.healthy100kids.org/	
Follow Me! Healthy Parents, Healthy Kids	Community	Laura Miller	Columbus OH	http://followmekids.org/index.html	Nationwide Children's Hospital
CATCH	School	U Texas at Houston	United States	http://www.sph.uth.tmc.edu/catch/	
Just for Kids! Obesity Workbook	School	Balboa Publishing Co	San Francisco CA	http://www.just-for-kids.org/	
PE4life	School	Phil Lawler	United States	http://www.pe4life.org/	
All 4 Kids: Happy, Active, and Fit	Community	U Nevada	Las Vegas NV	http://www.unce.unr.edu/programs/health/files/pdf/All4Kids.pdf	USDA

Program	Setting	Organization/Contact	Location	Website	Funding
WOW-Way to Optimal Weight	Clinic	Eastern Maine Medical Center	Bangor, Maine	http://www.emmc.org/pediatric_services.aspx?id=5802	
On The Move	Community	Michael Heim	New Orleans LA	http://www.elmwoodfitness.com/Club/Scripts/Home/home.asp	
Pediatric Fitness Clinic	Clinic	U Wisconsin SMPH	Wisconsin	http://www.uwhealth.org/pediatric-obesity/pediatric-fitness/11338	
Bienestar Health Program	School	Dr. Roberto Trevino	San Antonio TX	http://volunteer.truist.com/unitedwaysatx/org/304979.html	
Bike It	Community	Sustrans	England	http://www.sustrans.org.uk/assets/files/Bike%20It/Sustrans_Bike_It_an%20intro_081014.pdf	Bike Hub, Big Lottery Fund, multiple local contributors
Eat Well Be Active Community Partnerships	Community	Queensland Obesity Summit	Queensland, Australia	http://www.qld.gov.au/community-partnerships/	Queensland Health, Dept of Local Govt, Sport and Recreation
Together, Lets' Prevent Childhood Obesity	Community	EPODE European Network	France	http://www.epode-european-network.com/	Proteins

a suburb of Saint Louis, the Maplewood-Richmond Heights School District is educating young students about gardening and preparing healthier food choices. The Seed to Table program was started in 2006 with the help of graduate nutrition students from Saint Louis University. The program goals were to expose children to the world of gardening and emphasize healthy food and lifestyle choices. In 2008, the Missouri Foundation for Health awarded the school district with a grant that not only allowed expansion of the program to middle school students, but also enabled the hiring of full time staff. Pre-K through 1st graders spend one day a week in gardening and nutrition classes, and all 6th graders spend time rotating through the garden. An after-school program also gives more exposure to students by not only giving them chances to enhance their gardening skills but also allow them to learn how to make healthy meals from their harvest [1].

6.1.2 America Scores Program (Saint Louis, Missouri)

Another Saint Louis area program aimed at preventing obesity is the America Scores Program. Split into 10-week sessions in the fall and spring, the 20-week program engages 150 children between the ages of 8 and 11 from the Saint Louis Public Schools in both physical activity and education. The physical activity involves 6–8 hours of soccer practices, soccer games, and community service projects a week. Participants also learn about nutrition and healthy eating habits. The program also serves to enrich the vocabulary and literacy skills of children who may otherwise be struggling in school. BMI is measured before and after each 10-week session and charted to monitor progress [2].

6.1.3 Healthy Kids, Healthy Communities (Northern Mississippi)

It is certainly no secret that obesity rates are much higher in areas with high poverty rates and/or high populations of minority ethnic groups. The Robert Wood Foundation has set aside tens of millions of dollars to fund grants in the Healthy Kids, Healthy Communities project. Four-year grants up to $360,000 have been given to 50 communities across the country to support their established local efforts to give families "access to affordable healthy foods and opportunities for physical activities." Communities targeted include those with high crime, poverty, and traffic levels and also food deserts. The Healthy Kids, Healthy Communities program hopes to reverse the rise of childhood obesity by 2015 [3, 28].

One community recipient of the grant are the Counties of Desoto, Marshall, and Tate in Mississippi. Mississippi unfortunately has the distinction of being consistently among the "fattest states" in the USA. Tate County alone has an adult obesity rate of 74%. The Community Foundation of Northwest Mississippi is "spear-heading" the initiative. The main goal of this foundation is to get the people of the community to involve in more outdoor physical activities through developing areas around the Coldwater River watershed. The group hopes to develop parks, biking trails, and community gardens to get more people physically active and encourage healthier food choices by teaching gardening skills [4].

6.1.4   Healthy Schools Initiative (South Carolina)

South Carolina, often known for its high stroke rates, has aimed at childhood obesity by addressing all aspects of the child beyond the physical. Funded by the Centers for Disease Control (CDC), the South Carolina Healthy Schools Initiative has been working on "improving the culture and climate of schools and the academic achievement of children and adolescents by promoting strategies, programs, and services that encourage positive healthful behaviors." The CDC developed eight components of a healthy school which comprise the backbone of this initiative. The proposed components of a healthy school include: (1) providing and healthy school environment for students; (2) providing health education in school; (3) encouraging physical education; (4) ensuring proper nutrition when it comes to school meals; (5) improving family and community involvement in the student's education; (6) providing appropriate health services and clean environments for children; (7) providing social and mental health services as needed; and (8) promoting the health of staff members involved in student contact. South Carolina hopes that applying these measures can improve the long-term health of South Carolina both physically and mentally [5].

6.1.5   Healthy 100 Kids (Florida)

The Florida Hospital for Children opened a center dedicated to tackling childhood obesity. Being called Healthy 100 Kids, the center approaches childhood obesity from four areas. The first is a pediatrician who is specialized in obesity-related illnesses such as sleep apnea, hypertension, and type II diabetes mellitus. The second is a child psychologist who deals with issues of depression and other mental health issues which many obese children suffer with. They also counsel families on their dynamics and parenting skills which may contribute to the child's obesity. The third is a registered dietitian who aides families in selecting and preparing better food choices. The fourth is an exercise physiologist who helps children and families with routines and activities to help improve and increase physical activity. All specialists will be using evidence-based therapies and treatments along with conducting studies on new techniques to tackle childhood obesity [6].

6.1.6   Follow Me! Healthy Parents, Healthy Kids
(Columbus, Ohio)

Follow Me! Healthy Parents, Healthy Kids is a program comprised of volunteers whose primary goal is to work with parents to become role models for their children when it comes to healthy lifestyles [29]. One aspect of the program is the establishment of a summer activity series. There are free activities once a week for 2 hours available in a local park including gardening tips, fitness activities led by local professional fitness instructors and college athletes, and introduction of new healthy treats for the children. Parents are educated through various events and are provided with online resources which help push them to "lead by example." The organizers hope that if this program is successful, it can expand to cities across Ohio and beyond [7].

6.1.7   CATCH Program (Texas)

The Texas elementary school system has been participating in one of the largest studies in North America looking at ways to combat childhood obesity. *A Coordinated Approach to Child Health Program* (the CATCH program) offers a proven model for school systems looking to turn the tide against childhood obesity [30]. This program includes 2,500 elementary and middle schools across Texas and 7,000 other schools nationwide. Those schools have adopted guidelines encompassing four major components of student health. The first component is a classroom curriculum which teaches children about healthy food choices, smoking avoidance, and the importance of daily physical activity. The second component is physical education. When many school districts are cutting back on physical education, the CATCH program requires at least 30 min of physical activity a day by "blending fun and fitness." The third component is the requirement that all school cafeterias prepare their meals using "Eat Smart Guidelines," with less fat and sodium content in their meals. Family Fun Nights comprise the final component and invite families to come out and develop healthy eating lifestyles. The School Physical Activity and Nutrition (SPAN) population-based surveillance study showed that obesity prevalence rates in nine counties leveled off with significant reductions in obesity rates, most notably highest risk areas mostly located along the Texas–Mexico border [8–10].

6.1.8   Just For Kids! Obesity Workbook
(San Francisco, California)

The Just For Kids! Program is a workbook that has been developed for educators, individual families, physicians, and community activists to help combat childhood obesity. This 5–10-week program is aimed at helping children make changes in their diet, exercise, and communication skills. The program was developed by medical school faculty at The University of California at San Francisco who adopted it from SHAPEDOWN. It employs games, hands-on projects, and age-appropriate storylines that teach children about healthy foods, the importance of exercise, and also helps kids build up their self-esteem which can plague obese children.

In 1992, the developers designed a study to test the efficacy in 8–10-year-old children. Within four classrooms, 120 students were divided into two groups, control vs. intervention. Students were evaluated over a 10-week period. The investigators were looking for improvements in physical fitness, nutritional knowledge, BMI, skinfold thickness, blood pressure, and resting heart rate. Ninety-nine percent of the study participants self-identified as ethnic minorities. Data were collected before and after the intervention. Over the 10-week period, the investigators observed statistically significant differences in triceps skinfold thickness, blood pressure, and nutritional knowledge. BMI and physical fitness did not improve between the two groups. Though short in duration, this program holds promise to improve pediatric health [11].

6.1.9   PE4life

Physical education is being scaled down or even eliminated in many communities but one program is helping schools, businesses, and communities transform physical education with new and innovative ideas. PE4life is a program that has been used by 40 states and nine countries. This program includes seven core principles in physical education. The first principle is to make sure that all students are able to participate in the activity. The second principle is to incorporate a variety of activities so that students can find something that makes them happy and more willing to participate. The third principle is to make sure that the activities are safe. The fourth principle is to make sure that students are individually assessed in terms of their physical fitness and nutritional knowledge throughout the course of the program. The fifth principle is to use technology such as pedometers and calorie counters to give students the ability to monitor both their activity levels and caloric intake. The sixth core principle is to take "gym class" out of the gymnasium and into their respective communities and beyond. The last core principle is that physical education should be offered at least once a day. Nutrition is also addressed by equipping educators with tools to teach students about calories, calorie counting, and calorie balance [12].

6.1.10   All 4 Kids: Happy, Happy, Active, Fit program
             (Las Vegas, Nevada)

Habits are often formed from an early age and one program aims at attacking childhood obesity using that fact. *All 4 Kids* was created for 3–5-year-old children. Started in 2007, it uses dance, games, books, art, and food tasting to teach about healthy foods such as fruits and vegetables, and the importance of exercise. Program administrators go to daycares and preschools around the City of Las Vegas, and targets low-income and/or minority children. The program is three days a week over an 8-week period and has shown some promise in helping to increase the percentage of children who eat more fruits and vegetables. Recently, they received a million dollar grant from the National Institute of Food and Agriculture to study the effectiveness of their intervention and expand the program to other states [13, 14].

6.1.11   Way to Optimal Weight: WOW (Bangor, Maine)

WOW is a weight loss program aimed at children between the ages of 4 and 19 who have BMIs greater than the 85th percentile for age. The program uses a multidisciplinary approach involving a pediatrician, nurse, dietitian, psychologist, and personal trainer. This team works with patients and their families on the issues surrounding their problem with obesity, and develops ways to improve. Thirty minutes of physical activity is also included with the sessions [15].

6.1.12   On The Move (New Orleans, Louisiana)

The Elmwood Fitness Center in the greater New Orleans area has come up with an inventive program to help combat childhood obesity. *On The Move* serves children aged 9–13, teaches them the importance of exercise with group, noncompetitive fitness classes, and seeks to improve their nutrition by introducing them to new and exciting healthy foods. They have also invested in a mobile unit that goes out into the community to help educate children about the importance of exercise and provides demonstrations from a chef who introduces recipes that are healthy and tasty [16, 17].

6.1.13   Pediatric Fitness Clinic (University
             of Wisconsin School of Medicine)

The University of Wisconsin has started its Pediatric Fitness Clinic to help children develop healthy eating habits and increase physical activity. The team includes physicians, exercise physiologists, and registered dietitians. Children undergo individual assessments and a "health and fitness action plan" is developed for families to follow [18, 19].

6.1.14   Bienestar Health Program (San Antonio, Texas)

The Beinestar Health Program is aimed primarily at children of Hispanic descent but can certainly be used in any culture. *Bien estar* is Spanish for "being well." Plans with thirteen lessons address healthy living, diabetes, the food pyramid, and vitamins among other health topics. Students receive a workbook. The program begins with a pretest to assess baseline knowledge of general health. Each lesson is meant to be interactive as the teacher asks a series of questions and injects teaching points according to the lesson plan. Students then complete a worksheet on that specific topic to solidify the day's lesson. At the end of the series, a posttest is administered to evaluate comprehension and retention. The program is aimed for 4th grade level and above, providing a fantastic workbook that can be incorporated in any curriculum [20, 21].

6.2   INTERNATIONAL PROGRAMS

6.2.1   England

The UK's Faculty of Public Health created *Healthy Weight, Healthy Lives: A Toolkit for Developing Local Strategies* [22]. This resource provides a framework for communities to identify the root causes of childhood obesity and to coordinate resources to address these problems. Written for local public health commissioners, it provides information about improving daily exercise in children, promotion of breastfeeding and healthy food choices both at home and at school. *Cycling England* has worked toward getting more children biking safely to school, and the *Bike It* program (sponsored by Sustrans) works directly with local schools and trains cycling ambassadors to talk to parents, teachers, administrators, and children at schools about travel planning and safety [23, 24]. Finally, the Bikeability project works with local children to teach them how to safely handle a bike at three levels. The first level teaches children to properly control a bike. The second level teaches children how to control a bike in traffic. The third level targets secondary school students to control their bicycles in heavy traffic. These programs also encourage children to ride their bicycles to school.

6.2.2   Australia

The Eat Well Be Active Community Partnerships Program (CPP) is a joint initiative between the Department of Local Government, Sport and Recreation, Queensland Health and the Department of Recreation, Queensland Health and the Department of Education, Training and the Arts, which provides funding to support development and implementation of community-based health programs in Queensland [31]. These grants are available to any local government, tribal council, school or not-for-profit institution. Eligible projects include those that will improve accessibility to gyms and other places of physical exercise, assisting local governments in improving opportunities for physical activity and healthy food choices, and helping child-care institutions to develop physical activity and education programs for young children.

One recipient of the CPP funding was a kindergarten that organized a family game day where children would move from one station to another and perform physical tasks. These game-a-thons were held on weekends in order to involve more family members and siblings. As the children complete each activity, they receive a reward such as a badge or a sticker. The games have also been used as fundraisers where children earn money for each "lap" around the games. These activities encourage parents to be active with their children and also allow parents and teachers to monitor the children's physical progress [22].

6.2.3 France

EPODE (Together, Let's Prevent Childhood Obesity) is a methodology to prevent childhood obesity by involving multiple stakeholders in a partnership to prevent childhood obesity [25, 26]. Since starting at two towns in 1992, the program has expanded to include 167 cities across France. Each town is provided with a professional coach that works with local teams to implement programs that will improve the health of children. Private sponsors finance this coaching and also partially finance some of the initiatives, including flyers in local grocery stores about healthy eating, creation of bicycle and walking trails, and visits to farms and food factories. In the two pilot towns, there was no increase in obesity between 1992 and 2000, whereas in surrounding towns, the rate of obese children doubled. The key to the success of these programs is that they involve multiple levels of the child's environment – from the child's own family, school, local government(s), and private sponsors. Although the involvement of private corporations has been criticized, the EPODE model has been adopted by the EPODE European Network (EEN) and has been used as a model to create programs in other European cities. An example of one of the community-based initiatives developed in an EPODE city is the Tastes of the Season program, which allows children to taste new foods and provides them with recipe booklets to take home. Healthy recipe ideas are also available in childcare centers, schools, and grocery stores.

6.2.4 China

Li *et al.* recently examined the effect of a comprehensive school-based intervention strategy on childhood obesity [27]. The children received nutritional education with a cartoon pamphlet and six special lectures for the children and two lectures for parents. Children also participated in the Happy 10 program. This classroom-based physical activity intervention encourages children to engage in exercise twice daily for 10 min/episode, or once daily for 20 min at a time. Teachers, school cafeteria managers, and school administrators also participated in nutrition and health classes. To measure the effectiveness of this program, each child's height, weight, waist circumference, body composition, and pertinent laboratory measures will be compared to those at schools receiving only physical activity interventions, only nutritional interventions, or no interventions. Although the full results of this study are not yet available, the study design shows how community-based obesity interventions are being examined critically to validate or refute efficacy.

REFERENCES

1. http://www.mrhsd.org/gardens/index.html
2. http://www.americascores.org/#/stlouis/program/2280
3. http://www.healthykidshealthycommunities.org/about
4. http://www.healthykidshealthycommunities.org/communities/desoto-marshall-and-tate-counties-ms
5. http://www.scdhec.gov/health/chcdp/schools/healthy_schools.htm
6. http://articles.orlandosentinel.com/2010-06-23/health/os-children-obesity-20100623_1_childhood-obesity-obese-children-overweight
7. http://healthy100kids.org/
8. http://www.chronicdisease.org/files/public/SSS_TX_obesity_CATCH_WEB.pdf
9. http://www.sph.uth.tmc.edu/catch/PDF_Files/CATCH%20National%20Fact%20Sheet_2-8-10.pdf
10. Lupeker RV *et al.* (1996) Outcome of a field trial to improve children's dietary patterns and physical activity: The child and adolescent trial for cardiovascular health (CATCH). JAMA 275:768–777
11. http://www.just-for-kids.org/JFK_Links_Research.html
12. http://www.pe4life.org/
13. http://www.unr.edu/news/templates/details.aspx?articleid=5424&zoneid=33
14. http://www.emmc.org/pediatric_services.aspx?id=58902
15. http://www.bangordailynews.com/detail/140369.html
16. http://www.elmwoodfitness.com/club/scripts/library/view_document.asp?GRP=0&NS=KIDS&APP=80&DN=onthemove
17. http://www.ochsner.org/community/programs_childhood_health_and_education/
18. http://www.uwhealth.org/about-uwhealth/teen-fitness-program-targets-childhood-obesity-epidemic/12470
19. http://www.uwhealth.org/pediatric-obesity/pediatric-fitness/11338
20. http://www.sahrc.org/

21. http://volunteer.truist.com/unitedwaysatx/org/304979.html
22. Healthy Weight, Healthy Lives: A Toolkit for Developing Local Strategies. http://www.fphm.org.uk/resources/AtoZ/toolkit_obesity/2008/full_obesity_toolkit.pdf
23. Bike it Guide for Parents and Teachers. http://www.sustrans.org.uk/assets/files/Bike%20It/Sustrans_Bike_It_an%20intro_081014.pdf
24. Bike it Project Review 2010. http://www.sustrans.org.uk/assets/files/Bike%20It/Bike%20It%20Review%202010.pdf
25. EPODE European Network. http://www.epode-european-network.com/
26. Westley H (2007) Thin living. BMJ 335:1236–1237
27. Li Y, Hu X, Zhang Q, Liu A, Fang H, Hao L, Duan Y, Xu H, Shang X, Ma J, Xu G, Du L, Li Y, Guo H, Li T, Ma G, The nutrition-based comprehensive intervention study on childhood obesity in China (NISCOC): a randomised cluster controlled trial. BMC Public Health 2010;10:229–236
28. http://www.healthykidshealthycommunities.org/sites/default/files/HKHC_Release.pdf
29. http://followmekids.org/home2.html
30. Nader P et al. (1999) Three-year maintenance of improved diet and physical activity: The CATCH cohort. Arch Pediatr Adolesc Med 153:695–704
31. Eat Well Be Active Community Partnerships. http://www.qld.gov.au/community-partnerships/

7

Physical Activity Approaches to Pediatric Weight Management

Douglas L. Hill, Brian H. Wrotniak, and Kathryn H. Schmitz

Key Points

- Interventions to increase physical activity and to maintain healthier lifestyles are essential strategies to reduce and prevent both pediatric obesity and T2DM.
- Supervised physical activity, family based behavioral interventions, environmental/policy changes, and reinforcement interventions are effective ways to increase physical activity in the short term.
- Sustained multi-level approaches will be required to achieve long-term changes in physical activity and pediatric obesity.

Keywords: Physical Activity, Prevention, Pediatric Obesity

7.1 INTRODUCTION

This chapter reviews interventions designed to increase physical activity and reduce sedentary behavior among children in order to prevent or treat pediatric obesity. Interventions included range from individual approaches to upstream approaches that focus on changing environmental and policy factors that may influence pediatric obesity. We have organized the chapter under the topics of prevention and treatment with subtopics of school, family, community, and policy/environment. We conclude with a discussion of factors associated with successful interventions, emerging areas of research, and the importance of sustained, multilevel approaches to addressing

From: *Nutrition and Health: Management of Pediatric Obesity and Diabetes*,
Edited by: R.J. Ferry, Jr., DOI 10.1007/978-1-60327-256-8_7,
© Springer Science+Business Media, LLC 2011

pediatric obesity. This chapter updates previous reviews of the literature [1–5] by focusing on interventions published in the last 10 years.

In general, intensive family-based interventions have proven effective to treat obesity by changing health behaviors. The primary behaviors include healthy eating, physical activity, and sedentary behavior [5]. Some benefits for physical activity interventions have been reported; however, the interventions were limited mostly to the context of school-based physical education classes, and the amount of activity varied widely [1]. Benefits of school-based prevention programs with physical activity have been mixed [2]. Stronger evidence exists for the benefits of physical activity as part of an intervention to treat obesity [2]. One reviewer found insufficient evidence to endorse or recommend against behavioral counseling in primary care settings to promote physical activity [6]. Few data exist on maintenance of physical activity after the end of interventions for both children and adults [4], and no current reviews identify environmental or policy-based interventions to increase physical activity.

7.2 PHYSICAL ACTIVITY AND RECOMMENDATIONS

Physical activity is defined as bodily movement produced by the contraction of skeletal muscle that increases energy expenditure above the basal level [7]. Physical activity is associated with numerous health benefits for children, including reduced adiposity [8], improved fitness levels [9], lower blood pressure [10], reduced risk of insulin resistance [11–13], increased bone strength [14], enhanced motor proficiency [15, 16], and improved psychosocial outcomes – such as mood [17], body image satisfaction [18], self-efficacy, and self-esteem [17, 19]. In contrast, sedentary lifestyles and behaviors (like television watching and playing video games) are associated with being overweight [20–22] as well as diverse, negative health outcomes, including hypertension [23], decreased aerobic endurance [9], and poorer muscle strength [9]. Watching television [24], using computers [25], and playing video games [25] may also contribute to children getting less sleep, which may cause metabolic and endocrine changes that increase the risk of weight gain [26–28].

The current *Dietary Guidelines for Americans* recommends that children get at least 60 min of physical activity daily and limit inactive forms of play, such as television watching and computer games [29]. Healthy People 2010 recommends that adolescents engage in vigorous physical activity that promotes cardiorespiratory fitness on 3 days or more per week and for 20 min per occasion or more [30]. Many children do not meet these physical activity recommendations [7, 31], and youth become less physically active as they age [7, 31, 32]. Current health statistics on physical activity indicate that physical activity remains relatively unchanged in recent years [33], even though computer and video game use increased between 2005 and 2007 [34].

Barlow and Dietz [35] report recommendations for evaluation, treatment, and prevention of childhood obesity, including the role of physical activity in weight management. Clinicians should obtain a history of physical activity and sedentary behavior, identify deterrents to physical activity, identify opportunities for increasing physical activity and reducing sedentary behavior, and find out which caregivers are available to support physical activity of the child. Clinicians should also work with the family to help them learn to monitor behavior, set goals to change behavior, and create a supportive family environment for the child to be more active [35, 36].

7.3   LITERATURE SEARCH

To review recent literature and discuss its clinical and research implications, we searched PubMed using the terms "obesity" and "physical activity." The search was limited to English-language articles published during 1998–2008 (since pediatric obesity was not generally recognized or closely studied prior to that time), that studied children and adolescents (up to age 18 years), and that were either clinical trials or randomized control trials. The initial search yielded 235 articles. Articles were excluded if: 1) they dealt primarily with an older population (*e.g.*, the majority of participants were older than 18); 2) they addressed issues for specific diseases or conditions (*e.g.*, Prader Willi syndrome); 3) they presented observational data only; 4) no intervention was tested; or 5) there was no control condition for the intervention. Some authors cited other relevant articles that did not appear in the original PubMed search. These articles were also included in the final list.

Sixty-two articles met inclusion criteria. They were classified as either interventions to *prevent* pediatric overweight and obesity, or interventions to *treat* pediatric overweight and obesity. Studies were then subclassified based on the setting and whether the unit of analysis was individual or group. Based on this classification scheme, the search netted seven types of studies: school-based prevention (26 interventions), family-based prevention (6 interventions), community- or clinic-based prevention (2 interventions), environmental- or policy-based prevention (2 interventions), school-based treatment (6 interventions), family-based treatment (12 interventions), community- or clinic-based treatment (8 interventions). Although we identified two interventions based on environment or policy to prevent obesity, there were no treatments that met criteria as environmental- or policy-based.

Some interventions had elements of multiple categories (*e.g.*, a school-based intervention with a family component for parents). We classified such studies based upon which components of the intervention involved the majority of the contact with participants, were emphasized by the authors, and were covered in greatest detail in the text. For example, a prevention intervention consisting of regular meetings with students in a school setting (and a small number of meetings with parents and other family members) was classified as a school-based prevention intervention. Many interventions aimed to increase physical activity and reduce sedentary behavior as two strategies within a larger, multi-component intervention attempting to change eating habits and to increase other healthy behaviors. In the summary tables presented at the end of this chapter, we indicate components of all the larger, combined interventions.

The intensity of the overall interventions varied widely. Some interventions required just a few brief meetings, while others lasted for years. The nature of the physical activity interventions also varied, with many simply encouraging participants to be more active and others consisting of regular and supervised exercise sessions. Another subset of interventions focused on reducing sedentary behavior or replacing sedentary behavior with physical activity.

Interventions were presented in classrooms, behavioral groups, physical education classes, after school programs, by phone, over the internet, and through open and closed loop reinforcement systems. The tables summarize the major outcomes: physical activity and sedentary behavior (self-report or accelerometry data), anthropometry (body mass index or BMI, BMI Z scores, body fat percentage, skin fold thickness, or waist circumference), and fitness (VO_2 test, performance on physical tasks). Studies without specific anthropometric outcomes were included, because the association has been established between increased physical activity or decreased sedentary behavior and improved health outcomes, independently of weight loss and changes in BMI [7, 37]. In some cases, ongoing studies with promising pilot data are included, because they highlight potential new innovative ways for approaching physical activity strategies for weight control.

7.4   OBESITY PREVENTION PROGRAMS

Perhaps the most promising way to address the childhood obesity epidemic is through primary prevention strategies aimed at establishing healthy physical activity and nutrition behaviors prior to excess weight gain. Changing behaviors related to obesity in childhood potentially has a large return, as a lifetime of obesity-related health problems could be prevented or attenuated. Physical activity may be especially appropriate in prevention programs for two reasons. First, physical activity is more helpful for maintaining weight loss than generating weight loss. Second, once children gain weight, it becomes more difficult for them to become or to stay physically active.

7.4.1   School-Based Prevention Programs

The majority of interventions identified by our search were school-based programs to prevent obesity (Table 7.1). School-based interventions may be an effective way to reach at once a large number of children to improve their behaviors. However, school interventions can be difficult to implement as they require the cooperation of administrators and staff across multiple schools. In some cases, officials resisted random assignments of their schools to different conditions in a research study [38].

Some interventions in this category included family components (involving parents), but the central intervention took place in the schools. Investigators worked in sites ranging from nursery schools to high schools, yet the majority of these interventions occurred in elementary or middle schools. Most interventions were traditional classroom interventions integrated into the curriculum that presented students with information about healthy eating and encouraged them to be more physically active. A few interventions took the form of clubs that met during lunch or after school [39, 40]. Others took the form of an enhanced physical education program [41, 42]. Half these interventions (13 total) included some form of supervised physical activity. Several interventions focused exclusively on increasing physical activity, but fewer focused on reducing sedentary behavior. Several investigators targeted specific ethnic populations or females only. One study [43] incorporated treatment programs for overweight and obese students, in addition to obesity prevention strategies for youth with healthy weight.

Results of these studies demonstrate the difficulty of achieving measurable differences in physical activity and anthropometric outcomes, even with an intensive, ongoing prevention intervention. Interventions which had supervised exercise tended to be more successful in increasing physical activity (compared with less structured designs). However, the long-term effects of successful, supervised activity were limited if children returned to old habits after the intervention stopped [44]. Combined interventions that included healthy eating were sometimes effective in preventing weight gain, even if physical activity was not increased. Interventions that encouraged participants to increase physical activity alone were less likely to show measurable effects compared with a comprehensive approach that included dietary modification. One interesting comprehensive program was the Healthy Buddies program [45], in which older children were taught about healthy eating and physical activity so they could mentor a younger student. The 4th and 5th graders of the prevention arm had a significantly smaller BMI increase, compared to unmentored controls.

7.4.2 Family-Based Prevention Programs

Few family-based prevention studies exist. Of six interventions (Table 7.2), four were pilot studies of interventions with specific ethnic

Table 7.1
School-based Interventions to Prevent Obesity

Author (year)	Description of participants, sample size, setting	Intervention components	Combined intervention	Supervised PA	Length of intervention/ follow up	Primary outcome variables	Outcomes/findings	Results summary	Ref.
Robinson et al. 1999	San Jose, California 192 3rd and 4th grade students	18 lesson classroom intervention to reduce television, videotape, and videogame use	No	No	6 months	BMI TST WC Waist to hip ratio Hours per week of television Videogames	Adjusted difference between intervention and control (95% CI) -0.45 kg/m² (-0.73 to -0.17), **P = 0.002** -1.47 mm (-2.41 to -0.54), **P = 0.002** -2.30 cm (-3.27 to -1.33), **P < 0.001** -0.02 (-0.03 to -0.01), **P < 0.001** -5.53 (-8.64 to -2.42), **P < 0.001** -2.54 (-4.48 to -0.60), **P = 0.01**	Intervention was effective in reducing SB and found differences in BMI and adiposity between intervention and control	[92]
Sahota et al. 2001	Leeds 634 children ages 7-11 years 10 primary schools, randomized	APPLES Teacher training, modification of school meals. School action plans targeting the curriculum, physical education, food shops, and playground activities	Yes	No	11 month intervention/ 12 month follow up	BMI PA (self-report) SB (self-report)	Mean Difference between intervention and control (CI) 0 (-0.1 to 0.1) **NS** -0.2 (-0.4 to 0.1) **NS** 0.0 (-0.1 to 0.1) **NS**	No significant differences	[93]
Caballero et al. 2003	1,704 Native American students followed from second to fifth grade	Pathways: School based intervention with Native American population to improve nutrition and increase PA. Intervention included classroom, food service, physical education, and family environmental components	Yes	Yes	3 years	%Body fat BMI PA accelerometer for 1 day PA self-report	Intervention: 40.3) Control: 40.0 **P = 0.67** Intervention: 22.0 Control: 22.2 **P = 0.30** Intervention: 267.22 Control: 246.70, **P = 0.31** Intervention: 0.27 Control: 0.24, **P = 0.001**	Significant increase in self-reported PA	[79]

Study	Sample / Setting	Intervention			Length of intervention	Duration of exercise / Measure	Difference between intervention and control	Outcome	Ref
Frenn et al. 2003	Central City Middle School in US 117 students (6th–8th grade) Quasiexperimental Random assignment to "academic families"	Health Promotion/Trans theoretical Model intervention Four 45 min classroom interventions about fat, food choices, and exercise	Yes	No	Length of intervention not stated. No separate follow-up.	Duration of exercise (self-report: Child and Adolescent Activity Log)	Difference between Intervention and Control t = 2.02; df = 99, $P = 0.046$	Significant increase in self-reported duration of PA	[94]
Frenn et al. 2003	341 students (ages 12–15) from two urban low income middle schools	Internet and video version of a Health Promotion/ Transtheoretical model based intervention to improve diet, reduce fat intake, and increase PA	Yes	No	5–6 sessions (one school had peer led gym lab)	PA (Child and Adolescent Activity Log)	Significant group effect ($P = 0.002$)	Those with peer led gym lab reported higher PA.	[95]
Neumark-Sztainer et al. 2003	Twin Cities, Minnesota 201 high school girls (grades 9–12) with low PA levels 6 schools Randomly assigned by school	New Moves: multicomponent, girls only high school PE class 4 PE sessions per week, 1 social support/nutrition session every other week	Yes	Yes	16 weeks (one semester)/ 8 month follow up	BMI (kg/m²) PA (hours/week) SB (hours/week)	Intervention: 26.97 Control: 26.38, **P = 0.96** Intervention: 6.31, Control: 6.24, **P = 0.93** Intervention: 15.34, Control: 15.39, **P = 0.98**	No significant differences	[41]
Story et al. 2003	Minnesota 54 African-American girls (ages 8–10 years) from three schools	Minnesota GEMS Pilot Girlfriends for KEEPS (Keys to Eating, Exercise, Playing, and Sharing). Intervention designed to improve healthy eating and increase PA. Club meeting format 1 hour, twice a week after school. Included family component (handouts, phone calls, and two family nights)	Yes	No	12 weeks	BMI (kg/m²) WC (cm) PA (accelerometer counts/min)	Mean (SE) Intervention 21.7 (0.2) Control 21.5 (0.2), **P = 0 0.5** Intervention 72.0 (0.5) Control 70.7 (0.5), **P = 0.08** Intervention 503.7 (26.9) Control 446.2 (24.6), **P = 0.12**	No significant differences *Feasibility study with insufficient power to detect differences*	[39]

(continued)

Table 7.1
(continued)

Author (year)	Description of participants, sample size, setting	Intervention components	Combined intervention	Supervised PA	Length of intervention/ follow up	Primary outcome variables	Outcomes/findings	Results summary	Ref.
Warren et al. 2003	Oxford, England 213 children ages 5–7 years 3 primary schools Randomly assigned	Control (Be Smart), Nutrition (Eat Smart), Physical Activity (Play Smart), and Combined Nutrition and Physical Activity (Eat Smart Play Smart. Conducted in lunchtime clubs	Yes	No	20 weeks	Final (20 weeks) % overweight % obese % Running at morning break % Running at Lunch Break	BS: 7; ES: 14; PS: 11; ESPS: 2; NS BS: 0; ES: 7; PS: 2; ESPS: 2: NS BS: 90; ES: 88; PS: 85; ESPS: 91; NS BS: 66; ES: 54; PS: 72; ESPS: 68; NS	No significant differences	[40]
Kain et al. 2004	3 cities in Chile: Santiago, Curico, and Casablanca 5 primary schools 3,086 students (grades 1–8) Not randomly assigned	Nutrition education and Physical Activity intervention (90 minutes additional per week, behavioral PA program, active recess)	Yes	Yes	6 month intervention	Boys BMI (kg/m^2) BMIz TST (mm) WC 20 meter shuttle run test stages completed (SRT) Girls BMI (kg/m^2) BMIz TST (mm)	Change in Mean from Baseline to 6 month : Intervention: 0.0 Control: +0.3, **P < 0.001** Intervention: -0.12 Control: -0.02, **P < 0.001** Intervention: -0.5 Control: -0.8, **P = 0.14** Intervention: -0.9 Control: +0.9, **P < 0.001** Intervention: +1.04 Control: 0.0, **P < 0.001** Intervention: +0.3 Control: +0.2, **P = 0.6** Intervention: -0.04 Control: -.07, **P = 0.49** Intervention: +0.5 Control: +0.9, **P = 0.14**	Significant effect on adiposity and fitness for boys Significant effect only on fitness for girls *Not randomly assigned and initial rates of obesity higher in intervention condition. (School system required that schools with higher obesity rates be in intervention condition)*	[38]

Study	Description			Duration	Measures	Results	Outcomes	Ref
Simon et al. 2004	Bas-Rhin, France 954 adolescents (aged 11–12) Note: unusual outcome measures and anthro only at baseline. Intervention centered on adolescents physical activity and sedentary behavior (ICAFS) Multilevel Physical activity intervention to change knowledge, attitudes, social support, and environmental conditions	No	No	6 month	WC; 20 meter shuttle run test stages completed (SRT); **Girls** % participating in Leisure Organized PA (LOPA); % High SB; **Boys** % participating in Leisure Organized PA (LOPA); % High SB	Intervention: +0.8 Control: +1.1 **P = 0.18**; Intervention: +0.7 Control: -0.3, **P < 0.001**; Intervention: 83 Control: 50, OR 3.30 (1.42-8.05) **P < 0.01**; Intervention: 17 Control: 28, OR .54 (.38-.77) **P < 0.01**; Intervention: 81 Control: 66, OR 1.73 (1.12-2.66) **P < 0.01**; Intervention: 41 Control: 48, OR .52 (.35-.76) **P < 0.01**	Significantly increased leisure physical activity and reduced sedentary behavior for both boys and girls	[96]
Fitzgibbon et al. 2005	Chicago, Illinois 300 children (mostly low-income African-American) from 12 Head Start preschool programs. Hip Hop to Health Jr (African American) Healthy eating and exercise intervention. Often included hand held puppets. Also included some materials mailed to parents.	Yes	Yes	14 week (40 minutes, 3 times weekly) 2 year follow up	BMI change from baseline; PA (% ≥ 7 X week, parent report); TV (hours per day, parent report)	Intervention: 0.48 (0.14) Control: 1.14, **P < 0.008**; Intervention 39.2 (5.4) Control: 38.4, **NS**; Intervention 2.9 (0.2) Control: 3.1 (0.2), **NS**	Significant change in BMI, but not in PA or diet. May be because of insensitive self-report measures	[77]
Frenn et al. 2005	Midwestern urban public school 137 seventh graders from six classes. Computer/internet version of a Health Promotion/Transtheoretical model based intervention to improve diet, reduce fat intake, and increase PA. Included tailored feedback	Yes	No	8 forty minute sessions	PA (Child and Adolescent Activity Log)	Participants who completed more than half of intervention sessions: increase of 22 minutes. Control: decrease of 46 minutes **P = 0.05**	Significant increase in PA for those who completed more than half of sessions	[97]

(continued)

Table 7.1
(continued)

Author (year)	Description of participants, sample size, setting	Intervention components	Combined intervention	Supervised PA	Length of intervention/ follow up	Primary outcome variables	Outcomes/findings	Results summary	Ref.
Pate et al. 2005	South Carolina 2,744 high school girls, 24 high schools, group randomized	LEAP Comprehensive physical activity program to increase PA among girls	No	Yes	1 school year	% reporting 1 hour of moderate to vigorous PA per day; % reporting 30 min of vigorous activity; % ≥85th percentile BMI; % ≥95th percentile BMI	Adjusted means (SE) Intervention: 72.3 (2.2) Control: 70.3 (2.2) **P = 0.53**; Intervention: 44.5 (2.6) Control: 36.4 (2.9) **P = 0.05**; Intervention: 35.0 (0.9) Control: 33.9 (1.1) **P = 0.5**; Intervention: 17.7 (0.8) Control: 17.6 (1.0) **P = 0.97**	Significant increase in regular vigorous activity	[42]
Fitzgibbon 2006	331 students from 12 predominately Latino Head Start centers	Hip Hop to Health Jr (Latino) Healthy eating and exercise intervention. Often included hand held puppets. Also included some materials mailed to parents	Yes	No	14 week (40 minutes, 3 times weekly) 2 year follow up	BMI change from baseline; PA (% ≥ 7 X week, parent report); TV (hours per day, parent report)	Intervention: 0.46 (0.17) Control: 0.70, **P = 0.34**; Intervention: 28.6 (4.13) Control: 17.82 (4.32), **NS**; Intervention: 2.34 (0.12) Control: 2.34(0.12), **NS**	Intervention that was successful with African-American sample was not effective with Latino sample	[78]
Harrison 2006	Ireland 312 children age 10 (4th grade classes) Nine schools (five intervention, four control)	Switch Off-Get Active 10 lesson teacher led intervention to replace screen time with PA	No	No	16 weeks	PA (1 day Previous Day Physical Activity Recall); Screen time; BMI; 20 meter shuttle run test stages completed (SRT)	Adjusted Difference between Control and Intervention(CI) Increase of 0.84 (0.11-1.57) 30 min blocks in intervention, **P < 0.05**; Decrease of -0.41 (-0.93-0.12) 30 min blocks in intervention, **P = 0.13**; Decrease of -0.08 (-0.38-0.22) 30 min blocks in intervention, **P = 0.63**; Increase of 1.7 (-3.5-6.9) 30 min blocks in intervention, **P = 0.55**	Significant increase in moderate/ vigorous PA. Insignificant decrease in screen time.	[98]

Study	Sample/setting	Intervention			Duration	Outcome measures	Results	Conclusion	
Reilly et al. 2006	Glasgow, Scotland 545 children (mean age 4.2) from 36 nursery schools (preschools)	MAGIC (Movement and Activity Glasgow Intervention in Children) Enhanced physical activity program in nursery school plus home based health education to increase PA and reduce SB	No	Yes	Three 30 minute sessions a week over 24 weeks/follow up at 6 months and 12 months (BMI only)	BMI at 12 months (expressed as standard deviation score) PA (counts per minute) at 6 month (accelerometry) % monitored time sedentary at 6 months (accelerometers) % monitored time in MVPA	Intervention: 0.39 (0.98) Control: 0.41 (1.00), **P = 0.90** Intervention:732 (163) Control: 809 (209), **P = 0.18** Intervention: 69.3 (50.4 – 86.6) Control: 66.9 (45.6 – 88.7), **P = 0.08** Intervention: 2.6 (0.4 – 11.1) Control: 3.0 (0.3 – 13.0), **P = 0.05**	Insignificant increase in percentage time spend in moderate/ vigorous PA	[99]
Robbins et al. 2006	77 inactive girls grades 6–8 2 midwest middle schools Random assignment	Girls on the Move Individually tailored computerized PA program plus nurse counseling, telephone calls, and mailings	No	No	12 weeks	BMI Self-reported days of week of PA Mean (SD)	No differences Intervention 3.38 (1.44) Control: 3.4* (1.65) NS	No significant differences	[100]
Spiegel and Foulk 2006	1,013 students (4–5 grade) from 69 classes in four states (Delaware, Kansas, North Carolina, Florida). One intervention and one control class at each school	Wellness, Academics, and You Classroom intervention focused on BMI, fruit and vegetable consumption, and PA. Classroom teacher led intervention	Yes	No	1 school year	> 85th percentile BMI at post intervention Increase in PA (school day) Increase in PA (outside school)	Intervention 34.4 Control: 39.5 **P < 0.05** Intervention 43.5 min week Control: No reported NS Intervention 15.08 min week Control: No reported NS	Significant effect on BMI but no change in PA.	[101]

(continued)

Table 7.1
(continued)

Author (year)	Description of participants, sample size, setting	Intervention components	Combined intervention	Supervised PA	Length of intervention/ follow up	Primary outcome variables	Outcomes/findings	Results summary	Ref.
Eliakim et al. 2007	Oranit, Israel 101 preschool children, four preschool classes randomly assigned	Combined dietary–behavioral–physical activity intervention PA intervention was exercise training for 45 minutes a day (6 days a week)	Yes	Yes	14 weeks	PA (steps per day)	Mean ± SEM Intervention: 6,927 (± 364) Control: 5,489 (± 284), **P < 0.003**	Significant increase in PA. Significant reductions in BMI and Body fat percentage.	[102]
						BMI	Intervention: 15.7 (± 0.2) Control: 16.2 (± 0.3), **P < 0.05**		
						BMI percentile	Intervention: 50.3 (± 4.3) Control: 59.4 (± 4.5), **P < 0.05**		
						Body fat %	Intervention: 18.1 (± 0.8) Control: 18.8 (± 1.0), **P < 0.05**		
Jiang et al. 2007	Beijing, China 2,425 students from five primary schools	Children and parents involved in nutrition education and PA intervention. Extra meetings for parents of obese and overweight children Obese, overweight, and children who failed PE tests asked to run for 20 min after class Children who became overweight involved in additional intervention sessions	Yes	Yes (for overweight only)	3 years	% overweight	Intervention: 9.8% Control: 14.4%, **P < 0.01**	Significant reduction in BMI and % students overweight or obese. *Mixture of prevention and treatment*	[43]
						% obese	Intervention: 7.9% Control: 13.3%, **P < 0.01**		
						BMI	Intervention: 18.2 (± 2.6) Control: 20.3 (± 3.4), **P < 0.01**		

Study	Location, sample	Intervention			Duration / Measures	Results	Conclusions	Ref
Stock et al. 2007	British Columbia, Canada 383 school children (kindergarten – 7th grade) in two elementary schools	Healthy buddies Older students (4th–7th grade) given instruction (one 45-minute session per week) and then paired with younger student to act as teacher about nutrition, physical activity, and healthy body image (one 30-minute session per week). Each pair also had two 30-minute PA sessions per week	Yes	Yes	1 school year	BMI 9 minute fitness run	Comparison of change in intervention to control K – 3rd grade BMI change: no significant change, not reported NS Increase in 9 m n distance: Intervention: 147 meters (95% CI 102 – 192) Control: 108 (95% CI 56-160) NS 4-5th grade BMI change Intervention: 0.4 kg/m² (95% CI 0.5 – 0.9) Control: 0.7 kg/m² (95% CI 0.5 – 0.9) **P = 0.005** Increase in 9 min distance: Intervention: 75 meters (95% CI 32 – 118) Control: 81 (95% CI 43-118) NS	BMI increase was significantly smaller in intervention condition compared to the control condition for 4-5th graders	[45]
Gutin et al. 2008	Georgia, USA 18 schools randomly assigned 206 students followed from 3rd to 4th grade	Georgia FitKid Project After School PA intervention on aerobic fitness and % body fat Offered 5 days a week after school but did not have to attend all sessions	No	Yes	3 years Measured at beginning and end of each school year	Heart rate response to 3 minute exercise % body fat	Group by time interactions **(P < 0.01)** **(P < 0.01)**	Heart rates and percentage body fat were lower in intervention condition than control at end of each school year but Gains lost over summer each year	[44]

(continued)

Table 7.1
(continued)

Author (year)	Description of participants, sample size, setting	Intervention components	Combined intervention	Supervised PA	Length of intervention/ follow up	Primary outcome variables	Outcomes/findings	Results summary	Ref.
Martinez Vizcaino et al. 2008	Cuenca, Spain 1,044 children (mean age 9.4 years) 20 schools (10 control, 10 intervention) Random assignment of schools to condition	Movi program Recreational, noncompetitive PA program conducted at school after school hours	No	Yes	Three 20 minute sessions per week for 24 weeks 9 month follow up/endpoint	% overweight or obese BMI TST % Body fat	<u>Boys</u> % overweight change in intervention compared to control 0.72% (95% CI 0.39 to -1.31), **P = 0.28** BMI: change in intervention compared to control -0.07 (95% CI -0.12 to -0.27), **P = 0.45** TST change in intervention compared to control -1.14 mm (95% CI -1.71 to -0.57), **P < 0.001** % body fat change in intervention compared to control -0.37 mm (95% CI -0.86 to 0.13), **P = 0.15** <u>Girls</u> % overweight change in intervention compared to control .83% (95% CI 0.36 to 1.92), **P = 0.66** BMI: change in intervention compared to control -0.12 (95% CI -0.32 to .07), **P = 0.22** TST change in intervention compared to control -1.55 mm (95% CI -2.38 to -0.73), **P < 0.001** % body fat change in intervention compared to control -0.58% (95% CI -1.04 to -0.11) **P = 0.02**	Significant reduction in TST for boys and girls. Significant reduction in body fat % for girls	[103]

Author/Year	Sample/Design	Intervention		Duration		Outcomes	Results	Conclusions	Ref
Kipping et al. 2008	South Gloucestershire, England 679 children age 9–10 (year 5 in school) 19 primary schools Cluster randomized control trial	Active for life year 5 Pilot Study. Adaptation of Planet Health intervention Sixteen lessons on healthy eating (six lessons), physical activity (nine lessons), and reducing TV viewing (one lesson)	Yes	5 month intervention	No	Screen viewing on weekdays Screen viewing on Saturdays BMI	Mean difference (95% CI) at -11.6 (-42.7 to 19.4), **P = 0.42 NS**, -15.4 (-57.5 to 26.8), **P = 0.50 NS** Odds Ratio 0.10 (-0.27 to 0.46), **P = 0.58 NS**	No significant differences. Insignificant trend in reducing screen time	[104]
Salmon et al. 2008	Melbourne Australia 311 children (mean age 10 years, 8 months) from schools in low socio-economic areas Randomly assigned by class	Switch-Play Behavioral Modification group (BM) focusing on PA and SB, Fundamental movement skills (FMS), combined BM/FMS, Control BM and FMS both consisted of 19 lessons. Combined BM/FMS received 38 lessons (2 X 19)	No	1 school year (March to November)	Yes (FMS condition)	Overweight/ Obese BMI PA (accelerometer counts per day) TV viewing (minutes per week)	Odds Ratio (CI) BM/FMS to control 0.38 (0.16 – 0.89), **P < 0.05** Beta Coefficient (CI) BM/FMS condition to control -1.30 (-2.24 to -0.35), **P < 0.01** BM to control 47.0 (24.2 to 69.8) **P < 0.001** FMS to control 47.5 (24.6 to 70.4), **P < 0.001** BM to control 229.3 (16.6 to 442.0) **P < 0.05**	Combined intervention had significant decrease in being overweight and BMI, though no differences on PA and SB measures Separate BM and FMS conditions showed increase in PA, but BM condition also showed increase in TV.	[105]
Trost et al. 2008	Manhattan, Kansas 42 preschool children	Move and Learn Opportunities for PA integrated into preschool curriculum	No	10 weeks (first two weeks are baseline)	Yes	Classroom MVPA weeks 5-8 (accelerometers) Observed PA (OSRAP)	(P < 0.05) Intervention compared to control had significantly higher MVPA during circle time (OR 2.6, CI 2.2-3.0, **P < 0.05**). Free choice outdoor (OR 1.4, CI 1.2 – 1.8, **P < 0.05**), and Free choice indoor (OR 1.2, CI 1.1 – 1.3, **P < 0.05**)	Significantly higher classroom MVPA and VAP in weeks 5 -8. Significantly higher observed PA during specific class room activities	[106]

Physical Activity (PA), Sedentary Behavior (SB), Body Mass Index (BMI), Triceps skinfold thickness (TST), Waist circumference (WC)

Table 7.2
Family-based Interventions to Prevent Obesity

Author (year)	Description of participants, sample size, setting	Intervention components	Combined intervention	Supervised PA	Length of intervention/ follow up	Primary outcome variables	Outcomes/findings	Results summary	Ref.
Baranowski et al. 2003	Houston, Texas 35 African American girls (8 years old) and parents	Baylor GEMS pilot study Food, Fun, and Fitness Project (FFFP) 4 week summer day camp. 8 week internet intervention. Included healthy diet and PA	Yes	Yes	12 weeks	BMI (kg/m^2) WC (cm) PA (accelerometer counts/ min)	Mean (SD) Intervention: 24.6 (1.0) Control: 24.1 (1.1), **P = 0.72** Intervention: 74.1 (0.9) Control: 71.7 (1.0), **P = 0.10** Intervention: 369.9 (22.0) Control: 364.0 (25.8), P = 0.86	Feasibility study with insufficient power to detect differences. No significant differences in BMI or PA. Use of internet component low	[80]
Beech et al. 2003	Memphis, Tennessee 60 African-American girls (age 8–10 years) and parent/caregivers randomly assigned	Memphis GEMS Pilot study Social Cognitive based intervention to improve diet and increase PA 3 conditions: Child Intervention, Parent Intervention, and Control	Yes	Yes	12 weeks	BMI (kg/m^2) WC (cm) PA (accelerometer counts/ min)	Mean (SE) Child: 24.3 (0.2) Parent: 24.3 (0.2) Control: 24.7 (0.2), **P = 0.22** Child: 74.0 (0.6) Parent: 74.7 (0.6) Control: 75.0 (0.7), **P = 0.55** Child: 361.0 (17.3) Parent: 387.9 (17.2) Control: 347.3 (18.2), **P = 0.45**	Feasibility study with insufficient power to detect differences.	[81]

Study	Setting/Population	Intervention			Duration	Outcomes measured	Results	Conclusions	Ref
Robinson et al. 2003	East Palo Alto and Oakland, California 61 African-American girls (ages 8-10 years) and parents/caregivers randomly assigned	Stanford GEMS Pilot Study Dance and TV reduction Free dance classes offered 5 days a week at 3 community centers during 3 month study. Sisters Taking Action to Reduce Television (START) consisted of 5 home visits with families to reduce television use	No	Yes	12 weeks	BMI (kg/m^2) WC (cm) PA (noon–6pm) (accelerometer counts/min) TV, videotape, and videogame use (hrs/week) Total household TV use (0-4 scale)	Mean (SD) Intervention: 21.45 (5.49) Control: 22.28 (5.65), **P = 0.16** Intervention: 71.62 (14.43) Control: 72.12 (13.38), **P = 0.35** Intervention: 744.9 (239.2) Control: 750.8 (437.7), **P = 0.53** Intervention: 15.34 (11.66) Control: 21.33 (14.32), **P = 0.14** Intervention: 1.85 (0.90) Control: 2.41 (1.11), **P = 0.007**	Feasibility study with insufficient power to detect differences. Significant reduction in reported household TV use.	[82]
Harvey-Berino et al. 2003	New York State, US; Ontario and Quebec, Canada 43 Native American mothers (21–31 years old) and child (ages 14–30 months old) pairs	Obesity prevention plus parenting support (OPPS) compared to parenting support alone (PS). Intervention delivered one-on-one in homes by indigenous peer-educator. 16 OPPS sessions covered 11 parenting topics and 10 topics related to healthy eating, PA, and reducing SB	Yes	No	16 weeks (weekly sessions)	Weight for Height z scores PA (accelerometers)	Intervention change from baseline: -0.27 (± 1.1) Control change from baseline: 0.31 (±1.1 , **P = 0.06**) Intervention change from baseline: 840 (± 5,298) Control change from baseline: 1,627 (±5,776). **NS**	Marginal trend for weight for height z score	[47]

(continued)

Table 7.2 (continued)

Author (year)	Description of participants, sample size, setting	Intervention components	Combined intervention	Supervised PA	Length of intervention/ follow up	Primary outcome variables	Outcomes/findings	Results summary	Ref.
Rooney et al. 2005	Wisconsin, United States 87 families randomly assigned to one of three conditions	Growing Healthy Families Three conditions: Pedometer (P), Pedometer plus education (PE), and Control (C). Family members in P and PE groups wore pedometers and encouraged to walk 10,000 steps daily for 12 weeks. PE group also attended 6 sessions on healthy eating and exercise	Yes	No	12 weeks/9-month follow-up	Average BMI percentile at 9 months	P and PE combined: 80.9 Control: 84.3, **P = 0.33**	No significant changes in BMI *Control condition lost weight. Intervention was conducted in two waves and there were significant differences between the waves.*	[48]
Hakanen et al. 2006	Turku, Finland 1,062 infants (7 months old) assigned to intervention or control	STRIP Individualized counseling focused on healthy diet and physical activity. Counseling focused on parents initially and later on children as they became older	Yes	No	Received counseling biannually for 10 years	% overweight at age 10 for girls % overweight at age 10 boys	Intervention: 10.2% Control: 18.8%, **P = 0.04** Intervention: 11.6% Control: 12.1%, **P ≈ 1.00**	Intervention was effective in preventing overweight among girls	[49]

Physical Activity (PA), Sedentary Behavior (SB), Body Mass Index (BMI), Triceps skinfold thickness (TST), Waist circumference (WC)

groups. These studies lacked sufficient power to detect differences between the intervention and control groups, although they reported promising trends. Three were pilot studies for the Girls Health Enrichment Multi-site Studies (GEMS), a multicenter research program to develop interventions to prevent excess weight gain in adolescent African-American girls [46].

The remaining pilot study was a home visit intervention with Native American mothers and young children aged 14–30 months. These authors reported a marginal trend for lower weight-for-height Z scores in the intervention group, but no differences in physical activity [47]. Rooney and her colleagues conducted a study in which families either received pedometers, received pedometers and education, or received no treatment. The children's BMI did not differ among the groups at 3 and 9 months [48]. The lack of results for this intervention may be because the control condition lost weight, or may reflect differences between the two waves of the study. Finnish investigators assessed the effect of biannual counseling for 10 years, starting with parents and their infants. This chronic intervention effectively prevented overweight among girls, but not the boys [49].

7.4.3   Community- and Clinic-Based Interventions to Prevent Obesity

Only two prevention interventions were conducted recently in community or clinical settings (Table 7.3). Roemmich and colleagues [50] significantly increased physical activity and marginally reduced television time among 18 healthy weight children (aged 8–12 years) by having them wear an accelerometer and making television time contingent on accumulating physical activity counts. Their intervention consisting of 4 weeks of free Pilates classes for girls resulted in a small reduction in age and gender-specific BMI percentiles [51]. Unfortunately, most of this improvement was among girls with healthy baseline weights, as opposed to girls who were heavier at baseline [51].

Another potential approach is to conduct an intensive prevention intervention with children who are at risk of overweight in a primary care setting. At least one ongoing study uses this clinical approach [52, 53].

7.4.4   Policy and Environmental-Based Prevention Interventions

Two recent interventions focused on environment or policy (Table 7.4). The Wise Mind intervention [54] consisted of making changes in the school cafeteria (to offer healthier choices), giving boxes of toys to teachers

Table 7.3
Community- and Clinic-based Interventions to Prevent Obesity

Author (year)	Description of participants, sample size, setting	Intervention components	Combined intervention	Supervised PA	Length of intervention/ follow up	Primary outcome variables	Outcomes/findings	Results summary	Ref.
Roemmich et al. 2004	Buffalo, NY 18 children (ages 8–12) randomly assigned to intervention or control	Open Loop Feedback: children wore accelerometer. Accumulating PA counts gave children access to TV time	No	No	6 weeks	Minutes of PA Minutes of TV time Minutes of Sedentary behavior	Significant group × time interaction with intervention group having greater minutes of PA in weeks 3, 4, and 6, **P < 0.05** Intervention group watched less TV, but group × time interaction not significant (**P = 0.09**) Group X time interaction not significant (**P > 0.24**)	Significant increase in PA, marginal trend in reducing TV time, no effect on SB.	[50]
Jago et al. 2006	Houston, Texas 30 girls (11 years old) from two YMCA after school programs	Free 1 hour Pilates classes offered 5 days a week for 4 weeks	No	Yes	1 month	BMI change BMI percentile Waist Circumference	Intervention: -0.5 Control: -0.1, **p = 0.11** Intervention: -3.1 Control: +0.8, **p = 0.04** Intervention: -1.1 Control: +0.1, **p = 0.19**	Small change in BMI, mostly for girls who were healthy at baseline. Less change for girls with higher baseline BMIs.	[51]

Table 7.4
Interventions to Prevent Obesity Based on Policy and Environment

Author (year)	Description of participants, sample size, setting	Intervention components	Combined intervention	Supervised PA	Length of intervention/ follow up	Primary outcome variables	Outcomes/findings	Results summary	Ref.
Williamson et al. 2007	670 students (2 to 6th grade) from four schools	Wise Mind Environmental approach including changes in cafeteria, having teachers encourage brief periods of PA during class and PA during recess, giving out toys to encourage PA, and publicizing the PA program	Yes	Yes	2 academic years	Change in BMI Z scores; Weight gain prevention % body fat; Change in PA minutes (self-report); Change in SB minutes (self-report)	Not significant (values not reported) Intervention: 51% Control: 54 7%, NS; Not significant (values not reported); Intervention: 22 (± 4.8) Control: -3 (± 4.5), $p = 0.06$; Intervention: -20 (± 20.2) Control: 4 (± 20.4), $p = 0.49$	Overweight children tended to lose weight in both conditions and underweight tended to gain weight. Marginal effect for PA	[54]
Foster et al. 2008	Philadelphia, Pennsylvania 1349 students (grades 4-6) from 10 schools with ≥50% of students eligible for free or reduced price meals	School Nutrition Policy Initiative (SNPI) Multicomponent intervention including nutrition education, changes nutrition policy, social marketing, and family outreach, and a student challenge to be less sedentary, more active, and eat more fruits and vegetables	Yes	No	2 years	Overweight prevalence %; Overweight Incidence %; BMI Z score; PA (hour/week self-report); SB (hour/week self-report); TV (hour/weekday self-report)	Intervention: 14.61 Control: 20.0, OR 0.65 (0.54 – 0.79), $P < 0.001$; Intervention: 7.46 Control: 14.9, OR 0.67 (0.54 – 0.79), $P = 0.03$; Intervention: 0.80 Control: 0.76, $P = 0.80$; Intervention: 21.28 Control: 20.62, $P = 0.40$; Intervention: 104.42 Control: 108.93, $P = 0.005$; Intervention: 2.89 Control: 3.02, $P = 0.005$	Overweight prevalence and incidence was significantly lower in intervention condition. Self-reported Sedentary behavior and weekday television was also significantly lower in intervention. Physical activity was not significantly different.	[55]

(and encouraging their use to positively reinforce brief periods of physical activity during class and recess), and publicizing the physical activity program. The intervention marginally raised levels of physical activity, but the intervention and control groups showed similar BMI and similar prevention of weight gain. The School Nutrition Policy Initiative (SNPI) was a multicomponent intervention in which school personnel evaluated their current policies, made changes (in staff training, nutrition education, foods and beverages served in the school), and used social marketing and family outreach techniques to change student behaviors [55]. The intervention included a 2-1-5 challenge for students to be less sedentary (≤2 h per day of television and video games), more physically active (≥1 h per day) and eat more fruits and vegetables (≥ 5 per day). The 2-year intervention successfully reduced prevalence and incidence of overweight (in intervention schools vs. control schools) and reduced sedentary behavior. These two studies suggest that *broader interventions that address environmental and policy factors related to preventing obesity may be more effective than individual level approaches.*

7.5   OBESITY TREATMENT INTERVENTIONS

7.5.1   School-Based Treatments

All six of the recent, school-based treatments involved supervised physical activity (Table 7.5), and four of these included nutritional education. All six successfully improved BMI and other physical outcome measures by the end of the intervention. Only one study [56] included a follow-up measure after the study, and unfortunately, the investigators found that the observed differences were no longer significant at follow-up. These findings suggest that intense, supervised physical activity can help overweight children lose weight, but these effects may not endure beyond the intervention.

7.5.2   Family-Based Treatments

Family-based treatments (Table 7.6) were generally successful in helping overweight children reduce their BMI. Epstein and colleagues [57] performed much of the classic work on family-based interventions for weight loss, finding significant differences in treatment groups as long as 10 years later. However, some of Epstein's more recent studies are not included in Table 7.6, because they lack a standard negative control (group that receives no intervention). Golan's 2006 study comparing a "Parent Only" intervention

Table 7.5
School-based Treatments

Author (year)	Description of participants, sample size, setting	Intervention components	Combined intervention	Supervised PA	Length of interven-tion/follow up	Primary outcome variables	Outcomes/findings	Results summary	Ref.
Braet et al. 2003	Ghent, Belgium 76 obese (BMI ≥130%) children and adolescents aged 10 – 17 years	Residential inpatient treatment program which included a controlled diet (1500 – 1800 kcal/day), physical education (4 hours/week), behavior modification, and some parental involvement	Yes	Yes	10 months	Change in median adjusted BMI	Intervention: -48% (range -4 to -102%) Control: +6% (range -29% to +27%) Condition by time interaction, **P < 0.001**	Intervention condition had significantly lower median adjusted BMI at end of intervention. Data reported for 24 month fol-low-up, but no comparisons.	[107]
Carrel et al. 2005	Rural middle school, Wisconsin 50 overweight (BMI above 95th percentile) middle school children	Lifestyle-focused fitness oriented gym class (smaller class, less competition focused, more time being active) compared to standard gym class	No	Yes	9 months	BMI Fitness (VO$_2$max mL/kg per minute) % Body fat	Intervention: 33 ± 10 Control: 30 ± 5, **P = 0.10** Intervention: 34.5 ± 6.0 Control: 32.5 ± 6.0, **P < 0.001** Intervention: 32.6 ± 6.4 Control: 34.5 ± 5.8, **P = 0.04**	Significant reduction in body fat percentage and increase in fitness.	[108]

(continued)

Table 7.5
(continued)

Author (year)	Description of participants, sample size, setting	Intervention components	Combined intervention	Supervised PA	Length of intervention/follow up	Primary outcome variables	Outcomes/findings	Results summary	Ref.
Graf et al. 2006	Cologne, Germany 255 overweight and obese children (Grades 1–4) from seven schools (three intervention, four control). 40 participants completed intervention, 71 "nonparticipants" invited at intervention schools but did not participate. 144 participants at control schools.	STEP TWO Children participated in after school sessions to improve nutrition and increase PA. Also included 6 evening parent session and 2 family events	Yes	Yes	9-month program	BMI change BMI standard deviation score change WC change	Mean (SD) p value reported for intervention vs. control Intervention: 0.3 (1.3) Nonparticipants: 0.5 (1.3) Control: 0.7 (1.2), NS Intervention: -0.15 (0.26) Nonparticipants: -0.09 (0.31) Control: -0.05 (0.27), **p = 0.028** Intervention: -3.1 (5.7) Nonparticipants: -3.4 (4.6) Control: -4.6 (4.9), NS	Intervention condition had significantly greater decrease in BMI standard deviation score compared to control condition.	[109]

Study	Population	Intervention		Duration		Measure	Results	Conclusions	Ref
Johnston et al. 2007	Houston, Texas 80 Mexican-American children (6-7 grade) at risk for overweight or overweight (≥ 85th BMI percentile) Randomly assigned	Instructor-led intervention (ILI) or control self-help (SH). ILI condition included daily participation in school-based program which included nutrition education, PA, and behavioral modification. SH condition given self-help manual written in English called "Trim Kids"	Yes	12 weeks followed by monthly booster sessions (6 months)	Yes	Change in BMI Z score	Intervention: -0.16 Control: 0.05, **P < 0.001**	Significant reduction in BMI Z score. *Unbalanced random assignment so that more participants would be in Instructor led intervention.*	[110, 111]
Huang et al. 2007	Elementary school in south Taiwan 120 obese (BMI at 95th percentile or higher) 5th graders (age 10–13 years)	30 minute instruction twice a week on healthy foods, behavior change, regular physical exercise. PA intervention 3 times a week for 40 minutes consisting of noncompetitive aerobic activities	Yes	12 weeks	Yes	BMI kg/m^2 change Body fat % change Fitness (800 meter running time in seconds) change	Intervention: -1.1 ± 1.3 Control: 0.4 ± 1.5, **P = 0.047** Intervention: -1.6 ± 1.8 Control: 1.2 ± 2.6, **P = 0.008** Intervention: -17 ± 32 Control: 6 ± 26, **P = 0.025**	Significant changes in BMI, body fat, and fitness.	[112]

(continued)

Table 7.5
(continued)

Author (year)	Description of participants, sample size, setting	Intervention components	Combined intervention	Supervised PA	Length of intervention/follow up	Primary outcome variables	Outcomes/findings	Results summary	Ref.
Ildikó et al. 2007	Hungary 74 overweight and obese boys (7 years old). Nonrandom assignment	Intervention condition participated in 2 weekly 45 minute PE classes and three weekly 60 minute extracurricular aerobic physical activity including swimming, water games, folk dance, and soccer. Also met 10 times with child psychologist to discuss risks of being overweight.	No	Yes	35 weeks/ 11 month follow-up	BMI kg/m^2 Body fat (Sum of 5 skin folds mm) Fitness (400 m run seconds)	Mean (SD) Intervention: 25.12 (4.19) Control: 25.76 (3.97), NS Intervention: 128.25 (20.23) Control: 132.31 (25.89), NS Intervention: 130.54 (17.16) Control: 134.79 (19.02), NS	Significant differences on skin folds and fitness at end of intervention, but no longer significant at follow-up.	[56]

Physical Activity (PA), Sedentary Behavior (SB), Body Mass Index (BMI), Triceps skinfold thickness (TST), Waist circumference (WC)

Table 7.6
Family-based Treatments

Author (year)	Description of participants, sample size, setting	Intervention components	Combined intervention	Supervised PA	Length of intervention/ follow up	Primary outcome variables	Outcomes/ findings	Results summary	Ref.
Nemet et al. 2005	Kfar-Saba, Israel 46 obese children (age 6–16 years) Randomly assigned	Combined dietary physical activity intervention including 4 evening lectures, 6 meetings with a dietician, and 1 hour exercise sessions twice a week	Yes	Yes	3 months/ 1 year follow-up	BMI kg/m^2 BMI percentile (%) Body fat % (Skin fold tests) Screen time (hours per day) Physical Activity (self-report, units)	Intervention: 26.1 ± 4.7 Control: 23.6 ± 5.8, **P < 0.05** Intervention: 92.3 ± 3.0 Control: 96.1 ± 1.4, **P < 0.05** Intervention: 38.3 ± 12.5 Control: 44.4 ± 9.7, **P < 0.05** Intervention: 3.3 ± 1.2 Control: 3.4 ± 1.7, **NS** Intervention: 34.1 ± 21.1 Control: 18.9 ± 14.4, **P < 0.05**	Significant differences in BMI, BMI percentile, percentage body fat, and self-reported PA	[113]
Golan et al. 2006	Israel 32 families with obese children (age 6–11 years, BMI percentile > 85th). Random assignment	Parents exclusively vs. parents and children. Sixteen 1 hour support and education group sessions held for each condition	Yes	No	6 months	BMI Z score Overweight percentage PA (hours per day) TV viewing (hours per day)	Mean (SD) Parent only: 1.6 Parent and child: 2.0, **P < 0.05** Parent only: 37.5 (22.0) Parent and child: 46.1 (17.8), **P < 0.05** Parent only: 4.5 (1.7) Parent and child: 5.0 (1.7), **NS** Parent only: 3.0 (1.4) Parent and child: 2.9 (1.3), **NS**	Parent only intervention had lower BMI Z-scores and a lower percentage of overweight children compared to parent and child intervention. No differences in PA between conditions	[58]

(continued)

Table 7.6
(continued)

Author (year)	Description of participants, sample size, setting	Intervention components	Combined intervention	Supervised PA	Length of intervention/ follow up	Primary outcome variables	Outcomes/ findings	Results summary	Ref.
Reinehr *et al.* 2006	Datteln, Germany 240 obese (BMI > 97th percentile) children aged 6–14 years	Obeldicks program Combined physical exercise, nutrition education, and behavioral therapy for child and family	Yes	Yes	1 year program with exercise therapy once a week, 2 year follow-up	BMI BMI standard deviation score	Mean (CI) Intervention: 28.2 (27.4 – 29.0) Control: 29.0 (28.0 – 30.8), Intervention X Time $P = 0.013$ Intervention: 2.1 (2.1–2.2) Control: 2.3 (2.1–2.4), Intervention X Time $P = 0.007$	Intervention had significant effect on BMI and BMI standard deviation score at 2 years.	[114]
Gillis *et al.* 2007	Jerusalem, Israel 27 obese (BMI > 90th percentile) Ultra-orthodox Jewish children (age 7–16 years) Random assignment.	Minimal intervention. Half hour talk with physician repeated after three months, diaries, and weekly phone contacts. Ultra-orthodox children chosen because minimal exposure to TV or computers	Yes	No	6 months	BMI SDS	Intervention: 1.93 ± 0.37 Control: 2.23 ± 0.29, **P = 0.40**	Insignificant trend in reducing BMI	[115]

Golley et al. 2007	Adelaide, Australia 111 overweight children aged 6–9 years and families randomly assigned to one of three conditions	Parenting alone group (P): 6 month positive parenting program. Parenting skills and intensive lifestyle education (P+DA) positive parenting program and 7 additional nutrition and PA sessions.	Yes	No	6 month program, 12 month follow-up	BMI Z score WC Z-score	Mean Difference from baseline to 12 months P+DA: -0.24 ± 0.43, P: -0.15 ± 0.47, Control: -0.13 ± 0.57, **NS** P+DA: -0.31 ± 0.53, P: -0.17 ± 0.50 Control: -0.02 ± 0.58, **NS**	There were no significant group X time effects, but P+DA condition showed a greater reduction in BMI Z-scores. Post-hoc analyses found that boys in intervention groups had significant reductions in BMI and WC Z-scores	[116]
Kalavainen et al. 2007	Kuopio, Finland 70 obese (weight for height from 120 to 200%) children (age 7–9 years) Random assignment	Group treatment. 15 sessions separately for parents and children. Topics included healthy eating, physical activity, parenting strategy, and behavioral modification	Yes	No	6 months/ 1 year follow up	Change in weight for height % Change in BMI kg/m^2 BMI SDS (British reference)	Mean (SD) Intervention: -3.4 (7.7), Control: **1.8** (7.8), **P = 0.008** Intervention: 0.1 (1.2) Control: 0.8 (1.3), **P = 0.016** Intervention: -0.2 (0.3), Control: -0.1 (0.3), **P = 0.081**	Significant differences in weight for height percentage (Finnish standard) and BMI.	[117]

(continued)

Table 7.6
(continued)

Author (year)	Description of participants, sample size, setting	Intervention components	Combined intervention	Supervised PA	Length of intervention/ follow up	Primary outcome variables	Outcomes/ findings	Results summary	Ref.
McCallum et al. 2007	Melbourne, Australia 163 children from 29 general practices. Age 5–9 years, classified as overweight/mildly obese (excluded if BMI Z score ≥ 3.0). Random assignment.	LEAP (Live, Eat, and Play) Primary care intervention 4 consultations with physician over 12 weeks targeting nutrition, physical activity, and sedentary behavior	Yes	No	12 weeks/15 month follow-up	BMI UK BMI Z score PA (parent ratings of child activity)	Mean (SD) Intervention: 21.7 (3.1) Control: 21.2 (2.4), **P = 1.00** Intervention: 2.00 (0.68) Control: 1.92 (0.59), **P = 0.62** Intervention: 3.3 (0.5) Control: 3.2 (0.5), **P = 0.08**	Significant increase in parent ratings of child's PA. No differences in BMI.	[118]
Rodearmal et al. 2007	Denver, Colorado 192 families with at least one child (age 7–14 years) who was overweight or at risk for overweight. Random assignment.	America on the Move Families asked to walk additional 2,000 steps a day and eliminate 100 k/cal of sugar from their diet. Control condition asked to monitor PA with pedometer but not make changes	Yes	No	6 months	Change in BMI Z score Change in % body fat Change in WC % who maintained or reduced BMI % who increased BMI Steps per day	Intervention: -0.066 ± 0.166 Control: -0.039 ± 0.139, **P = 0.282** Intervention: -0.262 ± 2.633 Control: -0.072 ± 2.363, **P = 0.611** Intervention: -0.682 ± 4.385 Control: -0.219 ± 4.127, **P = 0.462** Intervention: 67 Control: 53, **P < 0.05** Intervention: 33 Control: 47, **P < 0.05** Intervention greater than control, **P < 0.001** (values not reported)	Significant differences in percentage of children who maintained BMI, percentage of children who increased BMI, and steps per.	[60]

Study	Intervention			Duration	Measures	Results	Outcome	Ref
Savoye et al. 2007	New Haven, Connecticut 209 overweight (BMI > 95th percentile) children (aged 8–16 years). 119 completed study	Yale Bright Bodies Weight Management Program Family based intervention for inner city minority children. Included nutrition, behavior modification, and exercise sessions	Yes	Yes	One year	BMI change Body fat % change	Mean (95% CI) Intervention: -1.7 (-2.3 to -2.1) Control: 1.6 (0.8 to 2.3), P < 0.001 Intervention: -4.0 (-5.2 to -2.8) Control: 2.0 (0.5 to 3.5), P < 0.001	Significant differences in BMI and Body fat %.	[119]
Shelton et al. 2007	Queensland, Australia 43 children (age 3–10 years) with BMI ≥ 85th percentile	Parent based group behavioral program. Four 2 hour group sessions covering nutrition, physical activity, and parenting strategies	Yes	No	3 months	BMI WC PA hours (parent report on 3 days of child PA) SB hours (Parent reported child media use)	Mean (SD) Intervention: 24.8 (3.2) Control: 26.5 (4.0), P < 0.05 Intervention: 82.74 (11.07) Control: 80.28 (10.24), NS Intervention: 2.19 (0.62) Control: 2.05 (0.74), NS Intervention: 1.76 (1.05) Control 3.05 (1.20), NS	Significant difference in BMI, but not in PA and SB	[120]

(continued)

Table 7.6
(continued)

Author (year)	Description of participants, sample size, setting	Intervention components	Combined intervention	Supervised PA	Length of intervention/ follow up	Primary outcome variables	Outcomes/ findings	Results summary	Ref.
Wilfley et al. 2007	San Diego, California 204 overweight children aged 7–12 years with at least one overweight parent.	All participants completed a standard 4 month family-based behavioral weight loss intervention and then either a 4 month: Behavioral Skills Maintenance intervention (BSM), a 4 month Social Facilitation Maintenance intervention (SFM), or no maintenance intervention (control)	Yes	No	4 months of standard intervention, 4 months of maintenance, 2 year follow-up	BMI Z score Percentage over-weight	Mean (SD) Combined maintenance: 2.11 (0.36), Control: 2.00 (0.49) **P = 0.04** Combined maintenance: 60.5 (24.9) Control: 64.8 (22.9), **P = 0.11**	There was a significant difference in the BMI Z scores between the combined maintenance conditions and the control condition. There was an insignificant trend for percentage overweight. The differences were larger at the end of the maintenance intervention, but faded over time.	[59]

| Nemet et al. 2008 | Tel Aviv, Israel 22 obese (>95th BMI percentile) children (ages 8–11 years) from obese families (parents with BMI ≥ 27 kg/m². Randomly assigned | Combined dietary, behavioral, and exercise program. Participants and parents met regularly with dietician. Participants had exercise session twice a week (1 hour each), were encouraged to do additional activity outside of session, and participated in an additional 45 minutes per week of movement therapy. | Yes | Yes | 3 months | BMI kg/m² BMI percentile (%) Body fat % (Skin fold tests) Screen time (hours per day) | Intervention: 25.9 ± 1.9, NS Control: 26.4 ± 1.4, NS Intervention: 95.8 ± 1.0 Control: 97.3 ± 0.5, **P < 0.05** Intervention: 31.7 ± 3.3 Control: 38.5 ± 1.6, NS Intervention: 1.9 ± 0.3 Control: 4.6 ± 0.5, **P < 0.05** | Significant differences in BMI percentile and screen time | [121] |

Physical Activity (PA), Sedentary Behavior (SB), Body Mass Index (BMI), Triceps skinfold thickness (TST), Waist circumference (WC)

to a "Parent and Child" intervention found that "parent only" was more effective, suggesting that parents play a critical role in the success of these interventions [58]. Wilfey and colleagues [59] found that children who completed a 5-month treatment program and then were randomly assigned to one of two maintenance interventions (Behavioral Skills Maintenance, or Social Facilitation Maintenance) maintained weight loss better than children who were assigned to a control condition (after completing treatment).

The success of intense family interventions to treat obesity suggests that a similar approach may have potential in the context of prevention, especially with high-risk populations. The ongoing GEMS studies are one example of a more intense, family-based approach to prevention. Another promising model for prevention is America on the Move [60], which asked families to walk an extra 2,000 steps daily and to eliminate 100 kcal (of sugar) daily from their diet. Such specific, small changes should prove easier to implement than a broader intervention.

7.5.3   Community-Based and Clinical Treatments

Of the eight recent studies in this category, only one was a prototypical community intervention (Table 7.7). Weintraub and colleagues [61] organized a soccer program after school for overweight children which successfully reduced BMI and increased physical activity. This supportive team sport approach to losing weight was also popular with the parents and children, so it warrants further pursuit. The other interventions were initiated in primary care or research settings. They were not family-based, although parents did play a role in some of them. One intervention consisted of 4 months of intense, supervised sessions of exercise [62]. Three were behavioral interventions conducted by phone and mail [63, 64] or by internet [65]. Three were interventions to reduce sedentary behaviors and to replace them with physical activity [66–68]. These interventions all showed beneficial outcomes for their participants, suggesting that various approaches help overweight children lose weight and improve their health.

Two important questions remain about community based interventions. Which of these approaches will be most effective in the long term? Which are most practical? For example, a particularly effective, long-term intervention could be organizing team sports for overweight children that allows some of them to transition onto teams in regular sports. A practical, low-cost approach may be a simple, open loop kit designed for parents with an accelerometer (or pedometer), a television code access device, and instructions. This appoach might allow parents to reduce the sedentary behavior of children without an intensive behavioral intervention conducted by trained staff.

Table 7.7

Treatments based in the community or clinic

Author (year)	Description of participants, sample size, setting	Intervention components	Combined intervention	Supervised PA	Length of intervention/ follow up	Primary outcome variables	Outcomes/ findings	Results summary	Ref.
Owens et al. 1999	Augusta, Georgia 74 obese children (age 7–11 years) Randomly assigned	Physical training 5 days a week for 40 minutes (20 minutes of exercise on machines and 20 minutes of games such basketball and dodgeball)	No	Yes	4 months	% Body fat change PA 7-day recall $kJ \cdot d^{-1}$ Fitness (heart rate on supine ergometer) Change in Visceral adipose tissue (VAT) cm^3 Subcutaneous abdominal adipose tissue (SAAT) cm^3	Mean (SE) Intervention: -2.2 Control: 0.0 (0.4), **$P < 0.01$** Intervention: 162 (141) Control: -363 (175), **$P = 0.02$** Intervention: -3.8 (1.8) Control: 0.2 (1.4), **$P = 0.04$** Intervention: 1.3 (8.3) Control: 20.9 (4.3), **$P = 0.02$** Intervention: -16.2 (27.1) Control: 48.9 (19.9), **$P = 0.03$**	Significant effects on percentage body fat, visceral adipose tissue, and abdominal adipose tissue.	[62]
Faith et al. 2001	New York, New York 10 obese (> 85th BMI percentile) children (age 8–12 years) who watch 2 hours or more of TV per day and do not get regular PA. Random assignment	Participants given TV linked to exercise bicycle. Intervention condition had to pedal in order to activate television.	No	No	12 weeks	TV time (average hours per week) Pedaling time (average minutes per week)	Intervention: 5.4 Control: 21.3, **$P < 0.001$** Intervention: 50.5 Control: 17.7, **$P = 0.01$**	Significant decrease in television time and increase in pedaling time.	[66]

(continued)

Table 7.7
(continued)

Author (year)	Description of participants, sample size, setting	Intervention components	Combined intervention	Supervised PA	Length of intervention/ follow up	Primary outcome variables	Outcomes/ findings	Results summary	Ref.
Saelens et al. 2002	Southern California 44 overweight (20 to 100% above median BMI percentile) adolescents (age 12–16 years) Randomly assigned	Healthy Habits Behavioral weight control program initiated in primary care and extended through telephone and mail contact. Usual care was a single session of physician weight counseling	Yes	No	4 months/ 7 month follow up	BMI Z scores PA 7 day recall (kcal/hg/d) SB self-report (min/d)	Mean (SD) Mean Z scores not reported, condition by time interaction **P < 0.03** Intervention: 6.3 (3.5) Control: 6.9 (3.6), **NS** Intervention: 281 (245) Control: 267 [117], **NS**	Significant difference in BMI Z scores at 7-month follow-up.	[63]
Deforche et al. 2005	Ghent, Belgium 20 obese children (age 11–18 years) who had completed 10 month residential treatment program Randomly assigned	Maintenance program to prevent relapse after completing weight loss program. Weekly contacts by mail or phone. Participants mailed diaries to therapist and discussed by phone. Incentive points for participating in physical activities	No	No	5 months	Weight regain PA structured interview SB structured interview	Significant time by group interaction such that intervention group weight regain was slower than control. **P < 0.05** Significant time by group interaction such that intervention PA increased while control PA decreased **P < 0.05** NS	Significant effect on rate of weight regain and physical activity.	[64]

Study	Setting/Sample	Intervention		Duration	Outcome	Results	Conclusion	Ref
Goldfield et al. 2006	Eastern Ontario, Canada. 30 overweight or obese (> 85th BMI percentile) children (ages 8–12 years) Randomly assigned	Open loop feedback intervention Children wore accelerometers. Counts of PA earned TV/VCR/DVD time Note: no dietary intervention	No	8 weeks	Daily PA counts (accelerometers) Minutes per day MVPA Minutes per day of TV BMI kg/m^2	Mean (SD), P, Group X Time Intervention: 407.8 (192.4) Control: 239.8 (130.2), **P = 0.019** Intervention: 23.8 (17.0) Control: 12.3 (8.9), **P = 0.050** Intervention: 44.4 (26.5) Control: 166.3 (102.7), **P = 0.001** Intervention: 28.3 (5.6) Control: 28.5 (3.1), **P = 0.037**	Small but significant change in BMI. Significant effects on physical activity and sedentary behavior.	[67]
Doyle et al. 2008	San Diego California, and St. Louis, Missouri 80 overweight (≥ 85th BMI percentile) adolescents (age 12–17 years) Randomly assigned	Student Bodies 2 Internet intervention targeting weight loss and eating disorder attitudes/behaviors. Cognitive behavioral based approach with nutrition, monitoring, PA, and body image components. Also received pedometer and guide to calorie and fat content of foods	Yes	16 weeks/ 4 month follow-up	BMI Z score	Mean (SD) Intervention: 2.10 Control: 2.15, **P = 0.289**	Significant differences on BMI Z-score at post intervention, but not at 4 month follow-up.	[65]

(continued)

Table 7.7
(continued)

Author (year)	Description of participants, sample size, setting	Intervention components	Combined intervention	Supervised PA	Length of intervention/ follow up	Primary outcome variables	Outcomes/ findings	Results summary	Ref.
Epstein et al. 2008	Buffalo, New York 70 children (age 4–7 years) with BMI percentile ≥ 75th percentile. Randomly assigned	Intervention to reduce TV and computer use by 50%. TV allowance device used so that child had to enter code number to use TV or computer. Reduced amount by 10% each month until reached 50% of baseline.	No	No	6 months/2 year follow-up	BMI Z score Change in TV and computer hours per week Change in PA counts per minute (accelerometer)	Mean (SEM) Intervention: -0.24 (0.32) Control -0.13 (0.37), **P < 0.05** Intervention: -17.5 (7.0) Control -5.2 (11.1), **P < 0.001** Intervention: 31.4 (275.4) Control -62.7 (189.7), **NS**	Significant differences for BMI Z score and sedentary behavior	[68]
Weintraub et al. 2008	Northern California, US 21 children (grades 4–5) with BMI ≥ 85th percentile Randomly assigned	After school soccer program 3 – 4 days a week. 75 minutes of activity at each session. Control condition participated in after school health education program	No	Yes	6 months	BMI Z score Total activity counts per minute (accelerometers)	Mean (SD) Intervention: 2.06 (0.50) Control: 2.22 (0.30), **P = 0.04** Intervention: 545.41 (97.92) Control: 412.69 (93.16), **P = 0.04**	Significant differences for BMI Z score and physical activity.	[61]

Physical Activity (PA), Sedentary Behavior (SB), Body Mass Index (BMI), Triceps skinfold thickness (TST), Waist circumference (WC)

7.6 CONCLUSION AND FUTURE CHALLENGES

Overall, the results of the studies reviewed here indicate that changing physical activity can be productive but also challenging, especially in prevention interventions. This conclusion is consistent with previous reviews [2]. As has been found with obesity in general, it is difficult to change people's health behaviors. Short-term interventions to educate children and families about the benefits of a healthier lifestyle behavior are usually inadequate to prevent or treat obesity. Huang and Glass [69] have argued that many approaches to the obesity epidemic have focused on the individual level and ignored other factors that create an obesogenic environment. They call for sustained, multilevel approaches that address individual, family, environmental, and policy levels.

As reported in other reviews of obesity interventions [70], interventions that incorporate structured and supervised physical activity sessions appear to be most successful for increasing physical activity, and may be an important consideration in developing future interventions. After-school programs with supervised, enjoyable, and safe opportunities for physical activity are most promising.

Large school prevention programs have the best potential to *prevent* obesity in large numbers of children, which may be more effective than treating already obese children. However, as reported in past [2], many of the large prevention interventions reviewed here failed to yield meaningful differences in BMI and other key outcomes.

Interventions to *prevent* obesity display two disadvantages or limitations compared with treatments. First, children in prevention programs are not necessarily overweight so they (and their parents) may be unmotivated to make or maintain any changes. Second, obesity interventions are often conducted with a subset of overweight children who are selected because they and their families are motivated and likely to succeed in the program (introducing ascertainment bias into the results). By contrast, prevention programs are often conducted with all children in a given school or class.

Environmental interventions hold the potential to influence behavior indirectly (*e.g.*, by offering healthy choices in cafeterias and creating more opportunities for physical activity). Two studies of policy/environmental interventions in a school setting showed promising results [54, 55], suggesting that school interventions which include these components may be more effective. These interventions are also good examples of multilevel approaches that attempt to make changes at the individual level and broader environmental and policy levels. Environmental factors – such as pedestrian friendly neighborhoods [71] and access to recreational areas [72] – can predict greater physical activity and lower obesity. However, the benefits of these environments may be limited by individual preferences for walking over driving [73]. Simply creating more opportunities for physical activity (by blazing new trails for hiking and biking) does not ensure that people will use them [74]. Neighborhood crime may be another factor limiting physical activity in some communities, but evidence for this remains unclear [75].

Interventions focused on reducing sedentary behavior may also be effective. These interventions can take the form of family-based behavior modifications. They can also be based on open loop systems or closed loop systems. Here, technology is used to track physical activity, and children are positively reinforced for increasing their physical activity. However, it is unclear whether there would be long-term benefits for interventions which require special equipment maintained by researchers. Perhaps these interventions can be adapted to provide families with the knowledge and structure to continue the behavior modification interventions on their own.

Some ethnic groups are at greater risk for obesity and the associated health problems [76]. Behavioral health interventions must be targeted to high risk groups and aimed to find and eliminate health disparities. Unique challenges abound. The "Hip Hop Jr." program for preschool students in Head Start programs significantly improved BMI for African-American children [77], but was ineffective with Latino children [78]. The "Pathways" intervention – a 3-year program following Native American students from 2nd through 5th grade – significantly increased the self-reported physical activity upon intervention, but did not improve BMI or adiposity [79]. The ongoing GEMS studies may offer more insight on how to successfully implement obesity prevention programs with specific groups, such as African-American girls [80–82].

Ongoing research focuses on applying new technology to increase physical activity and reduce sedentary activity. Emerging approaches use "active" video games [83] or media stations that require a user to walk while using an electronic device [84]. These approaches do increase physical activity among normal weight adolescents and hold potential for obesity prevention and treatment [85]. Still, no currently published studies show empiric benefits in terms of obesity prevention or treatment from active gaming or walking with media stations. Active games appear to be a healthier choice than regular sedentary video games, but may not have much long-term impact if children quickly lose interest [86] and return to their usual sedentary games. In addition, some children may simply replace other healthy physical activities with active gaming. Active gaming may most benefit those children with *extremely low* levels of activity who already play video games regularly.

Another possible application of technology is to help children and parents monitor their physical activity more accurately. Personal digital assistants (PDAs) [87] and web-based applications [88] can help adults record their energy intake. Similar approaches could be used for tracking physical activity. However, while PDA and web-based approaches were used successfully for recording energy intake, they were no more effective than traditional paper approaches [87–90]. There are currently no published studies on the use of smart phones for these purposes.

Additional research is urgently needed on how other factors influence physical activity. We need to define how chronic conditions may cause children to be less physically active. For instance, an asthmatic child with lower activity levels or frequent steroid use has a higher chance of becoming overweight, which in turn can further limit lung function [91]. Another important area is the cross-sectional link between motor coordination in childhood and the tendency to be more sedentary and less physically active [15, 16]. If asthma, poor motor proficiency, and other chronic conditions prove to be independent risk factors for excess weight gain in youth, early interventions aimed at these comorbidities represent essential approaches to obesity management.

In conclusion, current literature on physical activity as an approach to treat or prevent pediatric obesity discloses various, effective approaches in the short-term. It remains difficult to achieve lasting changes in physical activity and measurable differences in BMI. Prevention interventions may be more effective if they are large multicomponent programs that include healthy eating, increasing physical activity, reducing sedentary behavior, as well as environmental and policy changes. Supervised physical activity sessions and supportive organized sports programs may be particularly effective for increasing physical activity. Diverse reinforcement interventions can reduce sedentary behavior among children. In treatment programs, a combination of supervised physical activity and an intensive family-based intervention is most effective. It is premature to conclude that active gaming can exert a significant benefit for obesity prevention or treatment. Even interventions that successfully increase physical activity or reduce sedentary activity of individual children often lack lasting effects [4]. It is vital to move beyond individually targeted strategies and adopt a more comprehensive approach to obesity research, prevention, and treatment [69]. One key element of a comprehensive approach is identifying effective approaches at the community, environmental, and policy level [3, 69] that will exert lasting impacts on the physical activity levels of children and their families.

REFERENCES

1. Schmitz KH, Jeffery RW (2002) Prevention of obesity. In: Wadden TA, Stunkard AJ (eds) Handbook of obesity treatment. Guilford, New York, pp. 556–593
2. Barbeu P, Gutin B, Sothern M (2006) Physical activity and adiposity in children and adolescents. In: Goran MI, Sothern M (eds) Handbook of pediatric obesity: etiology, pathophysiology, and prevention. CRC/Taylor & Francis Group, Boca Raton, pp. 157–174
3. Schmitz MK, Jeffery RW (2000) Public health interventions for the prevention and treatment of obesity. Med Clin North Am 84:491–512, viii
4. Holtzman J et al (2004) Effectiveness of Behavioral Interventions to Modify Physical Activity Behaivors in General Populations and Cancer Patients and Survivors. Evidence Report/Technology Assessment No. 102 (Prepared by the Minnesota Evidence-based Practice Center, under Contract No. 290-02-0009.) AHRQ Publication No. 04-E027-2. Rockville MD: Agency for Healthcare Research and Quality
5. Wilfley DE et al (2007) Lifestyle interventions in the treatment of childhood overweight: a meta-analytic review of randomized controlled trials. Health Psychol 26(5):521–532
6. US Preventive Services Task Force, Behavioral Counseling in Primary Care to Promote Physical Activity: Recommendations and Rationale. July 2002, Agency for Healthcare Research and Quality: Rockville, MD
7. USDHHS (1996) Physical Activity and Health: A Report of the Surgeon General. U.S. Department of Health and Human Services, Centers for Disease Control and Prevention, National Center for Chronic Disease Prevention and Health Promotion: Atlanta, GA
8. Li L, Li K, Ushijima H (2007) Moderate-vigorous physical activity and body fatness in Chinese urban school children. Pediatr Int 49(2):280–285
9. Sallis JF, McKenzie TL, Alcaraz JE (1993) Habitual physical activity and health-related physical fitness in fourth-grade children. Am J Dis Child 147(8):890–896
10. Akimoto-Gunther L et al (2002) Effects of re-education in eating habits and physical activity on the lipid profile of obese teenagers. Clin Chem Lab Med 40(5):460–462
11. Kim ES et al (2007) Improved insulin sensitivity and adiponectin level after exercise training in obese Korean youth. Obesity (Silver Spring) 15(12):3023–3030
12. Balagopal P et al (2007) Reduction of elevated serum retinol binding protein in obese children by lifestyle intervention: association with subclinical inflammation. J Clin Endocrinol Metab 92(5):1971–1974
13. Kang HS et al (2002) Physical training improves insulin resistance syndrome markers in obese adolescents. Med Sci Sports Exerc 34(12):1920–1927
14. Nemet D et al (2006) A combined dietary-physical activity intervention affects bone strength in obese children and adolescents. Int J Sports Med 27(8):666–671
15. Williams HG et al (2008) Motor skill performance and physical activity in preschool children. Obesity (Silver Spring) 16(6):1421–1426
16. Wrotniak BH et al (2006) The relationship between motor proficiency and physical activity in children. Pediatrics 118(6):e1758–e1765
17. Daley AJ et al (2006) Exercise therapy as a treatment for psychopathologic conditions in obese and morbidly obese adolescents: a randomized, controlled trial. Pediatrics 118(5): 2126–2134
18. Huang JS et al (2007) Body image and self-esteem among adolescents undergoing an intervention targeting dietary and physical activity behaviors. J Adolesc Health 40(3): 245–251
19. Strauss RS et al (2001) Psychosocial correlates of physical activity in healthy children. Arch Pediatr Adolesc Med 155(8):897–902

20. Leatherdale ST, Wong SL (2008) Modifiable characteristics associated with sedentary behaviours among youth. Int J Pediatr Obes 3(2):93–101
21. Burke V et al (2006) Television, computer use, physical activity, diet and fatness in Australian adolescents. Int J Pediatr Obes 1(4):248–255
22. Horn OK et al (2001) Correlates and predictors of adiposity among Mohawk children. Prev Med 33(4):274–281
23. Pardee PE et al (2007) Television viewing and hypertension in obese children. Am J Prev Med 33(6):439–443
24. Owens J et al (1999) Television-viewing habits and sleep disturbance in school children. Pediatrics 104(3):e27
25. Oka Y, Suzuki S, Inoue Y (2008) Bedtime activities, sleep environment, and sleep/wake patterns of Japanese elementary school children. Behav Sleep Med 6(4).220–233
26. Van Cauter E (2008) K. Knutson, Sleep and the epidemic of obesity in children and adults. Eur J Endocrinol 159:s59–s66
27. Spiegel K et al (2005) Sleep loss: a novel risk factor for insulin resistance and Type 2 diabetes. J Appl Physiol 99(5):2008–2019
28. Landhuis CE et al (2008) Childhood sleep time and long-term risk for obesity: a 32-year prospective birth cohort study. Pediatrics 122(5):955–960
29. USDHHS and USDA (December 2005) Dietary Guidelines for Americans, 2010. 7th edn. Washington, DC: U.S. Government Printing Office.
30. USDHHS, Healthy People 2010. 2nd ed. With Understanding and Improving Healthy and Objectives for Improving Health. 2 vols. November 2000: Washington, DC: U.S. Government Printing Office.
31. Pate RR et al (2002) Compliance with physical activity guidelines: prevalence in a population of children and youth. Ann Epidemiol 12(5):303–308
32. DiNapoli PP, Lewis JB (2008) Understanding school-age obesity: through participatory action research. MCN Am J Matern Child Nurs 33(2):104–110
33. Adams J (2006) Trends in physical activity and inactivity amongst US 14-18 year olds by gender, school grade and race, 1993-2003: evidence from the youth risk behavior survey. BMC Public Health 6:57
34. National Center for Chronic Disease Prevention and Health Promotion, D.o.A.a.S.H., Trends in the Prevalence of Physical Activity: National YRBS: 1991-2007. 2008, Centers for Disease Control and Prevention: Atlanta, GA.
35. Barlow SE, Dietz WH (1998) Obesity evaluation and treatment: expert Committee recommendations. The Maternal and Child Health Bureau, Health Resources and Services Administration and the Department of Health and Human Services. Pediatrics 102(3):E29
36. Dietz WH, Robinson TN (2005) Clinical practice. Overweight children and adolescents. N Engl J Med 352(20):2100–2109
37. Leermakers EA, Dunn AL, Blair SN (2000) Exercise management of obesity. Med Clin North Am 84(2):419–440
38. Kain J et al (2004) School-based obesity prevention in Chilean primary school children: methodology and evaluation of a controlled study. Int J Obes Relat Metab Disord 28(4):483–493
39. Story M et al (2003) An after-school obesity prevention program for African-American girls: the Minnesota GEMS pilot study. Ethn Dis 13(1 Suppl 1):S54–S64
40. Warren JM et al (2003) Evaluation of a pilot school programme aimed at the prevention of obesity in children. Health Promot Int 18(4):287–296
41. Neumark-Sztainer D et al (2003) New Moves: a school-based obesity prevention program for adolescent girls. Prev Med 37(1):41–51

42. Pate RR et al (2005) Promotion of physical activity among high-school girls: a randomized controlled trial. Am J Public Health 95(9):1582–1587
43. Jiang J et al (2007) The effects of a 3-year obesity intervention in schoolchildren in Beijing. Child Care Health Dev 33(5):641–646
44. Gutin B et al (2008) Preliminary findings of the effect of a 3-year after-school physical activity intervention on fitness and body fat: the Medical College of Georgia Fitkid Project. Int J Pediatr Obes 3(Suppl 1):3–9
45. Stock S et al (2007) Healthy Buddies: a novel, peer-led health promotion program for the prevention of obesity and eating disorders in children in elementary school. Pediatrics 120(4):e1059–e1068
46. Kumanyika SK et al (2003) Phase 1 of the Girls health Enrichment Multi-site Studies (GEMS): conclusion. Ethn Dis 13(1 suppl 1):S88–S91
47. Harvey-Berino J, Rourke J (2003) Obesity prevention in preschool native-american children: a pilot study using home visiting. Obes Res 11(5):606–611
48. Rooney BL et al (2005) Growing healthy families: family use of pedometers to increase physical activity and slow the rate of obesity. Wmj 104(5):54–60
49. Roemmich JN, Gurgol CM, Epstein LH (2004) Open-loop feedback increases physical activity of youth. Med Sci Sports Exerc 36(4):668–673
50. Jago R et al (2006) Effect of 4 weeks of Pilates on the body composition of young girls. Prev Med 42(3):177–180
51. Stettler N (2005) Primary care obesity prevention: one or multiple targets. Grant # 5R01HL084056-04. 2005.
52. La Monica S et al (2007) Changing pediatric primary care providers' skill-proficiency in obesity prevention with intense behavioral training: the smart steps study. Obesity 15:165
53. Williamson DA et al (2007) Wise Mind project: a school-based environmental approach for preventing weight gain in children. Obesity (Silver Spring) 15(4):906–917
54. Foster GD et al (2008) A policy-based school intervention to prevent overweight and obesity. Pediatrics 121(4):e794–e802
55. Ildiko V et al (2007) Activity-related changes of body fat and motor performance in obese seven-year-old boys. J Physiol Anthropol 26(3):333–337
56. Epstein LH et al (1994) Ten-year outcomes of behavioral family-based treatment for childhood obesity. Health Psychol 13(5):373–383
57. Golan M, Kaufman V, Shahar DR (2006) Childhood obesity treatment: targeting parents exclusively v. parents and children. Br J Nutr 95(5):1008–1015
58. Wilfley DE et al (2007) Efficacy of maintenance treatment approaches for childhood overweight: a randomized controlled trial. JAMA 298(14):1661–1673
59. Rodearmel SJ et al (2007) Small changes in dietary sugar and physical activity as an approach to preventing excessive weight gain: the America on the Move family study. Pediatrics 120(4):e869–e879
60. Weintraub DL et al (2008) Team sports for overweight children: the Stanford Sports to Prevent Obesity Randomized Trial (SPORT). Arch Pediatr Adolesc Med 162(3):232–237
61. Owens S et al (1999) Effect of physical training on total and visceral fat in obese children. Med Sci Sports Exerc 31(1):143–148
62. Saelens BE et al (2002) Behavioral weight control for overweight adolescents initiated in primary care. Obes Res 10(1):22–32
63. Deforche B et al (2005) Post-treatment phone contact: a weight maintenance strategy in obese youngsters. Int J Obes (Lond) 29(5):543–546

64. Doyle AC et al (2008) Reduction of overweight and eating disorder symptoms via the Internet in adolescents: a randomized controlled trial. J Adolesc Health 43(2):172–179
65. Faith MS et al (2001) Effects of contingent television on physical activity and television viewing in obese children. Pediatrics 107(5):1043–1048
66. Goldfield GS et al (2006) Effects of open-loop feedback on physical activity and television viewing in overweight and obese children: a randomized, controlled trial. Pediatrics 118(1):e157–e166
67. Epstein LH et al (2008) A randomized trial of the effects of reducing television viewing and computer use on body mass index in young children. Arch Pediatr Adolesc Med 162(3):239–245
68. Huang TT, Glass TA (2008) Transforming research strategies for understanding and preventing obesity. JAMA 300(15):1811–1813
69. Whitlock EP et al. Effectiveness of weight management programs in children and adolescents. Evidence Report/Technology Assessment No. 170 (Prepared by the Oregon Evidence-based Practice Center under Contract No. 290-02-0024). AHRQ Publication No. 08-E014. September 2008, Agency for Healthcare Research and Quality: Rockville, MD
70. Frank LD et al (2008) A hierarchy of sociodemographic and environmental correlates of walking and obesity. Prev Med 47(2):172–178
71. Bjork J et al (2008) Recreational values of the natural environment in relation to neighbourhood satisfaction, physical activity, obesity and wellbeing. J Epidemiol Community Health 62(4):e2
72. Frank LD et al (2007) Stepping towards causation: do built environments or neighborhood and travel preferences explain physical activity, driving, and obesity? Soc Sci Med 65(9):1898–1914
73. Evenson KR, Herring AH, Huston SL (2005) Evaluating change in physical activity with the building of a multi-use trail. Am J Prev Med 28(2 Suppl 2):177–185
74. Foster S, Giles-Corti B (2008) The built environment, neighborhood crime and constrained physical activity: an exploration of inconsistent findings. Prev Med 47(3): 241–251
75. Gallagher D et al. Influence of Ethnicity on Obesity-Related Facots in Children and Adolescents, in Handbook of pediatric obesity : etiology, pathophysiology, and prevention, M.I. Goran and M. Sothern, Editors. 2006, CRC/Taylor & Francis Group: Boca Raton. p. 35-51.
76. Fitzgibbon ML et al (2005) Two-year follow-up results for Hip-Hop to Health Jr.: a randomized controlled trial for overweight prevention in preschool minority children. J Pediatr 146(5):618–625
77. Fitzgibbon ML et al (2006) Hip-Hop to Health Jr. for Latino preschool children. Obesity (Silver Spring) 14(9):1616–1625
78. Caballero B et al (2003) Pathways: a school-based, randomized controlled trial for the prevention of obesity in American Indian schoolchildren. Am J Clin Nutr 78(5): 1030–1038
79. Baranowski T et al (2003) The Fun, Food, and Fitness Project (FFFP): the Baylor GEMS pilot study. Ethn Dis 13(1 Suppl 1):S30–S39
80. Beech BM et al (2003) Child- and parent-targeted interventions: the Memphis GEMS pilot study. Ethn Dis 13(1 Suppl 1):S40–S53
81. Robinson TN et al (2003) Dance and reducing television viewing to prevent weight gain in African-American girls: the Stanford GEMS pilot study. Ethn Dis 13(1 Suppl 1):S65–S77
82. Mellecker RR, McManus AM (2008) Energy expenditure and cardiovascular responses to seated and active gaming in children. Arch Pediatr Adolesc Med 162(9):886–891

83. Mellecker, R.R., et al., The feasibility of ambulatory screen time in children. Int J Pediatr Obes, 2008: p. 1-6.

84. Pate RR (2008) Physically active video gaming: an effective strategy for obesity prevention? Arch Pediatr Adolesc Med 162(9):895–896

85. Madsen KA et al (2007) Feasibility of a dance videogame to promote weight loss among overweight children and adolescents. Arch Pediatr Adolesc Med 161(1): 105–107

86. Beasley JM et al (2008) Evaluation of a PDA-based dietary assessment and intervention program: a randomized controlled trial. J Am Coll Nutr 27(2):280–286

87. Beasley, J.M., A. Davis, and W.T. Riley, Evaluation of a web-based, pictorial diet history questionnaire. Public Health Nutr, 2008: p. 1–9.

88. Yon BA et al (2006) The use of a personal digital assistant for dietary self-monitoring does not improve the validity of self-reports of energy intake. J Am Diet Assoc 106(8):1256–1259

89. Yon BA et al (2007) Personal digital assistants are comparable to traditional diaries for dietary self-monitoring during a weight loss program. J Behav Med 30(2):165–175

90. Firrincieli V et al (2005) Decreased physical activity among Head Start children with a history of wheezing: use of an accelerometer to measure activity. Pediatr Pulmonol 40(1):57–63

91. Robinson TN (1999) Reducing children's television viewing to prevent obesity: a randomized controlled trial. JAMA 282(16):1561–1567

92. Sahota P et al (2001) Randomised controlled trial of primary school based intervention to reduce risk factors for obesity. BMJ 323(7320):1029–1032

93. Frenn M, Malin S, Bansal NK (2003) Stage-based interventions for low-fat diet with middle school students. J Pediatr Nurs 18(1):36–45

94. Frenn M et al (2003) Addressing health disparities in middle school students' nutrition and exercise. J Community Health Nurs 20(1):1–14

95. Simon C et al (2004) Intervention centred on adolescents' physical activity and sedentary behaviour (ICAPS): concept and 6-month results. Int J Obes Relat Metab Disord 28(Suppl 3):S96–S103

96. Frenn M et al (2005) Changing the tide: an Internet/video exercise and low-fat diet intervention with middle-school students. Appl Nurs Res 18(1):13–21

97. Harrison M et al (2006) Influence of a health education intervention on physical activity and screen time in primary school children: 'Switch Off–Get Active'. J Sci Med Sport 9(5):388–394

98. Reilly JJ et al (2006) Physical activity to prevent obesity in young children: cluster randomised controlled trial. BMJ 333(7577):1041

99. Robbins LB et al (2006) Girls on the move program to increase physical activity participation. Nurs Res 55(3):206–216

100. Spiegel SA, Foulk D (2006) Reducing overweight through a multidisciplinary school-based intervention. Obesity (Silver Spring) 14(1):88–96

101. Eliakim A et al (2007) The effects of nutritional-physical activity school-based intervention on fatness and fitness in preschool children. J Pediatr Endocrinol Metab 20(6):711–718

102. Martinez Vizcaino V et al (2008) Assessment of an after-school physical activity program to prevent obesity among 9- to 10-year-old children: a cluster randomized trial. Int J Obes (Lond) 32(1):12–22

103. Kipping RR, Payne C, Lawlor DA (2008) Randomised controlled trial adapting US school obesity prevention to England. Arch Dis Child 93(6):469–473

104. Salmon J et al (2008) Outcomes of a group-randomized trial to prevent excess weight gain, reduce screen behaviours and promote physical activity in 10-year-old children: switch-play. Int J Obes (Lond) 32(4):601–612

105. Trost SG, Fees B, Dzewaltowski D (2008) Feasibility and efficacy of a "move and learn" physical activity curriculum in preschool children. J Phys Act Health 5(1):88–103

106. Graf C et al (2006) Who benefits from intervention in, as opposed to screening of, overweight and obese children? Cardiol Young 16(5):474–480

107. Hakanen M et al (2006) Development of overweight in an atherosclerosis prevention trial starting in early childhood. The STRIP study. Int J Obes (Lond) 30(4):618–626

108. Braet C et al (2003) Inpatient treatment of obese children: a multicomponent programme without stringent calorie restriction. Eur J Pediatr 162(6):391–396

109. Carrel AL et al (2005) Improvement of fitness, body composition, and insulin sensitivity in overweight children in a school-based exercise program: a randomized, controlled study. Arch Pediatr Adolesc Med 159(10):963–968

110. Johnston CA et al (2007) Weight loss in overweight Mexican American children: a randomized, controlled trial. Pediatrics 120(6):e1450–e1457

111. Fullerton G et al (2007) Quality of life in Mexican-American children following a weight management program. Obesity (Silver Spring) 15(11):2553–2556

112. Huang SH et al (2007) Effects of a classroom-based weight-control intervention on cardiovascular disease in elementary-school obese children. Acta Paediatr Taiwan 48(4):201–206

113. Nemet D et al (2005) Short- and long-term beneficial effects of a combined dietary-behavioral-physical activity intervention for the treatment of childhood obesity. Pediatrics 115(4):e443–e449

114. Reinehr T et al (2006) Long-term follow-up of cardiovascular disease risk factors in children after an obesity intervention. Am J Clin Nutr 84(3):490–496

115. Gillis D, Brauner M, Granot E (2007) A community-based behavior modification intervention for childhood obesity. J Pediatr Endocrinol Metab 20(2):197–203

116. Golley RK et al (2007) Twelve-month effectiveness of a parent-led, family-focused weight-management program for prepubertal children: a randomized, controlled trial. Pediatrics 119(3):517–525

117. Kalavainen MP, Korppi MO, Nuutinen OM (2007) Clinical efficacy of group-based treatment for childhood obesity compared with routinely given individual counseling. Int J Obes (Lond) 31(10):1500–1508

118. McCallum Z et al (2007) Outcome data from the LEAP (Live, Eat and Play) trial: a randomized controlled trial of a primary care intervention for childhood overweight/mild obesity. Int J Obes (Lond) 31(4):630–636

119. Savoye M et al (2007) Effects of a weight management program on body composition and metabolic parameters in overweight children: a randomized controlled trial. JAMA 297(24):2697–2704

120. Shelton D et al (2007) Randomised controlled trial: a parent-based group education programme for overweight children. J Paediatr Child Health 43(12):799–805

121. Nemet D, Barzilay-Teeni N, Eliakim A (2008) Treatment of childhood obesity in obese families. J Pediatr Endocrinol Metab 21(5):461–467

8 Behavior Modification in Pediatric Obesity

Gerri A. Minshall, Fiona Davies, and Louise A. Baur

Key Points

- Psychologic factors must be considered while implementing interventions to promote healthier lifestyles.
- Child and adolescent obesity prevails in many countries and is associated with a range of medical and psychosocial complications. Early intervention is critical as childhood obesity tracks into adulthood.
- Effective management of pediatric obesity requires an understanding of family dynamics, a developmentally appropriate approach, long-term behavior change, long-term dietary change, increased physical activity, decreased sedentary behavior, and judicious consideration of use of pharmacotherapy in adolescents.
- Behavioral modification techniques should be used to treat pediatric obesity. Training in these techniques is recommended for all health professionals involved in obesity treatment, with the involvement of specialist staff wherever possible.
- The most successful behavioral strategies in pediatric obesity include self or parental monitoring, stimulus control, goal setting or contracting, reinforcement, contingency management, modeling, preplanning, problem solving, parent training, and cognitive restructuring. These strategies are aimed at changing obesogenic behaviors and altering energy balance.

From: *Nutrition and Health: Management of Pediatric Obesity and Diabetes*,
Edited by: R.J. Ferry, Jr., DOI 10.1007/978-1-60327-256-8_8,
© Springer Science+Business Media, LLC 2011

- Challenges in usual clinical practice include appropriate management of families with multiple psychosocial barriers and providing behavioral management where there is limited availability of a clinical psychologist.
- A multidisciplinary weight management service should provide a welcoming and destigmatizing environment, easy physical access for large people, and staff with good teamwork skills and a respectful attitude toward obese people.

Keywords: Behavioral modification, Prevention, Pediatric obesity

Abbreviation

RCT   Randomized controlled trial

8.1   INTRODUCTION

The need for effective treatment of children and adolescents affected by obesity is highlighted by the high prevalence of pediatric obesity in many countries. The broad principles of treatment are outlined in Table 8.1.

The 2009 Cochrane Review on treatment of pediatric obesity, which included 64 randomized controlled trials (RCTs), provides some guidance regarding the effectiveness of clinical interventions [1]. The authors of the review found it difficult to recommend one specific treatment program over another, due to the relative lack of quality data. However, meta-analyses showed that combined behavioral lifestyle interventions, compared to standard care or self-help, can produce significant short-term and long-term clinically meaningful reductions in overweight in children and adolescents. The rest of this chapter provides a rationale for why behavior modification techniques are uniquely useful in the treatment of pediatric obesity. The key techniques and suggestions for how they can be implemented by a health professional are described.

8.2   BEHAVIORAL MODIFICATION

Behavior modification is a definition given to a number of strategies which are used to strengthen or weaken a specifically defined and clearly observable behavior. A typical example would be for a family to reduce their child's time spent in front of an electronic screen from 5 h/day to 2 h/day. Behavior modification is the clinical application of learning theory. For more detailed definitions and a history of the field, see Martin and Pear [2].

Table 8.1
Basic principles of management of obesity in childhood and adolescence

Assess and treat medical or psychosocial co-morbidities

Family involvement

Developmentally appropriate approach

Preadolescent children: focus on parents

• Adolescents: consider separate sessions for the young person and parent(s)

Long-term behavioral change

Long-term dietary change

• Energy reduction

• Food choices that are lower in fat and have a lower glycemic index

• Reduction in high-sugar foods and drinks

• Water as the main beverage

Avoidance of severe dietary restriction

• Appropriate portion sizes

• Modified eating patterns (regular meals, eat together as a family, avoid eating while watching the television)

Increase in physical activity

• Incidental activity

• Active transport options (*e.g.*, walking, cycling, using public transport)

• Lifestyle activities

• Organized activities

• Improved access to recreation spaces and play equipment

Decrease in sedentary behavior

• Reduce television, computer, play-station, and other small-screen recreation

• Alternatives to motorized transport

Consideration of pharmacological therapy

• Consider use of sibutramine or orlistat in moderately to severely obese adolescents, as an adjunct to lifestyle modification

• Consider use of metformin in insulin-resistant obese adolescents

The application of behavior modification techniques is essential in helping children and adolescents lose weight. Effective treatment of child and adolescent obesity assumes a family-wide approach [3]. Therefore, the patients, and more usually the parents, need a "scaffold" or a way of implementing changes in several different domains such as diet, physical activity, or screen time (*i.e.*, time spent at the television, computer, or other forms of electronic screen-based entertainment). They will require techniques that help them to adhere to and follow through with a range of specific behavior changes. Behavior modification provides this support.

Indeed, there is a strong tradition of behaviorism being used in weight loss programs. The early work in this field is reviewed by Epstein *et al.* [4]. The previously mentioned 2009 Cochrane review described numerous studies that included a behavioral component. While often not well described in the included studies, these components ranged from "communication skills" to "behavior chains." Success in weight loss is associated with using more behavioral techniques in a program. In a systematic review of weight loss intervention studies in children and adolescents, McLean *et al.* found that studies using a greater number of behavioral techniques such as monitoring, goal setting, and problem solving were associated with greater weight loss in parents and children [5].

Packaged, manualized, and often researched-based weight loss treatments are almost always referred to as "behavioral programs" [6, 7]. While this term distinguishes a lifestyle treatment from a pharmacological or surgical intervention, it also shows the important role of behavior modification in the field of weight loss. Namely, that the "how" is as important as the "what." In other words, losing weight involves making many changes and how effectively a change is implemented by a family is probably as important as which specific recommendations they start with.

Evidence-based guidelines on pediatric treatment from many jurisdictions and professional groups all highlight the importance of including family-focused behavior modification in treatment [8, 9]. Expert opinion also frequently describes the importance of behavioral strategies [10, 11] and there is consensus that merely educating people about a healthy diet or recommended physical activity is not enough to effect change. Group weight loss treatments, in particular, have behavior modification infused throughout their session agendas and treatment structures. A lifestyle group program may involve activities such as reviewing self monitoring, checking progress towards goals, and planning for high-risk situations. See Melin and Rosner [12] for a description of this approach in adult groups and Brennan *et al.* [13] for a description of its use in individual adolescent treatment. The advantage of manualized and marketed programs is that they often make the behavior modification part clearer and more engaging for the participants. However, this should not deter an individual practitioner from using behavior modification techniques.

Certainly there are good reasons why behavior modification is so salient in the field of weight loss. First, the need for behavioral strategies is highlighted by the fact that the twenty-first century obesity-conducive environment includes societal cues to consume more kilojoules (bigger plates, larger portion sizes), barriers to physical activity (community attributes such as lack of safety, few footpaths, etc.), and poor stimulus control around screens, such as having a range of electronic screens within the home and having the television permanently on while at home. Secondly, there is a strong evidence base that changing behaviors such as increasing lifestyle activity or reducing screen time are associated with weight loss [14].

While the reasons are compelling, there can be difficulties in implementing behavior modification strategies in a clinical setting. These challenges include the jargon that permeates the field and the fact that many published studies and programs do not clarify exactly what has been done. Some commercial programs restrict access to their resources and health professionals are often not trained in behavior modification. Finally, clinicians may feel uncomfortable having to deal with specific noncompliance ("You have not brought in your screen time monitoring form") vs. general noncompliance ("It sounds like John is still watching a lot of TV").

Aside from the evidence-base, the treatment guidelines, and the expert recommendations, there are a number of additional reasons why behavior modification enhances family-based weight loss treatment. For example, it makes treatment specific and relevant to a family (goal setting); it gives a sense of awareness and control (reinforcement, planning, self monitoring, and stimulus control techniques); it allows analysis by the parent or the health professional (self-monitoring); and it increases the likelihood a new behavior will be initiated (shaping, positive reinforcement, stimulus control, and goal setting).

Behavior modification in pediatric obesity is similar to the domain of Parent Management Training where numerous behaviors, in this case child disruptive behaviors such as noncompliance and tantrums, are targeted by various techniques. Strategies such as praise, ignoring, and punishment ("time-out") are "taught" by health professionals and implemented by parents. We will turn now to the evidence and application of some specific behavior modification techniques to child and adolescent obesity.

8.2.1   Key Behavioral Modification Techniques

Three key techniques used in behavior modification are goal setting, stimulus control, and self-monitoring. These three methods were used in some form by the majority of the studies included in the recent Cochrane review on pediatric obesity [1] and are described in detail below. Other strategies are also commonly used in pediatric obesity and are outlined in Table 8.2.

8.2.1.1   GOAL SETTING

Goal setting is a behavior modification technique widely used in obesity treatment, and often takes the form of either outcome goals (such as weight loss)

Table 8.2
Behavior modification techniques commonly used in pediatric obesity

Behavior modification technique	Purpose of the technique	Demonstration of how the behavioral strategy might be used in a pediatric obesity treatment session
Positive reinforcement such as praise or reward systems.	Makes desirable weight loss behaviors more frequent.	The clinician speaks to parents about praising their child whenever they play outside. The child or adolescent earns "points" for engaging in physical activity. When enough points are obtained, they exchange these for a meaningful, nonfood reward. The clinician discusses and plans this system with the parents and brainstorms various reward ideas.
Shaping	Rewards successive approximations to the desired behavior when the ideal behavior cannot currently be performed.	The clinician realizes that an adolescent would not be able to reduce their daily screen time from 6 h to the recommended 2 h. Therefore, the clinician negotiates an intermediate goal of 4 h/day.
Modeling	Demonstrating a desired behavior. This is a component of behavioral contracting where the parent and child check on each other's monitoring, goal achievement, and "earning" of rewards.	The clinician talks to the parents about setting their own healthy lifestyle or weight loss goals. The child then observes the parents engaging in behaviors such as regular physical activity, eating healthy snacks, and so on.

Household rules	Technically a form of instruction, modeling, and stimulus control. Household rules are a behavior management "shortcut" which make desirable behaviors more likely to occur.	Guided by the patients' preferences, the clinician talks to the parents about relevant household rules which can be realistically enforced. Examples include: children should ask before going to the refrigerator, no eating with the television on, and only adults can switch the television on.
Problem solving or preplanning	Essentially this is a cognitive-behavioral technique that combines all of the behavior modification strategies so that patients are prepared for difficult situations.	The clinician is aware of a high-risk situation, such as a common festival involving feasting. They then work through all of the above techniques as they are relevant to the challenging situation. For example, the clinician may discuss at length and brainstorm solutions with the patient to the weight gain risk embodied by the Christmas holiday period.

or performance goals (such as lifestyle changes). Well-specified goals are a way of clearly articulating people's good intentions. However, some researchers have commented on the level of assistance families require to set these types of goals and the effort needed to assess goal achievement [13]. The assumption is that goal setting will inherently be motivating, but Brennan *et al.* [13] found that these goals had limited motivational value for the families involved in their obesity treatment program, although they were still a useful tool for assessing progress.

The broader literature on goal setting and motivation has also raised questions about the inherent motivational value of these types of goals, finding that intentions only account for 20–30% of the variation in behavior [15]. This suggests that good intentions (i.e., outcome or performance goals) do not generally translate into actions, and that past behavior is a better predictor of future behavior than good intentions [15]. A classic example, familiar to all, is the frequent outcome of a New Year's resolution, with the well-recognized phenomenon of slipping back into past behaviors after a brief period of motivation (*e.g.*, quitting smoking, losing weight, getting fit).

However, considerable work has now been done looking at how to harness good intentions in behavioral change, and this provides clinicians with some specific suggestions for improving goal attainment in their patients. One factor is the nature of the goals – research suggests goals that are challenging, specific, short term, and positively framed are more likely to be achieved than goals that are vague, long-term, or focused on avoiding negative consequences [15]. For example, parents or adolescent patients may express vague goals such as their desire to "be more active" or "eat healthier food." Clinicians can increase the likelihood that patients will achieve their goals by helping them to phrase those goals in a more productive way (see Table 8.3), and by continually revisiting those goals to check progress.

In pediatric obesity treatment it is critical to help people work out how to start behavior change, how to overcome barriers and solve problems, and how to persist with new behaviors over time. One way of doing this is by focusing on implementation intentions (similar to the idea of planning presented in Epstein's studies [16]). Implementation intentions, in the form of "if-then" plans, have a moderate to large effect on goal achievement [17].

Getting started with goals is made easier by specifying the "when, where, and how" of a behavior. People are often distracted from performing goals, and thus establishing a plan to deal with these distractions is essential. Similarly, the person's habitual behavior will also tend to take over, and, thus, having a plan to address high-risk situations (*e.g.*, parties, holidays) is also important. In health care, it is important that patients leave a consultation with strong intentions as well as goals that can be effectively translated into

Table 8.3
Examples of good intentions vs. well-specified goals in obesity treatment

Good intention	Well-specified (if-then) implementation goal
We all need to be more active as a family and walk a bit more	I will walk with the kids to school from home every morning. *If* it is raining, *then* I will take an umbrella. *If* anyone sleeps in, *then* I will walk them home from school instead
Every family member needs to eat breakfast	I will eat put a small bowl of muesli with fruit and yogurt on the table every morning at 8 a.m. I will wake the kids up 10 min earlier on school mornings. *If* they sleep in, *then* I will give them a container with their breakfast in it to take to school
We need to eat less junk food	I will not buy any biscuits, chocolates, or other energy-dense food during the weekly shop. In order to make this easier, I will not take the kids shopping with me. *If* the kids ask for junk food, *then* I will offer them some fruit or yogurt

action [17]. Table 8.3 provides examples of typical "good intentions" that may be expressed by the parents of children attending a weight management service, and corresponding well-specified implementation goals developed after consultation with a clinician. Goals such as these should be written down and kept by both the clinician and the family, and checked in subsequent appointments in order to assess progress, and identify and problem solve any barriers to goal achievement.

Another important way to enhance the likelihood of goal achievement is to change the environment in order to support behavior change by decreasing triggers to eat energy dense food and increasing triggers for exercise [15]. In the behavior modification literature this is referred to as stimulus control and helps to decrease the reliance on motivation as a way to ensure progress against goals. The following section on stimulus control provides further details on some of the specific types of environmental changes that research has shown to be helpful.

8.2.1.2 STIMULUS CONTROL

Stimulus control refers to environmental changes designed to either increase or decrease the frequency of target behaviors, without relying on motivation or drawing on self-regulatory capacity. In other words, it refers to designing or containing the environment so that it facilitates weight loss behaviors. Individual decisions about food, sedentary behaviors, and physical activity are influenced on a daily basis by the broader environment, and people are largely unaware of these influences or even of the number of decisions they make about food, screen time, and exercise [18]. In obesity treatment there is a substantial research base which provides a set of recommendations which are appropriate to a wide range of people and that help to mitigate the effects of the modern obesity-conducive environment. It is assumed that these stimulus control measures will also help children and adolescents who need to lose weight. A list of suggestions, particularly focusing upon eating behaviors, is provided in Table 8.4 and can be used to help decrease energy consumption. They can also be used to guide an interview with families, as well as being useful in goal setting and formulating household rules.

Wansink [22] argues that overeating is largely driven by two environmental factors – consumption norms and (lack of) consumption monitoring. How much people eat is influenced by a variety of environmental factors. The factors which tend to increase consumption include larger packages; larger serving sizes; and larger bowls, plates and spoons [22]. Consumption monitoring refers to people's ability to detect when they are satiated and the research suggests that this perception is driven to a large extent by environmental cues (*e.g.*, when the plate is empty, when others stop eating) rather than internal cues (such as feeling full) [22]. Therefore, interventions which lead to healthier consumption norms (such as smaller plates) and better focus on internal cues for consumption monitoring (such as not eating while

Table 8.4

Recommended environmental changes

- Use smaller plates, bowls, containers, serving platters, and spoons [19–22]
- Do not keep energy-dense food in the home and, if you do, keep it at the back of the fridge or cupboard in opaque containers [22]
- Food which takes more effort to eat will tend to lead to smaller portions (*e.g.*, unshelled nuts, using chopsticks) [22]
- Serve food in the kitchen rather than leaving serving platters on the table [22]
- Tall, thin glasses are better than short, wide glasses [23]
- Serve less variety in energy-dense foods and more variety in low energy density foods (*e.g.*, vegetables, salads) [24]
- Do not leave snack foods on the table (take a serving and put the rest away) [22, 24]
- Eat at the table, without the TV on [22, 24]
- Put utensils down and take a sip of water in between mouthfuls [24]

distracted) could be reasonably expected to lead to a decrease in calorie consumption and therefore in weight.

Environmental changes which support goals without drawing on self-regulatory capacity aid in goal achievement and should make weight loss easier. Ideally they should occur in the context of clear implementation goals and will likely be aided by self-monitoring. Self-monitoring has a rich tradition of research in obesity treatment, as will be discussed in the following section.

8.2.1.3 SELF-MONITORING

Self-monitoring is the most researched, single behavior modification technique in child/adolescent pediatric obesity. It is the detailed recording of a specific behavior. Traditionally, self-monitoring takes the form of a "food diary" where all food and beverages consumed are written down and calories or fat grams eaten are also tallied. However, self-monitoring can occur for other domains and can focus on almost any measurable behavior. A pedometer is essentially a form of monitoring because it records a clear and discrete behavior – the number of steps a person has taken. Self-monitoring is frequently used early in treatment; so the data collected can drive subsequent goal setting and changes to the environment.

Self-monitoring has several advantages for the treatment of pediatric weight loss. First, it provides information to the patient and the clinician on the antecedents and consequences of a behavior. For example, self-monitoring may clarify that an adolescent's excessive snack food consumption is triggered by boredom. There is also the potential for the magnitude of a behavior to become salient to the patient or parent, *e.g.*, "I had no idea that my children watched so many hours of television." Monitoring may also keep patients focused on the overall goal of weight loss. It is also a form of data collection and as such allows comparisons over time. For instance, is an adolescent engaging in less screen time since the new household rules have been implemented?

There is evidence that self-monitoring is related to better weight control in children and adolescents. Saelens and McGrath [25] found that recording food items consumed but not calories or total calories was related to better weight outcome. Another US-based study [26] found that minority children who self-monitored lost more weight at 6 months than those who did not self-monitor. Importantly, this technique's impact on child weight loss is greater when the parents also self-monitor; in such a situation, not only are the children more likely to self-monitor but also are more likely to lose weight [27].

Despite its described strength, self-monitoring can be a challenging technique to implement with patients. Parental adherence to self-monitoring has been reported as low as only 12% in a particular study, doing any form of monitoring at all [26]. In spite of this, it is worth a clinician pursuing even partial adherence. Compliance may be helped by a detailed rationale or orientation to the technique, a special form being provided, and the clinician and patient working through an example within the consultation (see Fig. 8.1 for an example of a form used to self-monitor screen time).

Table 8.5 gives some examples of the use of the three key behavioral modification techniques, with a focus on the health professional working in solo clinical practice.

8.2.2   Behavior Modification and New Technologies

The harnessing of new technologies means that behavior modification techniques can be delivered in different ways. Excellent reviews exist on e-health and online interventions in weight loss [28, 29]. Table 8.6 provides some examples of innovations which may make it easier for a health practitioner in solo practice to incorporate behavior modification tools into their treatment approaches with obese patients.

8.3   CHALLENGES IN TREATING CHILD AND ADOLESCENT OBESITY IN USUAL CLINICAL PRACTICE

The above overview of behavior modification in pediatric obesity provides an evidence base for a range of therapists as they seek to treat children and adolescents affected by obesity. However, there are challenges in translating such evidence into everyday clinical practice. For example, the 2009 Cochrane Review on treating child and adolescent obesity [1] highlights a range of gaps in the research evidence, including in relation to behavioral management, as summarized in Table 8.7.

Importantly, most of the studies looking at strategies for behavioral management of obesity in children and adolescents have typically been performed in white, middle-class, intact families where the degree of motivation for change is relatively high and where there are few, or no, associated psychosocial co-morbidities [1]. But the reality of pediatric obesity, in western societies at least, is that it is more common in families from lower socioeconomic groups, with single parents and often a range of associated psychological or social problems [30]. Likewise, many of the obesity behavioral management studies to date have taken place in tertiary level centers with highly skilled staff [1]. However, usual weight management services in many countries have a smaller complement of experienced staff and there may be little, or no, clinical psychologist input into the treating team.

Name..   Date................

What did you use the screen for? Circle one:				How long? Write in below
Morning				
TV	Video or DVD	Game	Computer	
TV	Video or DVD	Game	Computer	
TV	Video or DVD	Game	Computer	
Afternoon				
TV	Video or DVD	Game	Computer	
TV	Video or DVD	Game	Computer	
TV	Video or DVD	Game	Computer	
TV	Video or DVD	Game	Computer	
Evening				
TV	Video or DVD	Game	Computer	
TV	Video or DVD	Game	Computer	
TV	Video or DVD	Game	Computer	
TV	Video or DVD	Game	Computer	
Late at night (After 10.30 pm)				
TV	Video or DVD	Game	Computer	
TV	Video or DVD	Game	Computer	
TV	Video or DVD	Game	Computer	
TV	Video or DVD	Game	Computer	
			Total Time Today? Add hours here:	

Fig. 8.1. Example of a self-monitoring form used for monitoring screen time.

Table 8.5
Key behavior modification techniques and how they can be implemented in a pediatric obesity treatment session by a clinician in solo practice

Key behavior modification technique	*Example of how a clinician can apply this technique in a pediatric weight management session*
Goal setting	• Talk to the patient's parents about their preferred area to address (*e.g.*, diet, physical activity, screen time). • Use a discussion to turn broad intentions into measurable, specific activities. • The clinician also leads a discussion about whether the behavioral goal is realistic and what are the plans should problems/barriers occur. • Implementation goals are then written down for the patient and the clinician. • In subsequent sessions, the clinician can facilitate further goal setting and check on existing goals.
Stimulus control	• During the assessment, the clinician is alert to ways that the patient's home environment triggers unhelpful dietary practices, sedentary behavior, and low levels of physical activity. • The clinician will ask further questions and request agreement to change obesity-conducive factors in the home environment. • With the help of the clinician, the patient's parents may agree to form some new household rules which address the unhelpful environmental triggers. • Common examples include not eating in front of the television, only turning on the television when a family member plans to watch a particular show, or not using the family car to drive children to school on a regular basis.
Self-monitoring	• The clinician decides on a behavior (or group of behaviors) that contribute to obesity and of which the patient would benefit from becoming more aware. • The clinician shows the parent a monitoring form (see Fig. 8.1) and explains what they will monitor and for how long. • Together the patient and the clinician work through a retrospective example to learn how monitoring works. • The clinician covers details such as where the monitoring form will be kept and when is the best time for the parent to monitor. • In the following session, the clinician asks to see the form and is careful to praise any compliance.

(continued)

Table 8.5
(continued)

Key behavior modification technique	Example of how a clinician can apply this technique in a pediatric weight management session
	• The parent or adolescent patient is asked some basic questions about adherence to the self-monitoring ("Were you able to do it every day?," "Did you find it helpful?").
	• Through this discussion and the information gleaned from the monitoring forms, the clinician and the parent settle on a new behavioral goal of, for instance, reducing the child's screen time from approximately 5 h/day to 3 h/day. They discuss ways that this goal could be reached.
	• The parent is given new forms and asked to monitor for another week. The intention now is to collect data on whether this reduction is occurring. The clinician assures the parent that they will not have to monitor forever because it is more important to do it in the early stages of changing a very frequent behavior.

Table 8.6
Examples of new technologies used to deliver behavior modification

Technology	Behavior modification function
Short Message Service (SMS) or Multimedia Message Service sent to patient's mobile phone	Prompts behaviors by acting as a reminder. Patients can send replies to questions so that it makes very simple monitoring easier.
Internet monitoring	May be a more convenient form of monitoring for some patients. Some programs (such as those working out or totaling calories) provide instant feedback and so may increase adherence.
Monitoring forms available on the internet	Reminder for clinicians to incorporate behavior modification into their treatment. Encourages patient information gathering. Easy way to obtain self-monitoring forms. Examples can be found on: www.healthy-child.org

Table 8.7

Gaps in the evidence base for treating childhood obesity [1][a]

- What interventions are most effective at different levels of obesity severity and at different ages and developmental stages?
- What strategies are most effective for long-term maintenance of healthy weight or reduced weight following initial treatment of obesity?
- What are the family characteristics that promote success in the treatment of child and adolescent obesity?
- What interventions are most effective for specific ethnicities, religious groups, or culturally diverse populations?
- What is the role of psychological and social factors such as self-esteem and the family's capacity to change behavior in the treatment and management of child and adolescent obesity?
- What are the most cost- and resource-effective methods of treating child and adolescent obesity in different health care settings?
- What is the role of bariatric surgery in the treatment of severely obese adolescents?
- What are the potential harms as well as benefits of different interventions?

[a]Derived from the 2009 Cochrane review on treating obesity in children [1]

Table 8.8

Potential barriers to behavioral change in families attending obesity treatment programs

Barrier	Effect	Potential intervention strategy
Poverty	Limited access to healthy food	Focus on low-cost food alternatives
	Limited access to activities and recreation space	Provision of low-cost physical activity alternatives
Culturally and linguistically diverse patients	Service may not be provided in their first language	Use of interpreters
	Cultural practices may not fit with standard advice on diet and activity	Culturally sensitive weight management advice
Learning disabilities or developmental disorders	Limited ability to benefit from education about diet and activity	Greater family involvement Intensive practical intervention Involvement of specialist support services

(continued)

Table 8.8
(continued)

Barrier	Effect	Potential intervention strategy
Family in crisis (*e.g.*, domestic violence)	Child or family is at risk, and unable to focus on weight management	Crisis intervention Case management until the situation has stabilized Involvement of additional support services such as child protection or social work
Psychiatric disorders	Unable to attend treatment or focus on weight management Poor motivation At risk	Involvement of mental health treatment and support services Case management until the situation has stabilized
Physical health problems	May not be able to participate in physical activity due to functional limitations	Provide alternative options

Thus, the current evidence base of behavioral management of obesity will need to be adapted for use in such clinical situations. How do you provide services when patients have a range of psychiatric or social problems and where the therapists are unlikely to include a social worker or clinical psychologist? There is an urgent need for obesity management studies performed in such everyday "real-life" clinical situations.

REFERENCES

1. Oude Luttikhuis H, Baur L, Jansen H *et al.* (2009) Interventions for treating obesity in children. Cochrane Database Syst Rev (1):CD001872. DOI: 10.1002/14651858. CD001872.pub2
2. Martin G, Pear J (2010) Behaviour modification: what it is and how to do it, 9th edn. Simon and Schuster, Englewood Cliffs
3. Golan M, Crow S (2004) Targeting parents exclusively in the treatment of childhood obesity: long term results. Obes Res 12:357–361
4. Epstein LH, Myers MD, Raynor HA, Saelens BE (1998) Treatment of pediatric obesity. Pediatrics 101:554–570
5. McLean N, Griffin S, Toney K, Hardeman W (2003) Family involvement in weight control, weight maintenance and weight-loss interventions: a systematic review of randomised trials. Int J Obes 27:978–1005
6. Wing RR (2002) Behavioral weight control. In: Wadden TA, Stuckard AJ (eds) [*Handbook of Obesity Treatment*]. Guilford Press, New York, pp 301–316
7. Saelens BE, Sallis JF, Wilfley DE, Patrick K, Cella JA, Buchta R (2002) Behavioral weight control for overweight adolescents initiated in primary care. Obes Res 10:22–32

8. National Health and Medical Research Council of Australia (2003) Clinical practice guidelines for the management of overweight and obesity in children and adolescents. National Health and Medical Research Council, Canberra

9. National Institute for Health and Clinical Excellence (2006) Obesity: guidance on the prevention, identification, assessment and management of overweight and obesity in adults and children. National Institute for Health and Clinical Excellence, London. Available at http://www.nice.org.uk/nicemedia/pdf/CG43NICEGuideline.pdf. Accessed Aug 2010

10. Robinson TN (1999) Behavioural treatment of child and adolescent obesity. Int J Obes Relat Metab Disord 23(Suppl 2):S52–S57

11. Dietz WH, Robinson TN (2005) Overweight children and adolescents. N Engl J Med 352:2100–2110

12. Melin I, Rossner S (2003) Practical clinical behavioural treatment of obesity. Patient Educ Counsel 49:75–83

13. Brennan L, Walkley J, Lukeis S et al. (2009) A cognitive behavioural intervention for overweight and obese adolescents illustrated by four case studies. Behav Change 26:190–213

14. Epstein LH, Paluch RA, Gordy CC, Dorm J (2000) Decreasing sedentary behaviours in treating pediatric obesity. Arch Pediatr Adolesc Med 154:220–226

15. Gollwitzer PM (1999) Implementation intentions: strong effects of simple plans. Am Psychol 54:493–503

16. Epstein LH, Paluch RA, Gordy CC, Saelens BE, Ernst MM (2000) Problem solving in the treatment of childhood obesity. J Consult Clin Psychol 68:717–721

17. Gollwitzer PM, Oettingen G (2007) The role of goal setting and goal striving in medical adherence. In: Park DC, Liu LL (eds) Medical adherence and aging: social and cognitive perspective. American Psychological Association, Washington, pp 23–47

18. Wansink B, Sobal J (2007) Mindless eating: the 200 daily food decisions we overlook. Environ Behav 39:106–123

19. Wansink B, van Ittersum K, Painter JE (2006) Ice cream illusions: bowls, spoons, and self-served portion sizes. Am J Prev Med 31:240–243

20. Sobal J, Wansink B (2007) Kitchenscapes, tablescapes, platescapes, and foodscapes: influences of microscale built environments on food intake. Environ Behav 39:124–142

21. Wansink B, Kim J (2005) Bad popcorn in big buckets: portion size can influence intake as much as taste. J Nutr Educ Behav 37:242–245

22. Wansink B (2010) From mindlessly eating to mindlessly eating better. Physiol Behav 100:454–463

23. Wansink B, van Ittersum K (2005) Shape of glass and amount of alcohol poured: comparative study of effect of practice and concentration. Br Med J 331:1512–1514

24. Wansink B (2006) Mindless eating: why we eat more than we think? Bantam Del, New York

25. Saelens BE, McGrath AM (2003) Self-monitoring adherence and adolescent weight control efficacy. Child Health Care 32:137–152

26. Kirschenbaum DS, Germann JN, Rich BH (2006) Treatment of morbid obesity in low-income adolescents: effects of parental self-monitoring. Obes Res 13:1527–1529

27. Germann JN, Kirschenbaum DS, Rich BH (2007) Child and parental self-monitoring as determinants of success in the treatment of morbid obesity in low-income minority children. J Pediatr Psychol 32:111–121

28. Norman GJ, Zabinski MF, Adams MA et al. (2007) A review of ehealth interventions for physical activity and dietary behaviour change. Am J Prev Med 33:336–345

29. Baulch J, Chester A, Brennan L (2008) Treatment alternatives for overweight and obesity: the role of online interventions. Behav Change 25:1–14
30. Lobstein T, Baur L, Uauy R (2004) Obesity in children and young people: A crisis in public health. Report of the International Obesity TaskForce Childhood Obesity Working Group. Obes Rev 5:4–104

9 Surgical Approaches to Pediatric Obesity

Aayed Al-Qahtani

Key Points

- Strict patient selection, careful preoperative preparation, and close post operative care are critical to successful outcomes with bariatric procedures.
- Laparoscopic gastric banding appears to be the best available option currently for pediatric obesity, followed by sleeve gastrectomy.
- Bariatric surgery should be performed at highly specialized centers with substantial pediatric subspecialty and surgical expertise on site.

Keywords: Bariatric surgery, Pediatric obesity, Roux-en-Y gastric bypass, RYGB, Laparoscopic gastric banding, Sleeve gastrectomy, Obesity, Children, Adolescents, Preoperative evaluation, Postoperative management

9.1 INTRODUCTION

Bariatric surgery is the most effective and longest-lasting treatment for morbid obesity and many related conditions in selected patients. Surgery for severe obesity displays benefits beyond weight loss. Mounting evidence suggests that bariatric surgery is among the most effective treatments for metabolic complications of morbid obesity, including type 2 diabetes mellitus (T2DM), hypertension, hypercholesterolemia, nonalcoholic fatty liver disease (NAFLD), and obstructive sleep apnea (OSA) [1]. Surgery results in the complete remission or significant improvement of T2DM and other life-threatening diseases in most morbidly obese patients. Significant debate

From: *Nutrition and Health: Management of Pediatric Obesity and Diabetes*,
Edited by: R.J. Ferry, Jr., DOI 10.1007/978-1-60327-256-8_9,
© Springer Science+Business Media, LLC 2011

surrounds the risks and benefits of bariatric surgery in the adolescent population, yet contemporary studies demonstrate the success of this option for appropriate patients [2–4]. Up to 1% of patients who have received bariatric surgery are under age 18 years. Significantly, over 2,000 pediatric patients (ages 21 or younger) in the United States underwent bariatric surgery in 2004, and 75% of bariatric surgeons planned to perform adolescent bariatric surgery in 2005 [3, 4].

9.2 PATIENT SELECTION AND SURGICAL INDICATIONS

9.2.1 General Criteria

When considering weight loss surgery in children and adolescents, the indications, the type of procedure, and the age at which it can be performed remain controversial. A consensus panel convened by the U.S. National Institutes of Health has proposed indications for bariatric surgery in *adults* [5]. Generally, adults with body mass index (BMI) $\geq$40 kg/m^2 with or without comorbidities, or BMI $\geq$35 kg/m^2 with comorbidities, are considered candidates for bariatric surgery. This panel specifically avoided making a recommendation for the treatment of patients younger than 18 years.

A task force convened by the American Pediatric Surgical Association (APSA) addressed this issue and recommended more conservative indications for pediatric bariatric surgery than those for adults [6]. Evidence suggests that early surgical intervention in extreme obesity provides the best chance to reverse comorbidities [7–9].

However, the author argues that available data support more aggressive treatment of adolescent obesity by using established adult criteria. The primary rationale is threefold. First, children and adolescents tend to display relatively more obesity and comorbidities than adults at the time of clinical presentation. Second, children and adolescents stand to suffer a greater loss of life span and productivity from untreated obesity (than adults). Third, children and adolescents currently lack any effective medical alternatives for chronic weight maintenance or weight loss. Clearly, more medical research is needed for pediatric patients. Thus, our criteria to consider pediatric patients for surgery resemble those for adults, but also include a supportive family environment, being involved in a weight management program for at least 6 months, and willingness and motivation by the patient and patient's family both to undergo surgery and to follow strict postoperative instructions. Based on our clinical experience, an algorithm is suggested (Fig. 9.1).

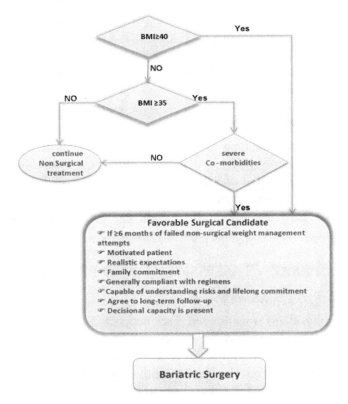

Fig. 9.1. Children and adolescent bariatric surgery decision making algorithm.

9.2.2 Early Intervention

Recently, adults with BMI ≥35 kg/m² (without comorbidity) have been accepted for bariatric surgery. For example, the nationwide Swedish Obese Subjects (SOS) study accepts men with BMI ≥34 kg/m² (without requirement of diagnosed comorbidity) [10]. One valid argument for early intervention is the fact that the duration of exposure to obesity decreases the likelihood of sustainable remission or cure [11]. In children and adolescents, the early but intense intervention of bariatric surgery should remain an exceptional plan of care for those few patients who are significantly impaired by their obesity.

9.2.3 Age Limits

Setting age limits for surgery is complex. A legitimate concern about bariatric surgery is potentially adverse growth sequelae. This concern can become reality for those procedures that result in significant malabsorption (*e.g.*, gastric bypass). However, in our experience, procedures like gastric banding and sleeve gastrectomy (SG) are relatively safe in younger patients. We have performed gastric banding on patients as young as 8 years of age who continued their normal growth until the end of adolescence. Long-term follow-up is mandatory to decide the cutoff age.

9.2.4 Predictors of Outcomes

Poor patient understanding of the surgical expectation and the required postoperative protocols will result in poor outcomes. Psychosocial issues impact treatment of obesity and its related problems. In addition, the abilities of the patient and family to comply with the treating team's instructions are mandatory for achieving acceptable weight reduction. Surgical and nutritional complications also predict poor outcomes from bariatric surgery [12].

9.3 PREOPERATIVE ASSESSMENT AND PREPARATION

9.3.1 Clinical Evaluation

Prudent physicians recommend and support a comprehensive team approach. An ideal team would be located within a children's medical center and encompass a minimum of four components: medical, nutritional, psychological, and surgical. This multidisciplinary team evaluates the patient before surgery and remains engaged in education and treatment after surgery. This evaluation promotes optimal medical, nutritional, and psychological care and facilitates good insight into the lifelong lifestyle changes required after bariatric surgery.

9.3.2 Surgical Assessment

Once the patient completes the preoperative medical, nutritional, and psychological evaluation and has achieved adequate metabolic control of any medical problems, he or she can be considered for bariatric surgery. The surgeon evaluates the patient's motivation and expectations, discusses the risks and benefits of different surgical interventions, excludes any absolute contraindications to surgery or anesthesia (Table 9.1), and recommends the most appropriate procedure for each individual patient.

9.3.3 Preoperative Work Up

Preoperative screening includes serum chemistry and lipid profiles, complete blood count, fasting blood glucose and insulin levels, glucose tolerance tests, hemoglobin A_{1C}, urinalysis, and thyroid function tests (typically serum thyrotropin and free T_4 levels). The preliminary evaluation may prompt consultation with a pediatric cardiologist, pediatric pulmonologist,

Table 9.1
Contraindications for bariatric surgery in children and adolescents

- Adolescents and children or their family do not comprehend risks and benefits of the intervention
- Adolescents and children are not autonomously motivated to consider operation
- Adolescents and children have unrealistic expectations for results of the surgical intervention
- Family/patients cannot commit strictly to comply with postoperative nutritional recommendations and long-term medical and nutritional monitoring
- History of noncompliance with treatment regimens or scheduled healthcare provider visits (although personal experience of the author suggests such families may become fairly compliant after surgery)
- Presence of a medically correctable cause of obesity (relative contraindication)
- Existence of a medical, psychiatric, or cognitive condition which may impair the ability of patient to assent to surgery or to adhere to postoperative dietary and medication regimen (relative contraindication)
- Illicit substance abuse in preceding year
- Current lactation, current pregnancy, or plans for pregnancy in upcoming 2 years
- Inability to provide informed assent (patient) and consent (family)

and pediatric endocrinologist. ACTH provocative testing, fasting morning serum cortisol, 24-h urinary free cortisol, serum FSH, serum LH, serum prolactin, or other endocrine evaluations are often needed to identify/ exclude underlying causes of obesity. Genetic consultation and genetic screening for common syndromes (*e.g.*, Prader-Willi) are indicated based on clinical judgment. Echocardiogram, sleep studies, and pulmonary function tests should be performed when clinically indicated (Table 9.2). Comorbidities guide extended preoperative testing, in accordance with recommendations from the American Society of Anesthesiologists (ASA) practice advisory on preanesthesia evaluation [13]. A preoperative evaluation by an anesthetist is recommended, preferably at least 1 month before surgery.

9.3.4 Preoperative Counseling

It is strongly recommended to have several counseling sessions with the patient along with their families prior to surgery. Our center conducts *three* preoperative sessions. Realistic expectations about various timelines, the possible complications, and their minimizing measures – along with a good understanding of the surgical procedure – go a long way toward appropriate

Table 9.2
Preoperative evaluation before pediatric bariatric surgery

Laboratory studies
Baseline studies must include current complete blood count (CBC),
   comprehensive serum chemistry panel, liver profiling (AST, ALT, GTT,
   albumin, total and direct bilirubin in all; consider hepatitis titers and
   serum ceruloplasmin for suspected comorbidities), thyroid function
   tests (serum thyrotropin and free T_4 levels), fasting serum lipid profile
   (cholesterol, HDL, LDL, triglycerides), fasting serum insulin, fasting
   blood dextrose, hemoglobin A_{1C} (optional), blood typing, urinalysis, serum
   total iron-binding capacity, ferritin, transferrin, vitamin B1, vitamin B12.
   Additionally, the following test can be indicated in some cases: ACTH,
   serum and/or 24-hour urinary free cortisol, FSH, LLH, Prolactin
Optional tests include
• A.M. 2-h oral glucose tolerance test (OGTT), performed with 25 g/kg
   Glucola PO with serum glucose and insulin values at baseline before
   Glucola, then 60 and 120 min post-Glucola
• *H. pylori* serology
Imaging studies
Ultrasonography of the gallbladder
In select patients, one or more of the following studies: plain chest radiog-
   raphy, bone age (plain anteroposterior radiograph of the nondominant left
   hand and wrist), echocardiography, DEXA scan
Diagnostic procedures
Electrocardiogram (if abnormal, perform Doppler echocardiography)
In select patients, pulmonary function test
If OSA suggested by history, perform sleep apnea study

compliance postoperatively. During these sessions, we distribute instructions
and demonstration booklets, explaining the procedures and the strict postoperative care and diet. The discussion weighs risks and benefits of the procedure and rationale for the choice of procedure to suit the individual patient.

9.3.5   Concurrent and Preoperative Medications

It is recommended that the patient's usual medications, except insulin
and oral hypoglycemics, be continued until the time of surgery. Antibiotic
prophylaxis reduces the otherwise increased risk of postoperative wound
infection [14, 15]. Anxiolysis, analgesia, and prophylaxis against both
aspiration pneumonia and deep vein thrombosis (DVT) should be addressed
during premedication. Oral benzodiazepines are reliable for anxiolysis and
sedation with little or no respiratory depression. Intravenous midazolam
can also be titrated in small doses for anxiolysis during the immediate

preoperative period. H_2-receptor antagonists and proton pump inhibitors reduce gastric volume, acidity, or both, thereby reducing the risk and complications of aspiration, and help in the healing of the gastric mucosa after SG. Morbid obesity is a major independent risk factor for sudden death from acute postoperative pulmonary embolism (PE) [16, 17]. Heparin administered before surgery and repeated every 12 h until the patient became fully mobile does reduce the risk of DVT [18]. Recently, low molecular weight heparins (LMWH) have gained popularity in thromboembolism prophylaxis, because of their bioavailability when injected subcutaneously [19]. In combination with subcutaneous heparin, we favor placement of pneumatic compression devices below the knee or full thigh length.

9.4 ANESTHETIC CONSIDERATIONS IN THE OBESE

9.4.1 Anesthesia for Bariatric Surgery

Anesthetic management of the obese, otherwise healthy, child can be challenging and has been reported to be associated with a higher incidence of critical incidents during anesthesia [20]. It is widely assumed that general anesthesia among obese adults is associated with an overall increased risk of peri-operative respiratory and cardiac complications. Pulmonary physiological derangements which accompany *adult* obesity include decreased functional residual capacity (FRC), forced vital capacity (FVC), and forced expiratory volume in 1 s (FEV1). *Pediatric* studies replicated these findings [21, 22]. During general anesthesia, obese adults are more likely to develop rapid oxygen desaturation during periods of apnea [23] and to exhibit lower tissue oxygen levels at a given arterial partial pressure of oxygen (pO_2) [24]. Minor respiratory complications following elective surgery are noted to be more common in obese adults compared with their lean counterparts [20, 25].

Obesity is also associated with increased intra-abdominal pressure and decreased lower esophageal sphincter tone. Although it has been widely perceived that obese patients are at increased risk for aspiration during anesthesia induction, this concept has been challenged. Warner *et al.* [26] found no correlation between obesity and pulmonary aspiration in a retrospective review of 215,488 general anesthetic episodes in *adults*. Similarly, in a retrospective review of 50,880 pediatric anesthetics, only one of the 52 patients who aspirated was obese, and this aspiration was of blood – not stomach contents – during dental surgery [27].

9.4.2 Sleep Apnea

It is imperative that while planning for surgery for obese patients, both the surgeon and the anesthetist are aware of the potential risks of pre- and postoperative complications in patients with OSA. Among obese adults presenting for gastric bypass surgery, as many as 70% displayed OSA on polysomnography that had not been diagnosed previously [28–31]. Patients with OSA are particularly sensitive to opioid and sedative medications, and many require continuous positive airway pressure (CPAP) at night. CPAP can complicate the postoperative course, because it is important to minimize pressure on the new anastomosis in cases of SG or gastric bypass.

9.4.3   Intraoperative Considerations

9.4.3.1   POSITIONING

Specially designed tables, or two regular tables joined together, facilitate safe anesthesia for bariatric surgery. Regular operating room tables support a maximum weight limit of ≈205 kg. Some operating tables can hold up to 455 kg, with a little extra width to accommodate the extra girth. Electrically operated or motorized tables facilitate maneuvering into various surgically favorable positions. Bariatric surgical patients are prone to slipping off the operating table during table position changes; therefore, they should be well strapped to the operating table. Particular care should be paid to protecting pressure areas, because pressure sores and neural injuries are more common in this group, especially in super obese and diabetic patients [32].

9.4.3.2   MONITORING

Standard ASA intraoperative monitoring protocols [13] include electrocardiogram, blood pressure, oxygen saturation, inspired oxygen concentration, and end-tidal carbon dioxide values. In addition, these cases require assessment of body temperature and measures to maintain normothermia during bariatric surgery. Physicians should use alternate sites for noninvasive blood pressure measurements (*e.g.*, the forearm). Invasive hemodynamic measurements should only be used when medically necessary.

9.4.3.3   INDUCTION, INTUBATION, AND MAINTENANCE OF ANESTHESIA

Concern about airway management in the obese patient is appropriate, but is probably less important than earlier thought. The vast majority of patients are easily managed with simple precautions. Anticipate the possibility of a difficult intubation. A towel or folded blankets under the shoulders and head can compensate for the exaggerated flexed position from posterior cervical fat [33]. The object of this maneuver, known as "stacking," is to position the patient so that the tip of the chin is at a higher level than the chest, which facilitates laryngoscopy and intubation.

9.4.3.4 PHARMACOLOGY/WEIGHT-BASED DOSING

Proper dosing of many medications for patients with severe obesity is uncertain. It is reasonable to base dosing close to the estimated lean body mass (approximately 120% of ideal body weight, IBW), then adjust as needed. Desflurane has been suggested as the inhaled anesthetic of choice in obese patients because of its rapid and consistent recovery profile [34]. Two different studies [35, 36] compared sevoflurane with isoflurane for use during bariatric surgery. These investigators favored sevoflurane for its rapid recovery, good hemodynamic control, infrequent incidence of nausea and vomiting, prompt regaining of psychological and physical functioning, early discharge from the hospital, and small cost. Rapid elimination and analgesia make nitrous oxide acceptable during bariatric surgery, but high oxygen demand in the obese limits its use. Obesity increases oxygen consumption and carbon dioxide production [37] due to excess metabolically active tissue and an increased workload on muscles and other supportive tissue.

Complete muscular relaxation is crucial during laparoscopic bariatric procedures to facilitate ventilation and to maintain an adequate working space for visualization and safe manipulation of laparoscopic instruments. Complete relaxation also facilitates the introduction of surgical equipment and extraction of excised tissues. Collapse of the intentional, iatrogenic pneumoperitoneum may be an early indication that muscle relaxation is inadequate, because muscle tone competes with the pressure limit set for the pneumoperitoneum. Tightening of the musculature around the surgeon's finger palpating the port site may also be a sign of inadequate paralysis. Tidal volumes >13 mL/kg IBW offer no added advantage during ventilation of morbidly obese patients during anesthesia [38, 39].

9.4.3.5 OTHER TECHNICAL ISSUES

Anesthesiologists help facilitate proper placement of an intragastric balloon and nasogastric (NG) tube during surgery to help the surgeon size the gastric pouch in bypass and gastric sleeve (GS). They also perform leak tests with saline and methylene blue (or air) to ensure anastomotic integrity. Care should be taken during injection of saline or methylene blue through the NG tube to ensure that the endotracheal tube cuff maintains a tight seal; otherwise, aspiration of methylene blue can occur, leading to chemical pneumonitis. It is important to completely remove all endogastric tubes (not just merely pull them back into the esophagus) before gastric division in gastric bypass surgery, to avoid unplanned stapling and transection of these devices. The anesthesiologist should *not* blindly reinsert the NG tube; in this situation, the monitor should be watched carefully while the NG tube is advanced, to avoid disruption of the anastomosis.

9.5   TYPES OF BARIATRIC SURGERY IN ADOLESCENTS AND CHILDREN

9.5.1   Current Procedures

Current bariatric surgical procedures can be classified by the mechanism of weight reduction: (1) *restrictive*, by decreasing the storage capacity of the stomach; (2) *malabsorptive*, through surgical bypass thus excluding intestinal loops; or (3) a combination of restrictive and malabsorptive. The restrictive procedures include laparoscopic gastric banding (LAGB), vertical banded gastroplasty (VBG), and sleeve gastrectomy (SG). The malabsorptive includes jejuno-ileal bypass (JIB), bilio-pancreatic diversion (BPD), and BPD with duodenal switch (BPD/DS). Gastric bypass has both restrictive and malabsorptive effects. Historically, both the JIB and the BPD were performed in adolescents in the 1970s and 1980s [40, 41]. Both have since been abandoned, due to the large malabsorptive component of these procedures and high risk of nutritional complications, morbidity, and mortality from bypassing the majority of the small intestine [41–43].

The modified BPD-DS preserves a cuff of duodenum and lengthens the common small intestinal channel. It has been performed in a small number of adolescents [44]; yet, it carries an increased risk of malabsorptive complications and requires lifelong nutritional supplementation. Therefore, it is rarely performed in adolescents with extreme BMIs. A small number of adolescents also received VBG in the 1990s [45] with modest weight loss and higher risk of postsurgical complications. This procedure is also no longer performed in adolescents. The three main surgical options for adolescents at present include the Roux-en-Y gastric bypass (RYGB), LAGB, and SG.

9.5.2   Roux-en-Y Gastric Bypass

RYGB (Fig. 9.2) remains the most commonly performed procedure in United States [46], comprising 90% of adolescent bariatric surgery cases in 2003 [4]. This procedure integrates restriction with altered absorption. RYGB has been used for surgical weight loss in adolescents since the 1980s [4, 47–49]. Technically, RYGB involves formation of a 15–20-mL gastric pouch plus fashioning of a Roux-en-Y gastrojejunostomy bypassing the fundus body of the stomach, the duodenum, and a variable length of proximal jejunum. The Roux limb is typically 75–150 cm in length and is anastomosed to the gastric pouch. This effectively reduces the size of meal that

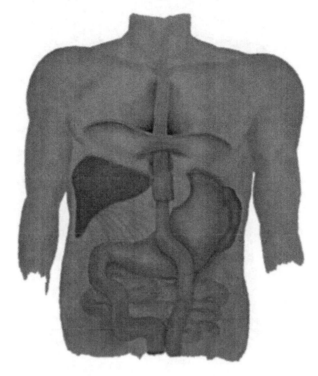

Fig. 9.2. The Roux-en-Y gastric bypass (RYGB).

the patient is able to ingest. Additionally, the bypass causes some degree of malabsorption and may have important physiologic consideration.

9.5.3 Laparoscopic Gastric Banding

LAGB (Fig. 9.3) is by far the most popular restrictive bariatric surgical intervention in Europe and Australia. LAGB is rapidly gaining popularity in the USA after receiving approval from the Food and Drug Administration in 2001 [50]. The procedure involves the placement of an inflatable band to form a 15–20-mL superior gastric pouch, with band position reinforced by the placement of anterior gastro-gastric sutures. The band connects to a self-sealing reservoir (*e.g.*, Portacath) implanted in the subcutaneous plane. This allows for adjustment of the stoma diameter to increase or reduce the rate of passage of food from the upper pouch into the body of the stomach. The LAGB is completely *reversible* as no part of the intestinal tract is divided.

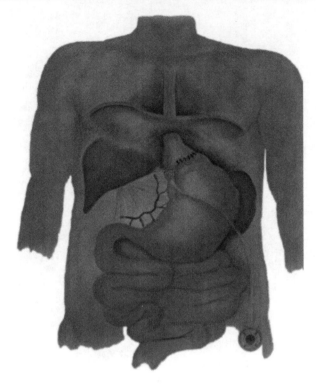

Fig. 9.3. Gastric banding.

9.5.4 Sleeve Gastrectomy

Also called greater-curvature, vertical, or longitudinal gastrectomy, SG is the first stage of BPD-DS. It is a form of unbanded gastroplasty involving sub-total (≈80%) gastric resection for creation of a long, lesser curve-based, gastric conduit (Fig. 9.4a–c). No portion of the intestinal tract is bypassed, but the fundus and greater curve of the stomach are removed. As an isolated procedure, the gastric pouch size usually varies from 60 to 120 mL, depending on the size of the bougie. We use a 36 French bougie to form a narrow lesser curve gastric tube that can be smaller or larger based on the size used. SG is gaining popularity due to a predictably lower risk of nutritional complications and weight loss performance that is potentially comparable to other procedures [44].

In 2003, SG was proposed as the first step of a two-stage laparoscopic Roux-en-Y gastric bypass (LRYGB) in adults [51]. Since then, many surgical teams adopted this procedure in adults with good results [52]. SG produces weight loss by two mechanisms. First, it produces early satiety as a purely restrictive procedure. Second, it reduces plasma ghrelin levels in addition to other physiological changes. We started offering laparoscopic SG for obese

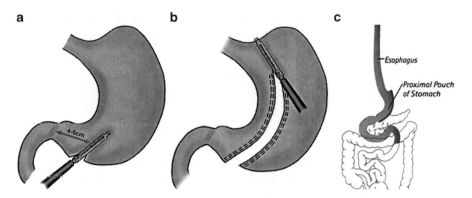

Fig. 9.4. (a) Starting gastric resection 4-6 cm from the pylorus (b) Completing the resection (c) The final look of the gastrointestinal tract after Gastric Sleeve.

children and adolescents in 2006. Forty-five candidates underwent LSG in our institution with a mean excess weight loss of 62% at 1-year follow-up. This outcome is encouraging and comparable to outcomes from other procedures.

9.5.5 *Choosing the Procedure*

For children and adolescents, the ideal bariatric surgical intervention is effective, safe, and applicable to all patients. Surgery must achieve considerable weight loss and resolution of comorbidity. Low operative morbidity and mortality is essential, with a short hospital stay, rapid return to normal activity, and – most important – reversible. The author opines that LAGB is now the *best* available option for pediatric obesity, followed by SG. Furthermore, gastric bypass should not be the first choice in children and adolescents. Certainly, all candidates are informed about all therapeutic options, including the advantages and disadvantages of each. SG is recommended for those unable to be very punctual with the banding adjustment protocol. Gastric bypass is very difficult to reverse in pediatric patients and can only be partially reversed.

9.6 PHYSIOLOGY OF BARIATRIC SURGERY

9.6.1 *Gastric Banding (LAGB)*

LAGB works by restricting the amount of food that can be eaten at a single meal, while also producing a feeling of fullness that persists between meals. Food fills and distends the small upper gastric pouch, producing a sensation of being full. By restricting the passage of food out of the pouch, the LAGB prolongs the feeling of fullness. This intrameal satiety is the key to making the LAGB effective. Additionally, esophageal and cardiac distention results in increased activity in areas of the brain that are involved in appetite regulation [53–55]. The other variable that has an impact on the function of the LAGB is the consistency of the food that fills the pouch.

Solid food achieves the best result because it effectively fills the pouch and slowly passes on to the distal stomach. Soft foods and liquids are less likely to achieve a good effect, because they empty from the pouch quickly and cannot produce prolonged satiety.

9.6.2 Gastric Sleeve

GS works by removing the storage capacity of the stomach. A subjective feeling of fullness results from a much smaller amount of food. Several studies on the amount of time it takes the new stomach to empty are somewhat in conflict; therefore, the stomach transit time is of doubtful reliability. A slower transit time would improve the feeling of fullness (satiety), but a faster transit time could help generate hormones that exert a negative effect on hunger (e.g., Peptide tyrosine tyrosine PYY, and Phosphoinositide PIP). These are generated in the duodenum, and their action is not yet well understood [56–59].

One intestinal hormone shown to be favorably affected by the GS operation is ghrelin. Ghrelin is produced in the part of the stomach that is removed, which is why circulating ghrelin level drops to a low level after the operation [56]. Ghrelin is important for how the brain perceives hunger, and low circulating ghrelin levels reduce hunger.

Due to a combination of the above factors, GS has demonstrated excellent weight loss for almost all patients. GS produces weight loss equal or superior to gastric banding, but without implantation of a foreign body and with the advantage to avoid some complications related to rearrangement of the intestinal tract (seen with the gastric bypass). These features make GS a very attractive option for obese children and adolescents.

9.6.3 Roux-en-Y Gastric Bypass (RYGB)

RYGB works by restricting the amount of food that can be eaten at a single meal. The small gastric pouch varies somewhere between 15 and 30 mL in size. This allows only a few ounces of solid food at a time. Eating too much volume will produce discomfort and eventually vomiting, both of which reinforce eating small amounts of food slowly. In addition, since no food will pass through the distal stomach and proximal intestine, there is a degree of malabsorption and little stimulation for the production of most intestinal hormones. For example, ghrelin stays at a very low level after RYGB [56]. As a result, most patients do not suffer wide swings in hunger shortly after eating, and the drive to eat is generally diminished.

9.6.4 Aspects Common to All Bariatric Surgery Procedures

Aspects of appetite control relevant to bariatric surgery are fatty acid secretion from lipolysis and ketone body formation from the catabolism induced by rapid weight loss. Free fatty acids and ketone bodies inhibit food intake in mammals [60]. Starvation *per se* results in increased cortisol levels and cytokines released from adipose tissue, both of which can exert centrally mediated appetite-reducing effects.

9.6.5 Eating Behavior Adaptation

In children and adolescents, maladaptive eating could predict failure of weight loss after bariatric surgery. Efforts should be directed towards good preoperative assessments and treatment of existing potential obstacles in order to normalize eating behavior and to identify the risk factors for development of maladaptive eating disorder postoperatively. Bariatric surgical procedures are excellent tools to change unhealthy eating behavior and teach the proper ones and must be reemphasized as such in all patients.

9.7 POSTOPERATIVE MANAGEMENT AND FOLLOW-UP PROTOCOLS

9.7.1 Postoperative Care on Priority

Obese children and adolescent patients require close postoperative observations. Patients with a history of OSA or other significant comorbidities should be admitted to a unit with strict postoperative monitoring (*e.g.*, intensive care unit). Some patients require the use of CPAP or bi-level positive airway pressure. Early postoperative ambulation and use of incentive spirometry should be initiated as soon as possible to reduce the pulmonary dysfunction and reduce the risk of DVT and PE. We always ask our patient to ambulate later on the day of surgery. Adequate analgesia is crucial in allowing early ambulation and restoring the pulmonary function. The nursing staff plays a vital role in the management of the obese child. Hospitals should be prepared to care for the obese patient population. Bariatric beds, transport devices to bring the patients to and from the operating room, should be large enough to accommodate the morbidly obese patient group. Radiological equipment, such as CT scanners and interventional radiology tables, should be capable of supporting these patients.

9.7.2 Follow-Up Protocol

Patients can plan on going home on the day of gastric banding or the next day, except patients who are living far away or having other medical problems. On the first postoperative day after SG, an optional hydro-soluble contrast study can confirm absence of gastric leaks. The dietician meets with each patient and family to review and instruct on the full postoperative diet protocol, based on the operation performed (Table 9.3).

Table 9.3

Recommendation for follow-up with the obesity management team after bariatric surgery

Postprocedure (years)	RYGB	LAGB	Sleeve gastrectomy
1	Months 1, 3, 6, 12	First visit at 2 weeks; q 4–6 weeks for 6 months, then q 3–6 months (if good weight loss)	First visit at 2 weeks; q 4–6 weeks for 3 months, then q 6 months
2	q 6 months	q 6 months	q 6–12 months
3	Annually	q 6 months	Annually
Long term	Annually	Annually	Annually

RYGB Roux-en Y gastric bypass; *LAGB* laparoscopic adjustable gastric banding

9.7.3 Postoperative Diet

Specific diet instructions and guidelines are very critical in achieving the goals of weight less and minimizing the complications (Tables 9.4 and 9.5).

9.7.4 Physical Activity

For laparoscopic procedures, there are minimal restrictions other than activities that cause pain. Patients are encouraged to walk frequently beginning the day of surgery and to breathe deeply and cough frequently. They are advised to make the long-term goal of 30–60 min of exercise daily.

9.7.5 Bathing

The patient may shower 2 days after surgery. However, baths and swimming should be avoided for at least 2 weeks.

9.8 COMPLICATIONS AND OUTCOMES

We will limit discussion to the most frequently performed or acceptable operations in children and the adolescent, namely gastric banding, SG, and gastric bypass (Table 9.6).

9.8.1 Complications of Laparoscopic Gastric Banding

The main complication of gastric banding is slippage. As this process progresses, regurgitation and vomiting during the night becomes a feature. The ultimate result is complete obstruction with signs of incarceration of the

Table 9.4

Postoperative diet following gastric banding

- Clear liquid diet for 24 h after surgery (examples: popsicles, Jell-O, chicken and/or beef broth, Crystal Light)
- Full liquids for the next 2 weeks (examples: protein shakes, low-fat yogurt, sugar-free pudding, skim milk, cream of wheat, etc.)
- Chopped/diced foods for following 3–4 weeks (examples: flaked tuna fish, finely chopped chicken and vegetables, diced fruits, etc.)
- Thereafter, regular diet as tolerated (ensure to continue with small bites and chew well).
- Take pills/tablets one at a time.
- Eat a minimum of 60–80 g of protein per day.
- Avoid drinking and eating at the same time; wait at least 30 min after a meal to resume drinking.
- Liquids will pass through the reduced stomach pouch quickly and will not make you feel full.
- Drinking liquids during or immediately after meals tends to flush food through the pouch, and you will not get the prolonged feeling of satiety needed to help you eat less.
- Staying hydrated throughout the day is important. Drink at least 6–8 cups of water per day, and make sure you consume them between meals.
- Many patients have a difficult time with solid foods during the morning hours. If this is the case for you, you can take a glass of liquid before your first meal.
- Too much food or big chunks of food can block the stomach pouch outlet. You can avoid this problem by chewing food well and eating small bits at a time. It is important to remember that your new stoma opening is approximately the size of a dime. Chew your food adequately so that it can easily fit through the opening.
- Eat only three small meals a day and make sure that these meals contain adequate nutrients. Your stomach can only hold about 1/4 cup of food or 2 oz at a time. Stop eating when your hunger is gone or when you feel comfortable.

proximal pouch. This results from the pressure generated in the proximal pouch from the ingested food. This pressure pushes the band downwards so that more gastric mass is trapped within the band. Pouch formation causes further vomiting and regurgitation. When the gastric mass surpasses its capacity – even if the balloon is completely deflated – pouch incarceration takes place. Slippage of the band can be minimized by following the dietary instruction and by taking a few sero-serosal sutures to the anterior gastric wall. Band erosion is a more gradual process in the wall of the stomach caused by trauma

Table 9.5
Postoperative diet following sleeve gastrectomy

General rules
- Eat slowly and chew thoroughly (at least 25 times).
- Avoid concentrated sugars, especially those in liquid form. They are filled with nonnutrient calories and slow down weight loss.
- Limit fats and fried foods; they are a concentrated source of calories.
- Remember the stomach can only hold 4–6 oz after surgery. You will probably feel satisfied after 2–3 tablespoons of food. Do *not* overeat! Over time your stomach will stretch, but it takes 6–9 months (possibly longer) for your new stomach size to stabilize and allow you to determine your normal meal amount.
- Stop eating when you feel comfortably satisfied. If ignored, vomiting will follow and you can stretch the size of the stomach.
- Drink at least 6–8 cups (8 oz) of fluid per day to prevent dehydration. Monitor for the following signs: headache, dizziness, nausea, lethargy, a whitish coating on the tongue, or dark urine.
- Stop drinking liquids 15 min before meals and resume 30–45 min after meals.
- Eat three small nutrient dense meals and one high-protein snack each day.
- Meals should contain protein first, then fruits and vegetables, and then whole grains.
- Introduce new foods one at a time in order to avoid intolerance. If a food is not tolerated, reintroduce it in 1 week.

Immediate (within 24 h)
Clear, sugar-free liquids
- You will be drinking water, tea, broth, or sugar-free Jell-O.
- Try to sip fluids at the rate of 1 oz/20 min (1–3 oz/h).
- Sipping fluids out of bottles or straws may cause gas. Gas is already a problem after surgery, so you will not want to make it worse.

Pureed liquid diet (week 1)
You will progress to a diet composed of pureed foods low in fat and without sugar. Foods allowed during this diet include: broth, low-fat/light yogurt, sugar-free Jell-O, sugar-free Popsicles, sugar-free fruit drinks, sugar-free pudding, sugar-free Sherbet, water, 1% milk or skim milk.
- To consume 60–80 g of protein per day, drink at least 3 high-protein supplements per day.

Soft diet (3–4 weeks)
- Blender-treated meat and poultry; soft poached eggs
- Low-fat cottage cheese, sugar-free puddings
- Unsweetened applesauce, pureed canned peaches (not in syrup), mashed ripe bananas

(continued)

Table 9.5
(continued)

- Blended soft cooked vegetables, or overcooked and mashed with a fork
- Oatmeal, grits, farina

Solid diet

If you can tolerate the items in the soft diet after 3–4 weeks, you will gradually advance to solids. This modified diet emphasizes lean protein, fruits/vegetables, and whole grains; it deemphasizes fat and sugar.

- This diet is very individualized. It is normal to experience food intolerances. Try to reintroduce that food a week later while focusing on eating slowly, chewing thoroughly, and not overeating.
- You will eventually be able to tolerate a variety of foods from each of the food groups.

Table 9.6
Complications of bariatric surgery

All bariatric procedures	Bypass	Banding	Sleeve
Atelectasis and pneumonia	Anastomotic leak Stomal stenosis	Band slippage band erosion esophageal dilatation	Gastric leak
Deep vein thrombosis	Marginal ulcers	Band or port infections	Obstruction
Pulmonary embolism	Staple line disruption	Port disconnection	Delayed gastric emptying
Wound infection	Nutrient deficiencies (iron, calcium, folic acid, vitamin B1 & B12)	Port displacement	Gastric reflux
Gastrointestinal bleeding	Dumping syndrome		Stricture
Gallstones	Small bowel obstruction		
Failure to lose weight	Internal hernia		
Intractable vomiting			

to the stomach wall during surgery or by the pressure of the band itself. This may occur with or without previous pouch dilatation. Tube disconnection can also occur, though uncommonly. Aneurysmatic balloon dilatation has also been reported in bands with a high pressure system. These complications could be minimized by using a low-pressure band placed by the pars flaccid route, as slippage is most frequently route-dependent [2, 61].

9.8.2 Laparoscopic Sleeve Gastrectomy

This procedure involves mobilizing the entire greater curvature of the stomach. This maneuver could damage the spleen, ranging from a segmental infarction to complete devascularization of the spleen, or resulting in a major hemorrhage necessitating splenectomy. Leakages from the staple line, stomach, or esophageal perforations are other possible complications. Gastric outlet narrowing or obstruction could be minimized by choosing a resection margin of the greater curvature 4–6 cm from the pylorus and using 32–36 Fr oral-gastric tube [62]. However, these complications are uncommon in our experience. To date, King Saud University Obesity Center has performed SG in over 72 children and adolescents without any of these major complications.

9.8.3 Gastric Bypass

Reported complications of this procedure include anastomotic leak, stricture formation, bowel obstruction, and malnutrition with micronutrient deficiency. Operative (30-day) mortality for gastric bypass when performed by skilled surgeons is ≈0.5%. The risk of dying in the first month after a RYGB from complications of the operation is ≈0.2–0.5% in expert centers. Studies have demonstrated that the mortality rate from hospitals with less experience with the procedure is far higher than that reported by expert centers.

Compared with open procedures, laparoscopic gastric bypass has a higher rate of intra-abdominal complications. However, patients benefit from shorter hospital stays, lower rate of wound complications, and higher postoperative comfort. Lifelong supplementation with vitamin B12, iron, folic acid, and calcium is recommended to avoid specific nutrient deficiency conditions and overt anemia [1, 63].

9.9 EFFECTS OF SURGERY ON COMORBID CONDITIONS

9.9.1 Obstructive Sleep Apnea

Studies with adults have reported a high success rate of OSA resolution after bariatric surgical weight loss [64–66]. Studies on the pediatric population also show a promising outcome of OSA after bariatric surgery.

Using an apnea hypopnea index (AHI) criteria of >10 events/h to define OSA, resolution occurred for all six adolescents with OSA after bariatric surgery in one series [67]. A similar result was seen in the Cincinnati bariatric cohort experience [68]. A significant reduction in sleep fragmentation (arousal index) and improvement in sleep architecture, in addition to a reduction in OSA severity, have been reported [69, 70].

9.9.2   Type 2 Diabetes Mellitus (T2DM)

Recovery from type 2 diabetes occurred in 76.8% of patients who underwent bariatric surgery [7, 71–76]. Improvement related to the surgical procedure and to duration of disease [74, 75]. This may be an important factor when considering appropriateness of bariatric surgery for younger diabetic patients. Several studies using homeostatic model assessment have reported improvements in insulin sensitivity and β-cell function [76, 77]. Interestingly, many patients become euglycemic well before the weight loss occurs with complete restoration of insulin resistance [11, 78, 79].

9.9.3   Hyperlipidemia

Improvement in dyslipidemias has been reported in ≈80% of surgical patients overall. In the Swedish Obesity Study, which compared 2,010 bariatric surgery patients to 2,037 matched controls receiving dietary management alone, hyperlipidemia incidence was tenfold lower at 2 years in the surgical treatment group [80]. In adolescents, significant improvements in total triglycerides and total cholesterol were documented 1 year after gastric bypass surgery. No significant changes were noted in high-density lipoprotein (HDL) or low-density lipoprotein (LDL) cholesterol [81].

9.9.4   Hypertension

Bariatric surgery has reduced prevalence of hypertension in obese adults. Among surgically treated patients, 62% of those with hypertension recovered normotension [73]. In children and adolescents, six studies (including our own series from Riyadh) reported resolution rates between 50 and 100% [82]. These are dramatic recovery rates, but in small studies.

9.9.5   Quality of Life

The Swedish Obesity Study and others reported dramatic improvements in the quality of life among patients after bariatric surgery, with a strong positive correlation between the degree of improvement in quality of life and the degree of weight loss [83, 84]. In an ongoing study, we observed similar results in our children and adolescents who underwent LAGB and SG where 75% reported better quality of life.

9.9.6 Hormonal Disturbance

In a study of 36 premenopausal women with polycystic ovary syndrome, those treated with bariatric surgery showed significantly improved hirsutism, insulin resistance, and ovulation and/or restoration of menstrual cycle [85].

9.9.7 Nonalcoholic Fatty Liver Disease

NAFLD refers to a wide spectrum of liver disease ranging from simple fatty liver (steatosis), to nonalcoholic steatohepatitis (NASH), to cirrhosis. All stages of NAFLD display fat infiltration. In NASH, the fat accumulation is associated with varying degrees of hepatitis and fibrosis. Up to 40% of obese children have ultrasound findings of NAFLD, and up to 83% have histology that suggests infiltration of the liver [86, 87]. In patients undergoing bariatric surgery, substantial weight loss is accompanied by a marked reduction in transaminases and a regression of fatty liver. However, rapid weight loss in this situation can also induce the occurrence of a fatty liver with liver inflammation [88]. The long-term outcome of untreated NASH acquired in childhood is under intense study, but the literature notes that 25% of adult patients who have NASH develop cirrhosis [89].

9.9.8 Long-Term Survival

Christou *et al.* and others reported lower mortality after bariatric surgery (*vs.* matched cohorts), resulting in 89% risk reduction of death over 5 years [90–94]. Most of the improvement was due to decreased diabetes, myocardial infarction, and cancer-related deaths.

9.10 SUMMARY

Morbid obesity is associated with multiple metabolic, physiological, and psychological abnormalities. These comorbidities markedly reduce the lifespan of the obese population. Bariatric surgery effectively reduces weight, but also resolves many comorbidities, thereby improving patients' quality of life. Different bariatric surgical techniques help achieve marked weight loss in morbidly obese patients.

At present, there is considerable interest in LAGB in pediatric patients, given its efficacy and relative safety. Loss of the excess weight usually peaks at 2–3 years after surgery. Three studies showed persistent weight loss at over 50% after 5 years. LAGB is also easier to perform than gastric bypass.

Although gastric bypass operations carry potential to achieve greater weight loss, this benefit is tempered by their increased risks of mortality and morbidity. Further, the bypass procedure is technically demanding, and surgeons must pass through a learning curve before embarking on bypass.

SG is a very suitable procedure in the adolescent population; however, long-term studies are not yet available. One factor should remain in the forefront when deciding the type of bariatric surgery in children and adolescents: reversibility when possible. Guidelines and protocols for pediatric obesity should be established by multidisciplinary experts and endorsed by professional societies. We present this work to support such efforts and propose such surgery be performed in specialized centers (as described in Table 9.7).

Table 9.7
Suggested institutional requirements for a bariatric surgery program for children and adolescents

1. Administrative support at the highest level of the institution/government
2. Bariatric surgeon(s) trained according to the American Society for Metabolic & Bariatric Surgery (ASMBS) recommendations
3. In addition to the surgeon, presence of a multidisciplinary team including a pediatrician, anesthesiologist, bariatric dietitian, bariatric nurse, and experienced office personnel. Additional clinical expertise should be at hand in case of need, such as pediatric cardiologist, pediatric pulmonologist, pediatric endocrinologist, and child psychiatrist.
4. Psychologist with expertise in bariatric patient evaluation
5. Qualified bariatric program coordinator
6. Various consultative services required for the care of morbidly obese surgical patients including the immediate availability of in-house critical care services
7. Availability of medical equipment and instruments for the care of bariatric patients throughout the hospital environment (including the clinic area, operating room, ICU, emergency room, and radiological facilities) suitable for the size and weights seen with extremely obese patients
   a. Hospital beds, gurneys, operating room tables, clinic exam room and waiting room furniture, scales, wheel chairs, and commodes need to be strong enough and extra wide to accommodate the extremely obese patient and family members.
   b. Patient movement/transfer systems for morbidly obese patients must be in place wherever the morbidly obese receives care.
   c. CT scanner, fluoroscopy tables, and nuclear medicine equipment with sufficient capacity to handle morbidly obese patients.
8. Program provides long-term medical follow-up of all patients, with formal monitoring and tracking system for outcomes' assessment.

REFERENCES

1. Buchwald H, Consensus Conference Panel (2005) Bariatric surgery for morbid obesity: health implications for patients, health professionals, and third-party payers. J Am Coll Surg 200:593–604
2. Al-Qahtani AR (2007) Laparoscopic adjustable gastric banding in adolescent: safety and efficacy. J Pediatr Surg 42:894–897
3. Schilling PL, Davis MM, Albanese CT et al. (2008) National trends in adolescent bariatric surgical procedures and implications for surgical centers of excellence. J Am Coll Surg 206:1–12
4. Tsai WS, Inge TH, Burd RS (2007) Bariatric surgery in adolescents: recent national trends in use and in-hospital outcome. Arch Pediatr Adolesc Med 161:217–221
5. Anon (1992) Gastrointestinal surgery for severe obesity: National Institutes of Health Consensus Development Conference Statement. Am J Clin Nutr 55(suppl 2): 615S.t–19S.t.
6. Inge TH, Krebs NF, Garcia VF et al. (2004) Bariatric surgery for severely overweight adolescents: concerns and recommendations. Pediatrics 114:217–223
7. Dixon JB, Dixon AF, O'Brien PE (2003) Improvements in insulin sensitivity and beta-cell function (HOMA) with weight loss in the severely obese, homeostatic model assessment. Diabet Med 20:127–134
8. Long SD, O'Brien K, MacDonald KG Jr et al. (1994) Weight loss in severely obese subjects prevents the progression of impaired glucose tolerance to type II diabetes: a longitudinal interventional study. Diabetes Care 17:372–375
9. Pories WJ, MacDonald KG Jr, Flickinger EG et al. (1992) Is type II diabetes mellitus (NIDDM) a surgical disease? Ann Surg 215:633–642
10. Sjostrom L, Larsson B, Backman L et al. (1992) Swedish Obese Subjects (SOS). Recruitment for an intervention study and selected description of the obese state. Int J Obes Relat Metab Disord 16:465–479
11. Pories WJ, Swanson MS, MacDonald KG et al. (1995) Who would have thought it? An operation proves to be the most effective therapy for adult onset diabetes mellitus. Ann Surg 222:339–350
12. Knol JA (1994) Management of the problem patient after bariatric surgery. Gastroenterol Clin North Am 23:345–369
13. ASA (2002) Practice advisory for preanesthesia evaluation. Anesthesiology 96:485–496
14. Derzie AJ, Silvestri F, Liriano E, Benotti P (2000) Wound closure technique and acute wound complications in gastric surgery for morbid obesity: a prospective randomized trial. J Am Coll Surg 191:238–243
15. Culver DH, Horan TC, Gaynes RP et al. (1991) Surgical wound infection rates by wound class, operative procedure and patient risk index: National Nosocomial Infections Surveillance System. Am J Med 91(suppl):152–157
16. Blaszyk H, Wollan PC, Witkiewicz AK, Björnsson J (1999) Death from pulmonary thromboembolism in severe obesity: lack of association with established genetic and clinical risk factors. Virchows Arch 434:529–532
17. Blaszyk H, Björnsson J (2000) Factor V Leiden and morbid obesity in fatal postoperative pulmonary embolism. Arch Surg 135:1410–1413
18. Kakkar VV, Howe CT, Nicolaides AN et al. (1970) Deep vein thrombosis of the leg: is there a "high risk" group? Ann Surg 120:527–532
19. Pineo GF, Hull RD (1998) Unfractionated and low-molecular weight heparin: comparison and current recommendations. Med Clin North Am 82:587–599

20. Smith HL, Meldrum DJ, Brennan LJ (2002) Childhood obesity: a challenge for the anaesthetist? Paediatr Anaesth 12:750–761
21. Inselma LS, Milanese A, Deurloo A (1993) Effect of obesity on pulmonary function in children. Pediatr Pulmonol 16:130–137
22. Lazarus R, Colditz G, Berkey CS et al. (1997) Effects of body fat on ventilatory function in children and adolescents: crosssectional findings from a random population sample of school children. Pediatr Pulmonol 24:187–194
23. Jense HG, Dubin SA, Silverstein PI et al. (1991) Effect of obesity on safe duration of apnea in anesthetized humans. Anesth Analg 72:89–93
24. Kabon B, Nagele A, Reddy D et al. (2004) Obesity decreases perioperative tissue oxygenation. Anesthesiology 100:274–280
25. Bryson GL, Chung F, Cox RG et al. (2004) Patient selection in ambulatory anesthesia – an evidence-based review: part II. Can J Anaesth 51:782–794
26. Warner MA, Warner ME, Weber JG (1993) Clinical significance of pulmonary aspiration during the perioperative period. Anesthesiology 78:56–62
27. Borland LM, Sereika SM, Woelfel SK et al. (1998) Pulmonary aspiration in pediatric patients during general anesthesia: incidence and outcome. J Clin Anesth 10:95–102
28. Benumof JL (2001) Obstructive sleep apnea in the adult obese patient: implications for airway management. J Clin Anesth 13:144–145
29. Frey WC, Pilcher J (2003) Obstructive sleep-related breathing disorders in patients evaluated for bariatric surgery. Obes Surg 13:676–683
30. O'Keeffe T, Patterson EJ (2004) Evidence supporting routine polysomnography before bariatric surgery. Obes Surg 14:23–26
31. den Herder C, Schmeck J, Appelboom DJ, de Vries N (2004) Risks of general anaesthesia in people with obstructive sleep apnoea. BMJ 329:955–959
32. Sawyer RJ, Richmond MN, Hickey JD, Jarratt JA (2000) Peripheral nerve injuries associated with anaesthesia. Anaesthesia 55:980–991
33. McCarroll SM, Saunders PR, Brass PJ (1989) Anesthetic considerations in obese patients. Prog Anesthesiol 3:1–12
34. Juvin P, Vadam C, Malek L et al. (2000) Postoperative recovery after desflurane, propofol, or isoflurane anesthesia among morbidly obese patients: a prospective randomized study. Anesth Analg 91:714–719
35. Sollazzi L, Perilli V, Modesti C et al. (2001) Volatile anesthesia in bariatric surgery. Obes Surg 11:623–626
36. Torri G, Casati A, Albertin A et al. (2001) Randomized comparison of isoflurane and sevoflurane for laparoscopic gastric banding in morbidly obese patients. J Clin Anesth 13:565–570
37. Luce MJ (1980) Respiratory complications of obesity. Chest 78:626–631
38. Cooper JR, Brodsky JB (1987) Anesthetic management of the morbidly obese patient. Semin Anesth 6:260–270
39. Bardoczky GI, Yernault JC, Houben JJ, d'Hollander AA (1995) Large tidal volume ventilation does not improve oxygenation in morbidly obese patients during anesthesia. Anesth Analg 81:385–388
40. Randolph JG, Weintraub WH, Rigg A (1974) Jejunoileal bypass for morbid obesity in adolescents. J Pediatr Surg 9:341–345
41. Organ CH Jr, Kessler E, Lane M (1984) Long-term results of jejunoileal bypass in the young. Am Surg 50:589–593
42. Hocking MP, Duerson MC, O'Leary JP, Woodward ER (1983) Jejunoileal bypass for morbid obesity. Late follow-up in 100 cases. N Engl J Med 308:995–999

43. Silber T, Randolph J, Robbins S (1986) Long-term morbidity and mortality in morbidly obese adolescents after jejunoileal bypass. J Pediatr 108:318–322

44. Prachand VN, Davee RT, Alverdy JC (2006) Duodenal switch provides superior weight loss in the super-obese (BMI ≥50 kg/m²) compared with gastric bypass. Ann Surg 244:611–619

45. Mason EE, Scott DH, Doherty C et al. (1995) Vertical banded gastroplasty in the severely obese under age twenty one. Obes Surg 5:23–33

46. Santry HP, Gillen DL, Lauderdale DS (2005) Trends in bariatric surgical procedures. JAMA 294:1909–1917

47. Rand CS, Macgregor AM (1994) Adolescents having obesity surgery: a 6-year follow-up. South Med J 87:1208–1213

48. Anderson AE, Soper RT, Scott DH (1980) Gastric bypass for morbid obesity in children and adolescents. J Pediatr Surg 15:876–881

49. Xanthakos SA, Inge TH (2006) Nutritional consequences of bariatric surgery. Curr Opin Clin Nutr Metab Care 9:489–496

50. Favretti F, Segato G, Ashton D et al. (2007) Laparoscopic adjustable gastric banding in 1,791 consecutive obese patients: 12-year results. Obes Surg 17:168–175

51. Regan JP, Inabnet WB, Gagner M et al. (2003) Early experience with two-stage laparoscopic Roux-en-Y gastric bypass as an alternative in the supersuper obese patient. Obes Surg 13:861–864

52. Mognol P, Chosidow D, Marmuse JP (2005) Laparoscopic sleeve gastrectomy as an initial bariatric operation for high-risk patients: Initial results in 10 patients. Obes Surg 15:1030–1033

53. Aziz Q, Andersson JL, Valind S et al. (1997) Identification of human brain loci processing esophageal sensation using positron emission tomography. Gastroenterology 113:50–59

54. Tataranni PA, Gautier JF, Chen K et al. (1999) Neuroanatomical correlates of hunger and satiation in humans using positron emission tomography. Proc Natl Acad Sci USA 96:4569–4574

55. Stephan E, Parado JV, Faris PL et al. (2003) Functional neuroimaging of gastric distention. J Gastrointest Surg 7:740–749

56. Dixon AF, Dixon JB, O'Brien PE (2005) Laparoscopic adjustable gastric banding induces prolonged satiety: a randomised blind crossover study. J Clin Endocrinol Metab 90:813–819

57. Kellum JM, Kuemmerle JF, O'Dorisio TM et al. (1990) Gastrointestinal hormone responses to meals before and after gastric bypass and vertical banded gastroplasty. Ann Surg 211:763–770

58. Alvarez-Bartolome M, Borque M, Martinez-Sarmiento J et al. (2002) Peptide YY secretion in morbidly obese patients before and after vertical banded gastroplasty. Obes Surg 12:324–327

59. Nijhuis J, van Dielen FM, Buurman WA et al. (2004) Ghrelin, leptin and insulin levels after restrictive surgery: a 2-year follow-up study. Obes Surg 14:783–787

60. Scharrer E (1999) Control of food intake by fatty acid oxidation and ketogenesis. Nutrition 15:704–714

61. Balsiger BM, Poggio JL, Mai J, Kelly KA, Sarr MG (2000) Ten and more years after vertical banded gastroplasty as primary operation for morbid obesity. J Gastrointest Surg 4:598–605

62. Lalor PF, Tucker ON, Szomstein S, Rosenthal RJ (2008) Complications after laparoscopic sleeve gastrectomy. Surg Obes Relat Dis 4:33–38

63. Sugerman HJ, Sugerman EL, Wolfe L et al. (2001) Risks and benefits of gastric bypass in morbidly obese patients with severe venous stasis disease. Ann Surg 234:41–46

64. Rasheid S, Banasiak M, Gallagher SF *et al.* (2003) Gastric bypass is an effective treatment for obstructive sleep apnea in patients with clinically significant obesity. Obes Surg 13:58–61
65. Guardiano SA, Scott JA, Ware JC, Schechner SA (2003) The long-term results of gastric bypass on indexes of sleep apnea. Chest 124:1615–1619
66. Scheuller M, Weider D (2001) Bariatric surgery for treatment of sleep apnea syndrome in 15 morbidly obese patients: long-term results. Otolaryngol Head Neck Surg 125:299–302
67. Sugerman HJ, Sugerman EL, DeMaria EJ *et al.* (2003) Bariatric surgery for severely obese adolescents. J Gastrointest Surg 7:102–108
68. Kalra M, Inge T, Garcia V *et al.* (2005) Obstructive sleep apnea in extremely overweight adolescents undergoing bariatric surgery. Obes Res 13:1175–1179
69. Charuzi I, Lavie P, Peiser J, Peled R (1992) Bariatric surgery in morbidly obese sleep apnea patients: short- and long-term follow-up. Am J Clin Nutr 55(suppl):594S–596S
70. Dixon JB, Schachter LM, O'Brien PE (2005) Polysomnography before and after weight loss in obese patients with severe sleep apnea. Int J Obes (Lond) 29:1048–1054
71. Sjostrom L, Lindroos AK, Peltonen M *et al.* (2004) Lifestyle, diabetes, and cardiovascular risk factors 10 years after bariatric surgery. New Engl J Med 351:2683–2693
72. Sjostrom L, Narbro K, Sjostrom CD *et al.* (2007) Effects of bariatric surgery on mortality in Swedish obese subjects. New Engl J Med 357:741–752
73. Buchwald H, Avidor Y, Braunwald E *et al.* (2004) Bariatric surgery: a systematic review and meta-analysis. JAMA 292:1724–1737
74. Polyzogopoulou EV, Kalfarentzos F, Vagenakis AG, Alexandrides TK (2003) Restoration of euglycemia and normal acute insulin response to glucose in obese subjects with type 2 diabetes following bariatric surgery. Diabetes 52:1098–1103
75. Schauer PR, Burguera B, Ikramuddin S *et al.* (2003) Effect of laparoscopic Roux-en Y gastric bypass on type 2 diabetes mellitus. Ann Surg 238:467–484
76. Dixon JB, O'Brien PE (2002) Health outcomes of severely obese type 2 diabetic subjects 1 year after laparoscopic adjustable gastric banding. Diabetes Care 25:358–363
77. Ballantyne GH, Farkas D, Laker S, Wasielewski A (2006) Short-term changes in insulin resistance following weight loss surgery for morbid obesity: laparoscopic adjustable gastric banding versus laparoscopic Roux-en-Y gastric bypass. Obes Surg 16:1189–1197
78. Guldstrand M, Grill V, Bjorklund A, Lins PE, Adamson U (2002) Improved beta cell function after short-term treatment with diazoxide in obese subjects with type 2 diabetes. Diabetes Metab 28:448–456
79. Muscelli E, Mingrone G, Camastra S *et al.* (2005) Differential effect of weight loss on insulin resistance in surgically treated obese patients. Am J Med 118:51–57
80. Sjostrom CD, Lissner L, Wedel H, Sjostrom L (1999) Reduction in incidence of diabetes, hypertension and lipid disturbances after intentional weight loss induced by bariatric surgery: the SOS Intervention Study. Obes Res 7:477–484
81. Lawson L, Harmon C, Chen M *et al.* (2006) One year outcomes of Roux en Y gastric bypass in adolescents: a multicenter report from the Pediatric Bariatric Study Group. J Pediatr Surg 41:137–143
82. ECRI Institute. Health Technology Assessment Information Service. Health Technology Assessment (2007) Bariatric surgery in pediatric patients. Retrieved 26 Feb 2008 from ECRI institute
83. Karlsson J, Sjostrom L, Sullivan M (1998) Swedish obese subjects (SOS) – an intervention study of obesity. Two-year follow-up of healthrelated quality of life (HRQL) and eating behavior after gastric surgery for severe obesity. Int J Obes Relat Metab Disord 22:113–126

84. Dixon JB, Dixon ME, O'Brien PE (2001) Quality of life after lap-band placement: influence of time, weight loss, and comorbidities. Obes Surg 9:713–721
85. Escobar-Morreale HF, Botella-Carretero JI, Alvarez-Blasco F, San Millan JL (2005) The polycystic ovary syndrome associated with morbid obesity may resolve after weight loss induced by bariatric surgery. J Endocrinol Metab 90:6364–6369
86. Must A (1999) Risk and consequences of childhood and adolescent obesity. Int J Obes Relat Metab Disord 23(suppl 2):S2–S11
87. Xanthakos S, Miles L, Bucuvalas J et al. (2006) Histologic spectrum of nonalcoholic fatty liver disease in morbidly obese adolescents. Clin Gastroenterol Hepatol 4:226–232
88. Roberts E (2003) Nonalcoholic steatohepatitis in children. Curr Gastroenterol Rep 5:253–259
89. Matteoni CA, Younossi ZM, Gramlich T et al. (1999) Nonalcoholic fatty liver disease: a spectrum of clinical and pathological severity. Gastroenterology 116:1413–1419
90. Christou NV, Sampalis JS, Liberman M et al. (2004) Surgery decreases long-term mortality, morbidity, and health care use in morbidly obese patients. Ann Surg 240:416–423
91. MacDonald KG Jr, Long SD, Swanson MS et al. (1997) The gastric bypass operation reduces the progression and mortality of non-insulin-dependent diabetes mellitus. J Gastrointest Surg 1:213–220
92. Flum DR, Dellinger EP (2004) Impact of gastric bypass operation on survival: a population-based analysis. J Am Coll Surg 199:543–551
93. Sjostrom L (2006) Soft and hard endpoints over 5 to 18 years in the intervention trial Swedish obese subjects. Obes Rev 7(S2):27 [abstract]
94. Peeters A, O'Brien P, Laurie C, et al. (2006) Does weight loss improve survival? Comparison of a bariatric surgical cohort with a community based control group. Obes Rev 7(S2):95 [abstract]

Part III
Diabetes: Clinical Assessments

10 Epidemiology of Type 2 Diabetes Mellitus in Pediatric Populations

Shreepal M. Shah

Key Points

- T2DM is directly related to obesity across the life span.
- Pediatric obesity and T2DM remain increasingly epidemic worldwide.

Keywords: Pediatric, Obesity, Type 2 diabetes mellitus, Epidemic

Diabetes mellitus has been among the leading causes of morbidity and mortality in developed countries since the end of World War II. Alarmingly, the incidence of type 2 diabetes mellitus (T2DM) has rapidly increased among children and adolescents since at least the late 1980s. Increasing urbanization, an epidemic of pediatric obesity, broad consumption of fructose corn syrup and other relatively cheap foods, increased economic pressures on families, and decreased physical activity – all these factors contribute to this problem.

Since T2DM is not a reportable disease in any jurisdiction, firm prevalence and incidence rates are unavailable. Still, the World Health Organization (WHO) has estimated the prevalence of diabetes in most countries. In 2000, WHO reported its estimate of diabetic adults as ~171 million worldwide. WHO projected that, during the 30-year period of 1995–2025, the adult diabetic subpopulation would increase by as much as 170% [1]. This projection included a 27% increase among developed countries and 42% in the underdeveloped countries. The American Diabetes Association (ADA) recently estimated the direct economic cost of diabetes

From: *Nutrition and Health: Management of Pediatric Obesity and Diabetes*,
Edited by: R.J. Ferry, Jr., DOI 10.1007/978-1-60327-256-8_10,
© Springer Science+Business Media, LLC 2011

for afflicted Americans to be over \$116 billion. Considering such indirect costs as loss of productivity, disability, and early mortality, the overall cost explodes, approaching \$174 billion in 2007 [2].

The rising prevalence of T2DM in children and adolescents was initially recognized in the United States in the 1990s. T2DM, which 15 years ago accounted for less than 3% of all cases of new onset diabetes in children and adolescents, today accounts for up to 45% of new onset cases among adolescents [3]. Table 10.1 presents nominal prevalence and incidence rates for T2DM in children and adolescents, based upon population-based studies in specific countries or regions. A heterogeneous group of disorders comprises ~90% of diabetic North Americans. As early as 1979, initial reports of a disturbing, upward trend for pediatric T2DM arose from longitudinal studies of Pima Indians living in the Western USA. Before 1980, >1% of Pimas had diabetes associated with obesity by age of 19. In this early report, five required insulin therapy, and four presented with diabetic ketoacidosis (DKA). By the 1990s, the prevalence of T2DM among Pima aged between 15 and 19 years had increased to 51%, and the disease had also emerged in the youngsters of 10–14 year age group (prevalence 0.22%) [4]. During the next 13 years after this initial report in 1979, numerous series of pediatric T2DM were published. Among native populations of Manitoba, Canada, 10–20% of those aged 5–14 years had T2DM [5, 6]. A similar observation came from Northwest Ontario among those younger than 16 years, but with higher age-specific prevalence of 2.5 per 1000 [7]. In Cincinnati, Ohio, one-third of all new cases of diabetes in the 10–19 year age group were classified as T2DM (age-specific incidence of 7.2 per 100,000 annually). T2DM comprised 2–4% of all childhood diabetes before 1992, but by 1994, T2DM accounted for 16% of all new cases in children [8]. Observers from Arkansas reported that African-Americans accounted for 70–75% of clinical T2DM there [9, 10]. Similar observations were reported from Cincinnati, Ohio.

Annual medical records were reviewed for all diabetic patients younger than 20 years at six Indian Health Service Facilities in Montana and Wyoming [11]. T2DM was diagnosed when a child had one or more of following characteristics: weight ≥95th percentile for age and gender, acanthosis nigricans, elevated serum C-peptide or insulin, family history of T2DM, treatment with oral agents (with or without insulin), or hypoglycemic therapy after 1-year of follow-up. From 1999 to 2001, 53% of prevalent cases and 70% of incident cases were diagnosed with T2DM. The average annual prevalence of probable T2DM was 1.3 per 1,000, and the incidence rate was 23.3 per 100,000, approximately four times higher than T1DM [12]. The prevalence of T2DM was high (20%) among Navajo tribe members over age 20, versus 0.4% in adolescent population, although an additional 3% displayed impaired glucose tolerance or impaired fasting glucose [13].

Table 10.1
Worldwide spread of type 2 diabetes mellitus in children and adolescents

Location	Race/ethnicity	Age group/mean age	Incidence per 100,000	Prevalence per 1,000	Newly diagnosed T2DM (%)	References
Tokyo, Japan	Japanese	Not specified	13.9	–	80.0	[17, 18]
Taipei, Taiwan	–	6–18 years	6.5	–	54.2	[46]
Singapore	–	12 years	–	–	10.0	[47]
Bangkok, Thailand	–	0–14 years	–	–	17.9	[48, 49]
Hong Kong	Chinese	<15 years	0.1	–	7.0	[50]
Shanghai, China	–	<18 years	–	–	2.4	[51]
India	Indian	<18 years	–	–	3.0	[52]
		<30 years			58.0	
New Zealand	Maori	15 years	–	–	35.7	[53]
Germany	–	14.0±2.0	–	–	1.5	[20]
Austria	–	<15 years	0.25	–	1.6	[54, 55]
England	–	<18 years	1.52	2.0		[56]
France	–	8.5–14.9 years	–	–	2.0	[57]
Sweden	–	0–18 years	–	–	0.5	[58]
Australia	White, Middle Eastern, Asian, Aboriginal	14.2±2.0	2.5	–	10	[59, 60]
Saudi Arabia	Saudis	<14 years	–	1.2	–	[61]
		14–29 years		7.9		
United Arab Emirates	–	0–18 years	–	–	12.5	[62]
Argentina	–	12.9±2.8	–	–	4.16	[63]

(continued)

Table 10.1
(continued)

Location	Race/ethnicity	Age group/mean age	Incidence per 100,000	Prevalence per 1,000	Newly diagnosed T2DM (%)	References
Arizona	Pima Indians	15–19 years	–	51	–	[4]
		10–14 years		22		
Montana and Wyoming	–	<20 years	23.3	1.3	70.0	[11]
Manitoba, Southwestern Quebec, Southwestern Ontario	First Nations	5–14 years	–	1–2.5	–	[6]
		15–19 years		2.3–3.5		
Northwestern Ontario	First Nations	<16 years	–	2.5	–	[5]
New York	–	<18 years	–	–	50.0	[15]
Florida	–	Not specified	–	–	20.0	[71]

A population-based surveillance for diabetes prevalence among black and non-Hispanic white youth younger than 19 was reported from South Carolina. The prevalence of T2DM among black patients was 26%, while 10% for the non-Hispanic whites. The total estimated cases of T2DM among youth over age 10 were 0.6 per 1,000 [14].

Investigators at Montefiore Medical Center (Bronx NY) reported a tenfold increase in their number of T2DM patients over a 10-year period. T2DM accounted for 12% of all new cases in their pediatric cohort by 1990, whereas by 2000 almost 50% of newly diagnosed patients had T2DM. This Bronx cohort was mainly black, Caribbean-Hispanic, and Asian Indian children. At presentation, t mean age was 14 ± 2.3 years; mean body mass index (BMI) was 34.4 ± 9 kg/m^2; female/male ratio was 1.6:1, and 89% possessed acanthosis nigricans. All were pubertal [15].

To estimate the incidence of T2DM among youth younger than 20, classified by race/ethnicity and diagnosis, CDC and NIH in 2002–2003 funded The SEARCH for Diabetes in Youth Study across ten sites in the USA. SEARCH sampled from a population of more than ten million during this period [16]. This multiregional database displayed that overall incidence rate of pediatric diabetes (all types) was 24.3%, highest among 10–14 year old youth and with higher rates in females (than males). On the basis of these data, about 15,000 youth in the USA would be newly diagnosed annually with type 1 diabetes, and about 3,700 youth with new onset T2DM annually. SEARCH reported the rate of new cases among youth was 19 per 100,000 each year for T1DM and 5.3 per 100,000 for T2DM annually [17]. Not surprisingly, for children in the two groups analyzed (up to age 4 years, and those between 5 and 9 years), the majority had T1DM regardless of race/ethnicity. Proportions of diabetic youth with T2DM were highest among American Indian groups (25.3% among 10–14 year olds and 49.4% among 15–19 year olds), followed by African-American (22.3 and 19.4% respectively), Asian/Pacific Islanders (11.8 and 22.7%, respectively), and Hispanic youth (8.9 and 17%, respectively). Non-Hispanic white youth had the lowest rates of T2DM (3.0 and 5.6%, respectively). The incidence rate was higher in females (than males) and was highest among 15–19 year old females across all racial/ethnic groups. Similar to other USA-based studies [18, 19], 21.2% of the SEARCH participants older than 10 years had positive glutamic acid decarboxylase (GAD65) antibodies. The majority of participants with T2DM and positive GAD65 titer were overweight, were of minority racial/ethnic background, but had GAD65 titer less than twofold the cut point used to define positivity.

The trend of rapidly accelerating incidence of pediatric T2DM has been observed worldwide. The incidence of T2DM among Libyan Arabs younger than 34 is 19.6 per 100,000 for males and 35.3 per 100,000 for females, in comparison with 9.4 and 8.5, respectively, for T1DM [20]. Among Japanese school children, the incidence of T2DM increased from 0.2 to 7.3 per 100,000 between 1976 and 1995. Among junior high school students, the incidence of T2DM was recently 13.9 per 100,000, compared to 2.07 per 100,000 for type 1 diabetes. Younger grammar school children in Japan had an incidence of T2DM of 2.0 per 100,000, comparable to 1.65 per 100,000 for T1DM. Japanese investigators have associated changing food patterns and rising obesity rates for increasing trend of T2DM in school children [21, 22]. An Italian study of 710 grossly obese children and adolescents (of various European origins) reported the prevalence of T2DM and insulin glucose tolerance as 0.1 and 4.5% respectively [23].

A small cohort of obese Caucasian children and adolescents living in Germany had 1.5% (eight subjects) with T2DM. All these were pubertal, and male:female ratio was 1:3 [24]. Analysis of multicenter database from 148 pediatric diabetes centers from Germany and Austria revealed 130 (0.6%) children of Caucasian origin with T2DM compared with 19,796 patients with type 1. Patients with T2DM were predominantly female, significantly older at the diagnosis and more over weight as compared to those with type 1 diabetes mellitus [25]. Data on the incidence of T2DM in children from Sweden found total of 31 cases (0.5%) of T2DM out of approximately 6,000 cases with diabetes. Out of them 55% were of ethnic minorities known to have high incidence of T2DM and male to female ratio was 1:2 [26].

The incidence in type 2 diabetes among children and adolescents has emerged in parallel with an alarming rise in number of youth who have become overweight or obese. Childhood obesity has reached epidemic levels in developed countries; 25% of children in the USA are overweight and 115% are obese. About 70% of obese adolescents grow up to become obese adults [27–29]. The prevalence of obesity has been increasing since 1971 in developed countries (Table 10.2). Worldwide approximately 22 million children under 5 years of age are overweight [30]. The highest prevalence rates of childhood obesity have been observed in the developed countries, although its prevalence is increasing in developing countries. The prevalence of obesity is high in the Middle East, Central and Eastern Europe [31]. Overweight and obese adults are at increased risk for morbidity and mortality associated with many acute and chronic medical conditions, including hypertension, dyslipidemia, coronary heart disease, diabetes mellitus, gallbladder disease, respiratory disease, cancer, gout and arthritis [32]. Data from NHANES surveys (1976–1980 and 2003–2006) show that the prevalence of obesity has increased among children and adolescents. The prevalence of obesity for children 2–5 years increased from 5 to 12.4%; for those aged 6–11 years, prevalence increased from 6.5 to 17% and for

Table 10.2

Change in prevalence of obesity in children and adolescents in the developed countries

Location	Age group	Year	Trend	References
USA	5–24	1973–1994	Twofold increase in prevalence of obesity	[64]
	6–19	1971–1974	Stable	[65]
	6–19	1976–1980	Stable	[65]
	6–19	1988–1994	Double to 11%	[65]
	6–19	1999–2000	Increased by 4%	[65]
Japan	6–14	1974–1993	Increased from 5 to 10%	[66]
UK	7–11		Increased from 8 to 20%	[67]
Spain	6–7	1985–1986	Increased from 23 to 35%	[68]
France	5–12	1992–1996	Increased from 10 to 14%	[69]
Greece	6–12	1984–2000	Increased by 7%	[70]

those aged 12–19 years, prevalence increased from 5 to 17.6% [33–36]. For 2003–2006, 11.3% of children and adolescents were at or above the 97th percentile of BMI for age from the 2000 CDC growth charts. For the same period, 16.3% of children and adolescents had a BMI for age at or above the 95th percentile of BMI for age and 31.9% were at or above the 85th percentile. Data showed that for children aged 6–11 years and 12–19 years the prevalence of overweight (BMI $\geq$ 85th percentile) was 33.3 and 34.1% respectively. Figure 10.1 and Table 10.3 show the trends in childhood overweight based on NHEAS data for various age groups, beginning with NHANES I 1963–1965 and ending with NHANES 2003–2006. Data from NHANES (2003–2006) showed prevalence of obesity was higher among adolescent Mexican American boys (22.1%) and then among non-Hispanic white boys (17.3%) and black boys (18.5%). Compare with the data from NHANES III (1988–1994), largest increase in the prevalence of obesity occurred among adolescent non-Hispanic black boys (7.8%) and Mexican American boys (8.0%) compared with non-Hispanic white boys (5.7%) (Tables 10.4, 10.5).

Prevalence of obesity in non-Hispanic black girls aged 12–19 years was highest (27.7%) compared with non-Hispanic white (14.5%) and Mexican American girls (19.9%) according to NHANES data (2003–2006). Data from NHANES III (1988–1994) through NHANES 2003–2006 showed that non-Hispanic black adolescent girls showed the largest increase in the prevalence of obesity (14.5%) compared with non-Hispanic white adolescent (7.1%) and Mexican American adolescent (10.7%) girls (Figs. 10.2, 10.3).

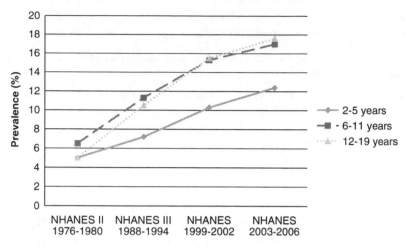

Fig. 10.1. Rising prevalence of obesity among North American children and adolescents.

Table 10.3
Trends in childhood obesity based on NHNEAS data for various age groups

	6–23 months (%)	2–5 years (%)	6–11 years (%)	12–19 years (%)
NHES 2 (1963–1965)	–	–	4.2	–
NHES 3 (1966–1970)	–	–	–	4.6
NHANES I (1971–1974)	–	5.0	4.0	6.1
NHANES II (1976–1980)	7.2	5.0	6.5	5.0
NHANES III (1988–1994)	8.9	7.2	11.3	10.5
NHANES 1999–2000	11.6	10.4	15.3	15.5
NHANES 2003–2006	–	12.4	17.0	17.6

Table 10.4
Trends in childhood obesity based on NHNEAS data for various age groups among boys

	6–23 months (%)	2–5 years (%)	6–11 years (%)	12–19 years (%)
NHES 2 (1963–1965)	–	–	4.0%	–
NHES 3 (1966–1970)	–	–	–	4.5
NHANES I (1971–1974)	–	5.0	4.3	6.1
NHANES II (1976–1980)	8.2	4.7	6.6	4.8
NHANES III (1988–994)	9.9	6.1	11.6	11.3
NHANES 1999–2000	9.8	9.9	16.0	15.5
NHANES 2003–2006	–	12.8	18.0	18.2

Table 10.5
Trends in childhood obesity based on NHNEAS data for various age groups among girls

Females	6–23 months (%)	2–5 years (%)	6–11 years (%)	12–19 years (%)
NHES 2 (1963–1965)	–	–	4.5	–
NHES 3 (1966–1970)	–	–	–	4.7
NHANES I (1971–1974)	–	4.9	3.6	6.2
NHANES II (1976–1980)	6.1	5.3	6.4	5.3
NHANES III (1988–1994)	7.9	8.2	11.0	9.7
NHANES 1999–2000	14.3	11.0	14.5	15.5
NHANES 2003–2006	–	12.1	15.8	16.8

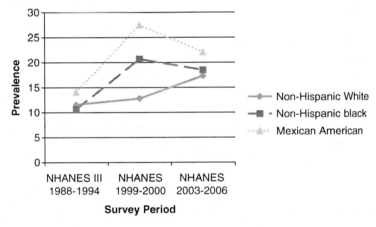

Fig. 10.2. Prevalence of obesity among adolescent boys in North America by race/ethnicity

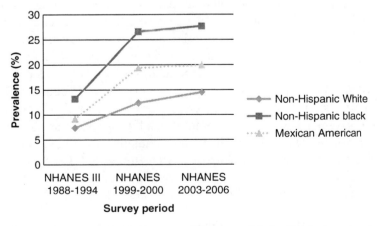

Fig. 10.3. Prevalence of obesity among adolescent girls in North America by race/ethnicity

Although children and adolescents representing all racial, ethnic and socioeconomical groups have been affected by the trend of obesity, Native Americans, Hispanics and African Americans have become particularly susceptible to the epidemic of obesity [37]. Along with T2DM, prevalence of hypertension among African-American and Hispanic children is also increasing, causing increased risk for developing cardiovascular disease [38]. Childhood obesity is directly linked to abnormalities in blood pressure, lipids, lipoproteins, and insulin levels in adults, as well as to the risk of both coronary artery disease and diabetes [39]. Becque and coworkers evaluated that 80% had elevated systolic blood pressure, diastolic blood pressure, or both in a group of obese adolescents [40]. They found that 97% had four or more of the following cardiovascular risk factors: elevated serum triglyceride levels (more than 100 mg/dL), low levels of high-density lipoprotein cholesterol levels (more than 200 mg/dL), elevated systolic blood pressure, diastolic blood pressure, or both (above the 90th percentile for age and sex), diminished maximal oxygen consumption (less than 24 mL per kilogram of body weight per minute), and a strong history in the immediate family of coronary heart disease, myocardial infarction, angina pectoris, or high blood pressure.

Insulin resistance is an almost inevitably associated with comorbidities of obesity and often precedes with development of type 2 diabetes. To determine the prevalence of glucose intolerance and insulin resistance, a multi-ethnic cohort involving 167 obese children and adolescents was studied at Yale Pediatric Obesity Clinic between 1999 and 2001 [41]. Impaired glucose tolerance was detected in 25% of the 55 obese children and 21% of the obese adolescents, silent T2DM was identified in 4% of the obese adolescents. This study showed that impaired glucose tolerance is highly prevalent among children and adolescents with severe obesity, irrespective of ethnic group. Impaired oral glucose tolerance was associated with insulin resistance while β cell function was still preserved. Besides documenting the high incidence of impaired glucose tolerance in severely obese children, in this study they all showed that insulin resistance and the fasting hyperproinsulinemia were the most important predictors of impaired glucose tolerance. All the children they studied were severely obese. In contrast, Sinaiko et al. have shown that, in adolescents, there is a significant correlation between body mass index and degree of insulin resistance as measured by the hyperinsulinemic–euglycemic clamp technique. Abdominal obesity and in particular increased visceral fat has been implicated as contributory to insulin resistance. A study of 32 overweight or obese Hispanic children without diabetes with a family history of T2DM indicated that increased visceral fat was independently related to both increased insulin resistance and decreased insulin secretion [42].

Epidemiological evidence from the past 20 years has demonstrated that the increasing incidence of type 2 diabetes in children parallels the increasing prevalence of obesity [43]. According to an International Obesity Task Force, more than 1.1 billion adults today worldwide are overweight, and 312 million of them are obese. This task force and the WHO have raised the definition of obesity to adjust for ethnic differences, and this broader definition may reflect an even higher prevalence with 1.7 billion people classified as overweight worldwide [44]. Approximately 197 million people worldwide have impaired glucose intolerance, due to obesity and associated metabolic syndrome. It is expected that this trend will increase to 420 million by 2025 [45].

Finally, in addition to well-recognized sequelae such as T2DM and metabolic syndrome, pediatric obesity appears to be associated with an increased risk of pseudotumor cerebri, orthopaedic diseases, and vitamin D deficiency. Each of these complications should be addressed by the appropriate specialists in the context of a comprehensive plan of care. Clearly, prevention among the pediatric and adolescent populations is key to these huge problems.

REFERENCES

1. King H, Aubert RE, Herman WH (1998) Global burden of diabetes, 1995–2025. Diab Care 21:1414–1431
2. American Diabetes Association (2008) Economic costs of diabetes in the US in 2007. Diab Care 31:596–615
3. Anonymous (2000) Type 2 diabetes in children and adolescents. American Diabetes Association. Diabetes Care 323:381–390
4. Savage PJ, Bennett PH, Senter RG, Miller M (1979) High prevalence of diabetes in young Pima Indians. Diabetes 28:937–942
5. Dean HE, Mundy RL, Moffatt M (1992) Non-insulin-dependent diabetes mellitus in Indian children in Manitoba. Can Med Assoc J 147:52–57
6. Dean H (1998) NIDDM-Y in First Nation children in Canada. Clin Pediatr 39:89–96
7. Harris SB, Perkins BA, Whalen-Brough E (1996) Non-insulin dependent diabetes mellitus among First Nations children: new entity among First Nations people of Northwestern Ontario. Can Fam Physician 42:869–876
8. Pinhas-Hamiel O, Dolan LM, Daniels SR, Standiford D, Khoury PR, Zeitler P (1996) Increased incidence of non-insulin-dependent diabetes mellitus among adolescents. J Pediatr 128:608–615
9. Scott CR, Smith JM, Cradock M, Pihoker C (1997) Characteristics of youth-onset non-insulin-dependent diabetes mellitus and insulin dependent diabetes mellitus at diagnosis. Pediatrics 100:84–91
10. Pihoker C, Scott CR, Lensing SY, Cradock MM, Smith J (1998) Non-insulin dependent diabetes mellitus in African American youths of Arkansas. Clin Pediatr 37:97–102
11. Harwell TS, McDowall JM, Moore K, Fagot-Campagna A, Helgerson SD, Gohdes D (2001) Establishing surveillance for diabetes in African Indian youths. Diab Care 24:1029–1032

12. Moore KR, Harwell TS, McDowall JM, Helgerson SD, Gohdes D (2003) Three-year prevalence and incidence of diabetes among American Indian youth in Montana and Wyoming, 1999 to 2001. J Pediatr 143:368–371
13. Kim C, McHugh C, Kwok Y, Smith A (1999) Type 2 diabetes mellitus in Navajo adolescents. West J Med 170:210
14. Oeltmenn JE, Liese AD, Heinze HJ, Addy CL, Mayer-Davis EJ (2003) Prevalence of diagnosed diabetes among African–American and non-Hispanic white youth. Diab Care 26:2531–2535
15. Grinstein G, Muzmudar R, Aponte L, Vuguin P, Saenger P, DiMartino-Nardi J (2003) Presentation and 5-year follow-up of type 2 diabetes mellitus in African-American and Caribben-Hispanic adolescents. Horm Res 60:121–126
16. Writing Group for the SEARCH for Diabetes in Youth Study Group, Dabelea D, Bell RA, D'Agostino RB Jr, Imperatore G, Johansen JM, Linder B, Liu LL, Loots B, Marcovina S, Mayer-Davis EJ, Pettitt DJ, Waitzfelder B (2007) Incidence of diabetes in youth in the United States. JAMA 297:2716–2724
17. National Diabetes Statistics (2007) http://diabetes.niddk.nih.gov/dm/pubs/statistics/index.htm. Accessed 26 February 2010
18. Brooks-Worrell BM, Greenaum CJ, Palmer JP, Pihoker C (2004) Autoimmunity to islets proteins in children diagnosed with new-onset diabetes. J Clin Endocinol Metab 89:2222–2227
19. Hathout EH, Thomas W, El Shahawy M, Nahab F, Mace JW (2001) Diabetic autoimmune markers in children and adolescents with type 2 diabetes. Pediatrics 107:E102
20. Kadiki OA, Reddy MR, Marzouk AA (1996) Incidence of insulin-dependent diabetes (IDDM) and non-insulin-dependent diabetes (NIDDM) (0-34 years at onset) in Benghazi, Libya. Diabetes Res Clin Pract 32:165–173
21. Kitagawa T, Owada M, Urakami T, Tajima N (1994) Epidemiology of type 1 (insulin-dependent) and type 2 (non-insulin-dependent) diabetes mellitus in Japanese children. Diabetes Res Clin Pract 24(Suppl):S7–S13
22. Kitagawa T, Owada M, Urakami T, Yamauchi K (1998) Increased incidence of non-dependent diabetes mellitus among Japanese school children correlates with an increased intake of animal protein and fat. Clin Pediatr 37:111–115
23. Invitti C, Guzzaloni G, Giraldinini L (2003) Prevalence and concomitants of glucose intolerance in European obese children and adolescents. Diab Care 26:118–124
24. Wabitsch M, Hauner H, Hertrampf M, Muche R, Hay B, Mayer H, Kratzer W, Debatin KM, Heinze E (2004) Type II diabetes mellitus and impaired glucose regulation in Caucasian children and adolescents with obesity living in Germany. Int J Obes Relat Metab Disord 28:307–313
25. Grabert M, Krause U, Rami B, Scober E, Schweiggert F, Thon A (2003) Prevalence and clinical characteristics of patients with non-type -1-diabetes in pediatric age range: analysis of multicenter database including 20 401 patients from 148 centers in Germany and Austria (Abstract). Diabetologia 46(Suppl 2):26
26. Zachrisson I, Tibell C, Bang P, Ortquist E (2003) Prevalence of type 2 diabetes among known cases of diabetes aged 0-18 years in Sweden (Abstract). Diabetologia 46(Suppl 2):56
27. Nicklas TA (2001) Eating patterns, dietary quality and obesity. J Am Coll Nutr 20:599–608
28. Parsons TJ, Power C, Logan S, Summerbell CD (1999) Childhood predictors of adult obesity: a systemic review. Int J Obes Relat Metab Disord 23:S1–S107
29. Whitaker RC, Wright JA, Pepe MS, Seidel KD, Dietz WH (1997) Predicting obesity in young adulthood from childhood and parental obesity. N Engl J Med 337:869–874
30. Strauss RS, Pollock HA (2001) Epidemic increase in childhood overweight, 1986–1998. JAMA 286:2845–2848

31. James PT (2004) Obesity: the worldwide epidemic. Clin Dermatol 22:276–280
32. Pi-Sunyer FX (1993) Medical hazards of obesity. Ann Intern Med 119:655–660
33. Ogden CL, Flegal KM, Johnson CL (2002) Prevalence and trends in overweight among U.S. children and adolescents, 1999–2000. JAMA 288:1728–1732
34. Hedley AA, Ogden CL, Johnson CL, Carroll MD, Curtin LR, Flegal KM (2004) Prevalence of overweight and obesity among us children, adolescence and adults, 1999–2002. JAMA 291:2847–2850
35. Ogden CL, Carroll MD, Flegal KM (2008) High body mass index for age among US children and adolescents, 2003–2006. JAMA 299:2401–2405
36. NHANES Surveys (1976–1980 and 2003–2006). http://www.cdc.gov/obesity/childhood/prevalence.html. Accessed 4 March 2010
37. American Diabetes Association (2000) Type 2 diabetes in children and adolescents. Diab Care 23:381–389
38. Sorof JM, Lai D, Turner J, Poffenbarger T, Portman RJ (2004) Overweight, ethnicity and the prevalence of hypertension in school-aged children. Pediatrics 113:475–482
39. Freedman DS, Khan LK, Dietz WH, Srinivasan SR, Berenson GS (2001) Relationship of childhood obesity to coronary heart disease risk factors in adulthood: the Bogalusa heart Study. Pediatrics 108:712–718
40. Becque MD, Katch VL, Rocchini AP, Marks CR, Moorehead C (1988) Coronary risk incidence of obese adolescents: reduction by exercise plus diet intervention. Pediatrics 81:605–612
41. Ranjana S, Gene F, Barbara T, William VT, Bruna B, Karin A, Mary S, Vera R, Sara T, Gina B, Robert S, Sonia C (2002) Prevalence of impaired glucose tolerance among children and adolescents with marked obesity. N Engl J Med 346:802–810
42. Cruz ML, Bergman RN, Goran MI (2002) Unique effect of visceral fat on insulin sensitivity in obese Hispanic children with a family history of type 2 diabetes. Diab Care 25:1631–1636
43. Fagot-Campagna A (2000) Emergence of type 2 diabetes mellitus in children: epidemiological evidence. J Pediatr Endocrinol Metab 13:11395–11402
44. Haslam DW, James WP (2005) Obesity. Lancet 366:1197–1209
45. Wild S, Roglic G, Green A, Sicree R, King H (2004) Global prevalence of diabetes: estimates for the year 2000 and the projections for 2030. Diab Care 27:1047–1053
46. Wei JN, Sung FC, Lin CC, Lin RS, Chiang CC, Chuang LM (2003) National surveillance for type 2 diabetes mellitus in Taiwanese children. JAMA 290:1345–1350
47. Lee WR (2000) The changing demography of diabetes mellitus in Singapore. Diabetes Res Clin Pract 50:S35–S39
48. Likitmaskul S, Tuchinda C, Punnakanta L, Kiattisakthavee P, Chaichanwattanakul K, Angsusingha K (2000) Increase of type 2 diabetes in Thai children and adolescents in Thailand. J Pediatr Endocrinol Metab 13:1209
49. Likitmaskul S, Kiattisathavee P, Chaichanwatanakul K, Punnakanta L, Angsusingha K, Tuchindra C (2003) Increasing prevalence of type 2 diabetes mellitus in Thai children and adolescents associated with increasing prevalence of obesity. J Pediatr Endocrinol Metab 16:71–77
50. Likitmaskul S, Kiattisathavee P, Chaichanwatanakul K, Punnakanta L, Angsusingha K, Tuchindra C (2000) Epidemiology of diabetes mellitus in children in Hong Kong: the Hong Kong childhood diabetes registry. J Pediatr Endocrinol Metab 13:297–302
51. Zhi D, Shen S, Luo F, Zhao Z, Hong Q (2003) IDF WPR childhood and adolescence, Diabcare survey 2001 in Shanghai (Abstract). O-25, ISPAD, Saint-Malo
52. Narayan KM, Fagot-Campagna A, Imperatore G (2001) Type 2 diabetes in children: a problem lurking for India? Indian Pediatr 38:701–704

53. Hotu S, Carter B, Watson PD, Cutfield WS, Cundy T (2004) Increasing prevalence of type 2 diabetes in adolescents. J Paediatr Child Health 40:201–204

54. Schober E, Rami B, Nachbauer E, Waldhor T, and the Australian Diabetes Incidence Study Group (2002) Type 2 diabetes is rare but not absent in children <15 years in Austria (Abstract). The 9th European workshop on pediatric endocrinology, Slovakia

55. Rami B, Schober E, Nachbauer E, Waldhor T (2003) Austrian Diabetes Incidence Study group. Type 2 diabetes mellitus is rare but not absent in children under 15 years of age in Austria. Eur J Pediatr 162:850–852

56. Ehtisham S, Kirk J, McEvilly A, Shaw N, Jones S, Rose S (2001) Prevalence of type 2 diabetes in children in Birminghham. BMJ 322:1428

57. Ortega-Rodriguez E, Levy-Marchal C, Tubiana N, Czernichow P, Polak M (2001) Emergence of type 2 diabetes in a hospital based cohort of children with diabetes mellitus. Diabetes Metab 27:574–578

58. Zachrisson I, Tibell C, Bang P, Ortqvist E (2003) Prevalence of type 2 diabetes among known cases of diabetes aged 0-18 in Sweden (Abstract). 18th International Diabetes Federation Congress, Paris, France

59. Davis E (2002) Incresing type 2 diabetes in children and adolescents in Western Australia (Abstract). Australian Diabetes Society and Australian Diabetes Educators Association. p 336

60. Harkin N (2002) Increasing recognisation of Type 2 diabetes in adolescents (Abstract). Australian Diabetes Society and Australian Diabetes Educators Association, p 171

61. El-Hazmi MAF, Warsy AS, AL-Swailem AR, Al-Swailem AM, Sulaimani R (1998) Diabetes mellitus as a health problem in Saudi Arabia and its complications. Eastern Mediterr Health J 4:58–67

62. Punnose J (2002) Childhood and adolescent diabetes mellitus in Arabs residing in the United Arab Emirates. Diabetes Res Clin Pract 55:29–33

63. Ramos O, Ferraro M, Andres ME, Arce L (2003) Type 2 diabetes in youth, an increasing problem in Buenos Aires? (Abstract). 18th International Diabetes Federation Congress, Paris, France

64. Freedman DS, Shrinivasan SR, Valdez RA, Williamson DF, Berenson GS (1997) Secular increase in relative weight and adiposity among children over two decades: the Bogulusa Heart Study. Pediatrics 99:420–426

65. Zametkin AJ, Zoon CK, Klein HW, Munson S (2004) Psychiatric aspects of child and adolescent obesity: a review of the past 10 years. J Am Acad Child Adolesc Psychiatry 43:134–150

66. Kotani K, Nishida M, Yamashita S, Funahashi T, Fujioka S, Tokunaga K, Ishikawa K, Tarui S, Matsuzawa Y (1997) Two decades of annual medical examination in Japanese obese children: do obese children grow into obese adults? Int J Obes Relat Metab Disord 27:912–921

67. Lobstein TJ, James WP, Cole TJ (2003) Increasing levels of excess weight among children in England. Int J Obes Relat Metab Disord 27:1136–1138

68. Moreno LA, Sarria A, Popkin BM (2002) The nutrition transition in Spain: a European Mediterranean country. Eur J Clin Nutr 56:992–1003

69. Rolland-Cachera MF, Deheeger M, Thibault H (2001) Epidemological basis of obesity. Arch Pediatr 8(Suppl 2):287–289

70. Krassas GE, Tzotzas T, Tsametis C, Konstantinidis T (2005) Prevalence and trends in overweight and obesity among children and adolescents in Thessaloniki, Greece. J Pediatr Endocrinol Metab 14:1319–1365

71. Macaluso CJ, Bauer UE, Deeb LC, Malone JI, Chaudhari M, Silverstein J et al. (2002) Type 2 diabetes mellitus among Florida children and adolescents, 1994 through 1998. Public Health Rep 117:373–379

11 Nutrition for the Diabetic Child

Catherine M. Champagne

Keypoints

- Integration of a licensed, registered dietitian into the team caring for the diabetic child or adolescent is essential.
- The majority of nutritional benefit for pediatric T2DM derives from family-based education on healthier lifestyle choices and on appropriate portion size.
- Dietary education is an ongoing process for families affected by pediatric obesity and T2DM.

Keywords: Type 2 diabetes mellitus, Nutrition, Dietitian, Education, Lifestyle

11.1 INTRODUCTION

Proper nutrition, coupled with lifestyle change, is an ideal way to prevent or manage diabetes. It helps to keep blood-sugar at near-normal levels, controls weight, and provides necessary nutrients. It helps reduce, or eliminate, the use of oral diabetes medications, and may prevent complications of diabetes. The way a child with diabetes should eat is exactly the way everyone in this country should eat – for good health! The entire family can benefit from following a well-balanced diet, so there is no need for a child to feel singled out.

From: *Nutrition and Health: Management of Pediatric Obesity and Diabetes*,
Edited by: R.J. Ferry, Jr., DOI 10.1007/978-1-60327-256-8_11,
© Springer Science+Business Media, LLC 2011

11.2 GENERAL DIETARY GOALS WITH PREDIABETES OR DIABETES

The main focus of nutrition in diabetes is to achieve tighter control of blood-sugar levels. For overweight children, the goal is to reduce the rate of body weight gain while allowing for proper growth and development. Children grow at different rates. For individuals with diabetes, who are on insulin or oral medication, calorie intake must be coordinated with medication or insulin administration, exercise, and other variables to control blood glucose levels. Nutrition and medication work hand in hand. Good nutrition also:

- Protects the heart by improving lipid (cholesterol and triglycerides) profile and controlling blood pressure. High blood pressure may even be seen in children.
- Helps achieve and maintain a reasonable weight.
- Helps manage or prevent complications of diabetes. A person with diabetes, whether Type 1 or 2, is at risk for a number of medical complications, including heart and kidney disease.
- Enhances overall health which results in a better quality of life.

There is not really one "diabetic" diet, because one size does not fit all. Proper nutrition should be individualized to help meet health and diabetic self-care goals. The diets with the most science behind them are the diets used in the Diabetes Prevention Program (DPP) and the tested diets of the Dietary Approaches to Stop Hypertension (DASH) trials. DASH is now thought to provide a sound way of achieving proper nutrition that will reduce blood pressure, improve lipid risk profiles, reduce cancer risk, and enable one to improve diabetes risk. What these diets do have in common, however, is that they are built around healthy choices within nutrient categories of carbohydrates, protein, fats, vitamins, and minerals. While both of these trials were carried out in adults, the focus is on health and what diabetic individuals (both young and old) should be consuming as part of an overall healthy diet. All nutrients play a specific role in preventing or managing diabetes.

11.2.1 Carbohydrates

Carbohydrates are present in vegetables, fruits, grains, cereals, breads, sugars, and to some extent in dairy foods. Simple carbohydrates, found in sweets, white bread, cakes, candy, and other foods containing simple sugars, are quickly digested by the body and cause a rapid rise in blood glucose. Complex carbohydrates, on the other hand, particularly those rich in fiber, do not normally elicit the same kind of quick response. The speed at which glucose is released into the bloodstream by a particular carbohydrate is termed its "glycemic index." Some suggest that we can use this index to choose foods that might better control blood-sugar swings; however, not all agree. Natural, unprocessed carbohydrates, typically complex ones, are worth choosing because they are high in many nutrients that can help to prevent or control diabetes. One of these is fiber, the material that gives strength and support to plant tissues, as well as texture. Although it is primarily made up of carbohydrates, fiber does not have a lot of available calories. High fiber foods break down into glucose more gradually, keep the stomach from emptying too quickly, and are absorbed more slowly into the bloodstream. There are two types of fiber in foods: soluble and insoluble. Insoluble fiber adds bulk to the diet, which helps maintain intestinal health and may help in some cancers. It does not dissolve in water and is mainly found in vegetables (particularly the skin), fruit pulp and the bran layer of grains. Soluble fiber attracts water during digestion and slows the rate of nutrient absorption. It is found in oat bran, seeds, beans, and certain fruits and vegetables. Table 11.1 summarizes the fiber recommendations from The American Academy of Pediatrics [1].

11.2.2 Protein

Protein from any number of sources – plant protein or animal protein – is part of a healthy diet to prevent, control, or manage diabetes. Generally, its role is to support the growth, repair, and maintenance of body tissues. The amount of protein needed in a day depends on the diabetic condition. The average American diet contains approximately 12–15% of daily caloric intake from protein, but a protein intake of as much as 20% of daily calories may be considered. In diabetic nutrition, protein is an important part of the diet and, when combined with carbohydrates and fat in a meal, helps to maintain a normal

Table 11.1
American academy of pediatrics fiber recommendation

	Fiber intake (g)
Ages 1–3 years – all children	19
Ages 4–8 years – all children	25
Ages 9–13 years – females	26
Ages 9–13 years – males	31
Ages 14–18 years – females	29
Ages 14–18 years – males	38

Table 11.2
Estimated average requirements (EAR) and recommended
dietary allowance (RDA) protein recommendations

	EAR (g/kg/day)	RDA
1–3 years	0.88	1.10 g/kg/day or 13 g/day
4–8 years	0.76	0.95 g/kg/day or 19 g/day
9–13 years	0.76	0.95 g/kg/day or 34 g/day
14–18 years		
Males	0.73	0.85 g/kg/day or 52 g/day
Females	0.71	0.85 g/kg/day or 46 g/day

blood-sugar level. Table 11.2 summarizes the estimated average requirement (EAR) and recommended dietary allowance (RDA) protein recommendations according to age and gender [2].

11.2.3   Fats

For decades, most health experts agreed that the healthiest diets were those low in the percentage of calories coming from fat. But now we know that there are good and bad types of fat. The good fats – found in foods like fish, olive oil, avocados, and many nuts – actually improve cholesterol levels in the blood and may significantly reduce the risk of heart disease. Interest in the Mediterranean diet approach to weight loss with its positive benefits on lipids and other blood variables suggests that its use in the treatment is worthy of consideration. The main fat source in the Mediterranean diet is olive oil, which is consumed in varying amounts. Total fat ranges from 28% to as much as 40% of energy. As for the bad fats, there are two types. Saturated fats – typically found in red meat, butter, ice cream, and tropical oils – increase the risk of heart disease by increasing total cholesterol levels in the body. With the Mediterranean diet, saturated fat in particular was low at approximately 7–8% of energy [3, 4]. The other bad fat is called "trans fat," found primarily in processed foods, such as stick margarines and many commercially baked or fried foods. Trans fat may be even worse than saturated fat, and should be avoided. They may elevate LDL cholesterol and lower beneficial HDL cholesterol. Overall, the current recommendation is that 25–35% of daily calories should come from fat (keep in mind that the number of calories consumed is of utmost importance), and less than 10% of those calories should be from saturated fats. Trans fats should be avoided as much as possible. Food labels now contain information on trans fat. Intake of cholesterol should be less than 300 mg daily [5].

Table 11.3
American Diabetes Association recommendations for children with diabetes

- Eat at least five servings of fruits and vegetables every day, including a variety of colors such as green, yellow, orange, and red.
- Aim for six servings of breads, cereals, and starchy vegetables. Starchy vegetables include peas, corn, potatoes, and dried beans such as pinto or kidney beans.
- Choose two to three servings of low-fat dairy products, like skim or 1% milk or nonfat yogurt.
- Choose lean meats, chicken, and fish. Pick meats without visible fat and remove skin from chicken and other poultry. Try to include two to three servings of fish a week. Avoid fried meats.
- Cut back on sweets and desserts. Most desserts are high in calories and do not contain many vitamins and minerals.

Table 11.4
Serving size equivalents

A serving of ...	Equals ...
Fresh fruit or vegetables	1 cup
Canned fruit or cooked vegetables	½ cup
Starchy vegetables or dried beans	½ cup
Bread	1 slice
Dry cereal	¾ cup
Cooked cereal	½ cup
Rice or pasta	1/3 cup
Dairy products	1 cup
Lean meats, chicken and fish	3 ounces
Oil, margarine, or butter	1 teaspoon

11.3 AMERICAN DIABETES ASSOCIATION RECOMMENDATIONS [6]

Table 11.3 summarizes the recommendations made by the American Diabetes Association for children with diabetes. Table 11.4 presents serving size equivalents.

11.4 THE DIABETES PREVENTION PROGRAM

Scientists involved in the DPP study found that the lifestyle change could sharply reduce the chances that a person with prediabetes would actually develop diabetes. The best success was with the lifestyle group, who received intensive training in diet, exercise, and behavior modification. By eating less fat and fewer calories and exercising for a total of 150 min a week, the aim was to lose 7% of their body weight and maintain that weight loss [7]. Again, while this was in adults, it is clear that dietary improvements and increasing physical activity are realistic goals for children to adhere to.

In DPP, healthy eating involved eating less fat. There is a lot of science showing that eating too much fat makes us fat and is related to heart disease and diabetes. Fat is essentially the most fattening thing we eat and contains more than twice the calories as the same amount of sugar, starch, or protein.

Fat is related to heart disease and diabetes. Research has shown that eating a lot of fat can increase cholesterol levels [8, 9]. Cholesterol is one type of fat in your blood. The higher the cholesterol, the greater the chances are of having a heart attack. Research has also shown that eating a lot of fat may increase chances of getting diabetes. Much of the fat we eat, actually more than half of it, is hidden in foods.

The fat gram goal or budget is something to be figured out or calculated on an individual basis. As an example, if a person needs to eat only 1,200 calories per day and the desirable percent of calories from fat is 30%, then that is $(1,200 \times 0.3)$ or 360 calories. One gram of fat has 9 calories, therefore $360 \div 9 = 40$ g of fat. That would be the goal; pretty simple to figure out.

The DPP focused on three ways to eat less fat. First, eat high-fat foods less often. For example, French fries should not be eaten every day. Second, smaller amounts of high-fat foods should be eaten because cutting back even a little can make a big difference. Third, just eat lower fat foods instead.

A key concept in the DPP was looking at the Food Guide Pyramid and making wise choices. We now have new guidelines for what children should eat and a new pyramid, called MyPyramid for Kids. This can be found at the following website: http://teamnutrition.usda.gov/resources/mpk_tips. pdf. The main suggestions for families are summarized in Table 11.5.

11.5 THE CALORIE BALANCE

Remember that calories count. The DPP Lifestyle Balance Program involved: healthy eating, including eating less fat and more grains, fruits, and vegetables. It also included being active. Both relate to weight loss. Both are part of the "calorie balance." Calories in food come from fat, starches and sugars, or protein, with fat highest in calories per gram. Calories also measure the energy used up in daily life activities. Weight is a result of the balance between food (calories in) and activity (calories out).

Table 11.5
Recommendations from My Pyramid for kids

Eat right
- Make half your grains whole. More often choose whole-grain foods, such as whole-wheat bread, oatmeal, brown rice, and low-fat popcorn.
- Vary your "veggies." Go dark green and orange with your vegetables – eat spinach, broccoli, carrots, and sweet potatoes.
- Focus on fruits. Eat them at meals and at snack time, too. Choose fresh, frozen, canned, or dried fruits. Minimize fruit juice.
- Get your calcium-rich foods. To build strong bones, serve low-fat and fat-free milk and other milk products several times a day.
- Go lean with protein. Eat lean or low-fat meat, chicken, turkey, and fish. Also, change your tune with more dry beans and peas. Add chick peas, nuts, or seeds to a salad; pinto beans to a burrito; or kidney beans to soup.
- Change your oil. We all need oil. Get yours from fish, nuts, and liquid oils, such as corn, soybean, canola, and olive oil. Avoid lard.
- Do not sugarcoat it. Choose foods and beverages that do not have sugar or caloric sweeteners as one of the first ingredients. Added sugars contribute calories with few, if any, nutrients.

Exercise
- Set a good example. Be active and get your family to join you. Have fun together. Play with the kids or pets. Go for a walk, tumble in the leaves, or play catch.
- Take the President's Challenge as a family. Track your individual physical activities together and earn awards for active lifestyles at www.presidentschallenge.org
- Establish a routine. Set aside time each day as activity time – walk, jog, skate, cycle, or swim. Adults need at least 30 min of physical activity most days of the week; children need 60 min every day or most days.
- Have an activity party. Make the next birthday party centered on physical activity. Try backyard Olympics, or relay races. Have a bowling or skating party.
- Set up a home gym. Use household items, such as canned foods, as weights. Stairs can substitute for stair machines.
- Move it! Instead of sitting through TV commercials, get up and move. When you talk on the phone, lift weights or walk around. Remember to limit TV watching and computer time.
- Give activity gifts. Give gifts that encourage physical activity – like active games or sporting equipment.

Remember that food and being active work together. To lose weight, it is best to eat less and be more active. That way, it changes both sides of the balance at once. Then, over time, a new balance can be reached at a new, lower weight.

11.6   MANAGING DIABETES WITH THE DASH EATING PLAN

One of the healthiest diets today resulted from a government-funded study called the DASH. This study was designed to look at the effects of certain dietary patterns on reducing blood pressure. The diet was effective on blood pressure control, but also found to be an appropriate diet for cardiovascular disease, cancer prevention, and is promoted as one way to help in diabetes prevention and diabetes care [10, 11].

Restricting sodium improves results. The diet appears to have antioxidant effects and may help lower LDL cholesterol levels, although beneficial HDL levels also decline. This diet is not only rich in important nutrients and fiber but also includes foods that contain far more electrolytes, potassium, calcium, and magnesium, than are found in the average American diet.

The dietary pattern is what it is all about. More information can be found online at http://www.nhlbi.nih.gov/health/public/heart/hbp/dash/new_dash.pdf. This website provides menus and more information for adhering to the DASH diet. The DASH diet recommendations are summarized in Table 11.6.

The DASH diet can be incorporated into any diet for those with diabetes. It emphasizes an eating plan that is low in saturated fat, cholesterol, and

Table 11.6
Recommendations from the DASH dietary pattern

- Reduce saturated fat, but include calcium-rich dairy products that are nonfat or low-fat.
- When choosing fats, select monounsaturated oils, such as olive or canola oils.
- Choose whole grains over white flour or pasta products.
- Choose fresh fruits and vegetables every day. Many of these foods are rich in potassium, fiber, or both which may help lower blood pressure. In one study, increasing intake of fruits and vegetables on DASH diet dropped blood pressure after 6 months.
- Include nuts, seeds, or legumes (dried beans or peas) daily.
- Choose modest amounts of protein (preferably fish, poultry, or soy products).

total fat and higher in fruits, vegetables, and low-fat dairy foods. It also is lower in sodium than many dietary patterns.

11.7 SUMMARY

The diets outlined here will certainly help to improve overall health and assist in preventing or managing diabetes in children. In some, the symptoms of diabetes may diminish; in others, medication requirements could be adjusted downward or eliminated; and in some others, complications may be improved or prevented altogether.

Motivation in children is the key to success and it is important that the parent, teacher, and medical professional enable the child to reach that success. Some important things to enable that level of motivation are included in Table 11.7. Following the recommendations and strategies presented in

Table 11.7
Recommendations for increasing motivation in children

- Help the child to stay aware of the benefits that can be achieved.
- Recognize childrens' successes. What changes in their eating and activity do they feel proudest of? Keep visible signs of progress.
- Encourage children to
  - Post weight and activity graphs on the refrigerator door.
  - Mark their activity milestones on a map toward a particular goal.
  - Measure themselves (waist, belt size) once a month.
  - Keep track of childrens' weight, eating and activity.
- Encourage children to
  - Record their activity daily.
  - Record what they eat (realize that this is a difficult task for them).
  - Record their weight regularly.
- Recommend adding variety to a routine. How have they varied their activity? What meals, snacks, or foods are they most bored with? Can they think of some ways to vary this part of their eating?
- Help children set new goals and rewards for themselves when they meet each goal.
  - Specific, short-term goals, just enough to challenge.
  - Clear rewards as something they will do or buy – if and only if – they reach their goal.
  - Try nonfood rewards that children can reward themselves for reaching a goal (movies, stickers, new games, etc.)
- Encourage children to involve friends, family, and others to help them stay motivated. Suggest that they call others for encouragement and support when needed.

this chapter will be helpful in achieving a quality of life for which we all strive. Lifelong changes toward a healthier life mean a better quality of life for children as they venture into adulthood.

REFERENCES

1. Gidding SS, Dennison BA, Birch LL *et al.* (2006) Dietary recommendations for children and adolescents: a guide for practitioners. Pediatrics 117:544–549
2. Food and Nutrition Board, Institute of Medicine (2005) Dietary reference intakes for energy, carbohydrate, fiber, fat, fatty acids, cholesterol, protein, and amino acids (macronutrients). The National Academies Press, Washington
3. de Souza RJ, Swain JF, Appel LJ, Sacks FM (2008) Alternatives for macronutrient intake and chronic disease: a comparison of the OmniHeart diet with popular diets and with dietary recommendations. Am J Clin Nutr 88:1–11
4. Champagne CM (2009) The usefulness of a Mediterranean-based diet in individuals with type 2 diabetes. Curr Diab Rep 9:389–395
5. U.S. Department of Health and Human Services and U.S. Department of Agriculture (2005) Dietary Guidelines for Americans, 6th edn. U.S. Government Printing Office, Washington
6. American Diabetes Association (2000) Nutrition recommendations and principles for people with diabetes mellitus. Diabetes Care 23(Suppl 1):S43–S46
7. Diabetes Prevention Program Research Group (2002) The diabetes prevention program (DPP): description of lifestyle intervention. Diabetes Care 25:2165–2171
8. Lichtenstein AH, Kennedy E, Barrier P, Danford D, Ernst ND, Grundy SM, Leveille GA, Van Horn L, Williams CL, Booth SL (1998) Dietary fat consumption and health. Nutr Rev 56(5 Pt 2):S3–S19
9. Hegsted DM, McGandy RB, Myers ML, Stare FJ (1965) Quantitative effects of dietary fat on serum cholesterol in man. Am J Clin Nutr 17:281–295
10. Appel LJ, Moore TJ, Obarzanek E, Vollmer W, Svetkey LP, Sacks F, Bray G, Vogt TM, Cutler JA, Simons-Morton D, Lin PH, Karanja N, Miller ER III, Harsha DW (1997) A clinical trial of the effects of dietary patterns on blood pressure. New Engl J Med 338:1117–1124
11. Liese AD, Nichols M, Sun X, D'Agostino RB Jr, Haffner SM (2009) Adherence to the DASH Diet is inversely associated with incidence of type 2 diabetes: the insulin resistance atherosclerosis study. Diabetes Care 32:1434–1436

ADDITIONAL RESOURCES

http://teamnutrition.usda.gov/resources/mpk_tips.pdf
http://www.nhlbi.nih.gov/health/public/heart/hbp/dash/new_dash.pdf
http://www.presidentschallenge.org
Royner AJ, Nansel TR (2009) Are children with type 1 diabetes consuming a healthful diet? A review of the current evidence and strategies for dietary change. Diabetes Educ 35:97–107

12 Pharmacologic Approaches to Type 2 Diabetes and Obesity in Children and Adolescents

Patama Pongsuwan

Key Points

- Few pharmacologic agents commonly used to manage pediatric obesity and type 2 diabetes mellitus (T2DM) have been studied rigorously in pediatric populations.
- Although not the mainstay of prevention and risk reduction, pharmacologic agents have proven effective in treating acute sequelae of pediatric T2DM.

Keywords: Metformin, Thiazolidinedione, Insulin, Sulfonylurea, Glargine, Detemir, Lispro, Aspart, Glulisine, GLP-1 agonist, PPAR-gamma agonist

Abbreviations

ADA	American Diabetes Association
BMI	Body mass index
DPP-IV	Dipeptidyl peptidase-IV
EASD	European Association for the Study of Diabetes
EMA	European Medicines Agency
FDA	US Food and Drug Administration
GIP	Glucose dependent insulinotropic peptide
GLP-1	Glucagon-like peptide 1

From: *Nutrition and Health: Management of Pediatric Obesity and Diabetes*,
Edited by: R.J. Ferry, Jr., DOI 10.1007/978-1-60327-256-8_12,
© Springer Science+Business Media, LLC 2011

HbA$_{1C}$ Hemoglobin A$_{1C}$
HTN   Hypertension
NYHA   New York Heart Association
PCOS   Polycystic ovarian syndrome
PPAR   Peroxisome proliferator-activated receptor
SGLT   Sodium-glucose cotransporters
T1DM   Type 1 diabetes mellitus
T2DM   Type 2 diabetes mellitus
TZD   Thiazolidinedione

12.1   CASE

A 12-year-old boy has been referred to you for evaluation. He reports feeling fatigue over the past year and his parents report that he "eats all the time." They deny food-seeking behaviors at night, enuresis, or poor academic performance. His weight is 60 kg (95th percentile for age), with body mass index (BMI) of 30 kg/m^2. Acanthosis nigricans is present at the posterior and lateral folds of his neck (visible anteriorly, but not circumferential) and also extends to but not beyond the axillary borders. His testicular volume is 5 mL bilaterally (Tanner stage II). His fasting blood glucose is 160 mg/dL, and hemoglobin A$_{1C}$ (HbA$_{1C}$) is 8%. His primary-care provider diagnosed T2DM. He is accompanied by his parents, who would like to know "all options" for his plan of care. What would you recommend to this patient and his family?

12.2   INTRODUCTION

Obesity and T2DM have emerged over the past 20 years as critical, common health issues in children and adolescents. Dominant risk factors for insulin resistance and T2DM in youth include low level of physical activity, unhealthy eating habits, family history of obesity or T2DM, specific ethnicities, puberty, and low birth weight [1–7]. Obesity and insulin resistance in youth, akin to metabolic syndrome and T2DM in adults, are highly associated with increased risk of cardiovascular disease [8–13]. Improved glycemic control and maintenance of healthy weight are essential to improve long-term outcomes. This chapter reviews available data on the pharmacological management of pediatric T2DM. Table 12.1 summarizes clinical management recommendations for pediatric T2DM, and Table 12.2 summarizes glycemic control goals for adult and pediatric patients with diabetes. The reader is referred to other chapters of this text, since these public health problems demand multidisciplinary approaches by the family, clinician, and, indeed, their community.

Table 12.1
Clinical management and therapeutic goal of pediatric T2DM [34, 116, 163]

Clinical management of pediatric T2DM
- Lifestyle modification is central to management. Behavioral modification should be the first line-treatment of T2DM, before medication, depending on the signs and symptoms and the degree of hyperglycemia at presentation. Weight reduction and increased levels of physical activity play important roles to decrease insulin resistance and improve glycemic control. Pharmacologic intervention does *not* replace lifestyle modifications.
- Other than metformin and insulin, hypoglycemic agents on the market have not been approved by the FDA for use in children or adolescents.

Therapeutic goals for pediatric T2DM and obesity [116]
- To maintain fasting glucose levels 80–130 mg/dL and HbA$_{1C}$<7.0%
- To prevent complications of T2DM, both macro- and microvascular diseases
- To prevent and treat other comorbidities, such as hyperlipidemia and hypertension, if indicated

Table 12.2
Goals of glycemic control in pediatric and adult T2DM [114]

	Fasting plasma glucose (mg/dL)	*HbA$_{1C}$*
Adult	70–130	<7%
Toddler and preschooler (0–6 years)	100–180	<8.5% (but >7.5%)
School age (6–12 years)	90–150	<8%
Adolescents and younssg adults (13–19 years)	90–130	<7.5%

12.2.1 Pharmacological Agents for T2DM

The pathophysiology of T2DM in children and adolescents resembles that in adults (Fig. 12.1) [14–19]. Gungor *et al.* demonstrated in adolescents with T2DM that insulin sensitivity declines 50%, together with a decrease of 75% in the first-phase insulin response, when compared to nondiabetic adolescents [16]. Generally, the degree of insulin resistance is considered to be more severe in adolescents, when compared to adult diabetic patients due to their higher circulating levels of pubertal steroids. In fact, some adolescents experience a rapid acceleration of loss of pancreatic β-cell function [16, 20].

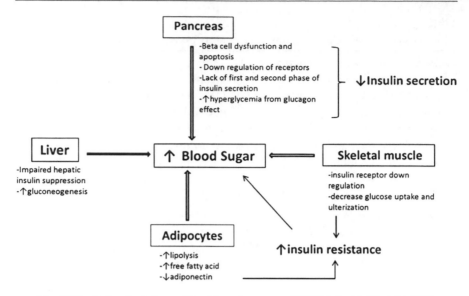

Fig. 12.1. Pathophysiology of insulin resistance and T2DM [1, 14, 21, 186, 187].

Owing to the paucity of published data regarding the long-term outcomes and efficacy of treatments for pediatric T2DM, most pharmacological options are based on clinical studies performed in adults and anecdotal pediatric experience. Table 12.3 suggests the indications for using pharmacological treatment in children and adolescents with T2DM. Figure 12.2 and Table 12.4 summarize the mechanisms of action, efficacy, side effects, and dosing recommendations for available agents.

12.3   INSULIN SECRETAGOGUES

12.3.1   Sulfonylureas (Glyburide, Glipizide, and Glimepiride)

Sulfonylureas are one of the most commonly used oral hypoglycemic agents in *adults*. Sulfonylureas acts by binding to the sulfonylurea receptor, which results in a calcium influx and a stimulation of insulin secretion [21, 22]. Sulfonylureas are considered to be very effective in controlling blood sugar as monotherapy or in combination with insulin sensitizers [23–26]. The information on currently available sulfonylureas and their recommended dosages is summarized in Table 12.4.

Table 12.3
Indications for pharmacologic treatment for pediatric T2DM [116]

Indications for pharmacologic therapy

Failed intensive attempts to modify lifestyle and diet in asymptomatic patients

Morbid signs or symptoms at presentation, such as diabetes ketoacidosis (DKA), symptomatic hyperglycemia (polyuria and polydipsia), or severe hyperglycemia (*e.g.*, hyperglycemic hyperosmolar nonketotic coma [HHNK])

When doubtful about diagnosis (T2DM vs. other disease), insulin therapy should be initiated for presumptive T1DM to control blood glucose, until T2DM has been confirmed

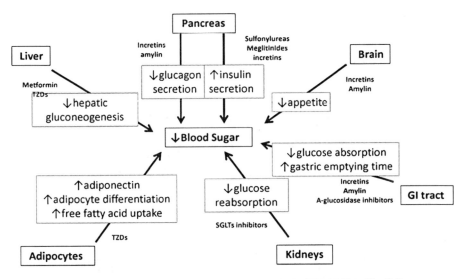

Fig. 12.2. Action sites of medication treatment in T2DM [21, 22, 130].

12.3.2 Meglitinides (Repaglinide and Nateglinide)

Meglitinides are short-acting oral hypoglycemic agents. Their action are similar to sulfonylureas by increasing insulin secretion through ATP-dependent K channels in pancreatic beta-cell [21].

Data on the use of sulfonylureas and meglitinides in pediatrics are still limited, and neither class of medication has regulatory approval for use in the pediatric population. In one small study in children with cystic fibrosis,

Table 12.4
Medications for treatment in pediatric T2DM [20, 21, 63]

Medication	Dose	Mechanism of action	Expected decreased in HbA_{1C} as monotherapy	Side effects
Sulfonylurea (adult dose, unlabeled use, no specific dose for pediatric patients)				
Glyburide	2.5–20 mg/day, once or twice daily in single or divided doses	Bind to sulfonylurea receptor, which is a component of ATP-dependent K Channels in pancreatic beta cell, resulting in calcium influx and stimulating insulin secretion	1.0–2.0%	Hypoglycemia
Glimepiride	1–4 mg once daily			
Glipizide	5–20 mg/day, once or twice daily			
Meglitinide (adult dose, unlabeled use, no specific dose for pediatric patients)				
Repaglinide (Prandin)	0.5–4 mg with each meal, with maximum dose of 16 mg/day	Short-acting, bind to different receptor from sulfonylureas but also results in increasing insulin secretion through ATP-dependent K Channels	0.6–2%	Hypoglycemia (lesser incidence when compare to sulfonylureas)
Nateglinide (Starlix)	60–120 mg, twice daily (before meal)			

	Dose	Mechanism of action		Side effects/contraindications
Biguanide				
Metformin	500–2,000 mg, once or twice daily	Enhances insulin binding to insulin receptor, increases peripheral glucose utilization, reduces hepatic gluconeogenesis, decreases free fatty acid and increases lipogenesis	1.0–2.0%	GI side effects, lactic acidosis Metformin is contraindicated in renal insufficiency, hepatic insufficiency, congestive heart failure
Thiazolidinediones (adult dose, unlabeled use, no specific dose for pediatric patients)				
Rosiglitazone (Avandia), may become unavailable	4–8 mg, once daily	Facilitate glucose transporter activity → increase rate of muscle glycogen synthesis and glucose oxidation	1.0–2.0%	Weight gain, peripheral edema, fluid retention. Rosiglitazone associated with macular edema. Association between TZDs and decreased bone mass and increased risk of fractures in adults
Pioglitazone (Actos)	15–45 mg, once daily	Promote fatty acid uptake and storage Regulate adipocyte differentiation		Contraindicated in heart failure by NYHA class III-IV and in active liver disease

(continued)

Table 12.4
(continued)

Medication	Dose	Mechanism of action	Expected decreased in HbA_{1C} as monotherapy	Side effects
α-glucosidase inhibitors (adult dose, unlabeled use, no specific dose for pediatric patients)				
Acarbose (Precose)	25 mg PO before large meals (3 times daily)	Inhibit pancreatic α-amylase and intersitnal α-glucosidase enzymes which convert carbohydrates into monosaccharides → delay glucose absorption and slower postprandial hyperglycemia	0.5–0.8%	GI disturbances: flatulence, bloating, diarrhea, abdominal discomfort
Incretin therapy (adult dose, unlabeled use, no specific dose for pediatric patients)				
Exenatide (GLP-1 agonist)	5–10 μg, subcutaneous injection, twice daily	Enhance glucose-dependent insulin stimulation effect and restore first and second phase insulin response to glucose, suppress postprandial glucagon secretion, delay gastric emptying time, and reduce food intake and body weight	0.7–0.9% [164]	GI side effects (especially nausea), increased risk of hypoglycemia when combined with sulfonylurea

Drug	Dose	Mechanism	A1C reduction	Comments
Liraglutide (modified long acting GLP-1 agonist)	1.2 or 1.8 mg, subcutaneous injection, once daily	Inhibit dipeptidyl peptidase IV enzyme, thus decreased the degradation of endogenous GLP-1	1.0–1.5% [165]	There are some reports of the association between exenatide and acute pancreatitis, and liraglutide with thyroid C-cell tumors in rodents
Sitagliptin (DPP-IV inhibitor)	100 mg, oral, once daily		0.5–0.7% [166]	
Saxagliptin (DPP-IV inhibitor)	2.5–5 mg, oral, once daily		0.5–0.7% [167]	
Amylin (adult dose, unlabeled use, no specific dose for pediatric patients)				
Pramlintide	Initial 60 µg, then gradually increase to 120 µg, 3 times/day before meal	Delays gastric emptying time, suppresses glucagon secretion, decreases appetite and food intake	0.2–0.4%	GI side effects; nausea, vomiting, anorexia Gradually dose titration along with insulin dose adjustment might required to prevent hypoglycemia Unknown long-term safety, expensive, 3 times/day injection

sulfonylureas may have improved glucose tolerance in the children [27]; however, there are still some concerns of hypoglycemic events in the sulfonylurea-treated group.

A randomized single-blind study compared glimepiride and metformin in pediatric patients with T2DM suggested that glimepiride is safe and effective for the treatment of T2DM in youth [28]. The reduction in HbA_{1C} levels in subjects treated with glimepiride was similar to that observed with metformin without significant differences in hypoglycemic events between the two groups. Nevertheless, sulfonylureas are not approved for the treatment of pediatric patients with T2DM. Further clinical trials using insulin secretagogues in children and adolescents with T2DM are warranted.

12.4   INSULIN SENSITIZER

12.4.1   Biguanides (Metformin)

Metformin improves insulin resistance by increasing peripheral utilization of glucose and reducing hepatic glucose production. Data from adult studies indicate that metformin is clinically effective in reducing insulin resistance and in promoting weight loss [24, 29–31]. In 1977, Lutjens and Smit first described a beneficial effect on weight and insulin levels in obese children treated with metformin [32]. Several later studies in children and adolescents also indicated that metformin is well tolerated and effective in improving glycemic control and in decreasing insulin resistance in children with T2DM and nondiabetic obese patients [33–36].

Metformin is the *only* oral hypoglycemic agent currently approved by the US Food and Drug Administration (FDA) and the EMA (European Medicines Agency) for treatment of T2DM in children aged 10 years and older. The recommended starting dose of metformin is 500 mg orally twice daily, with gradual titration to an effective dose up to a maximum dose of 2,000 mg/day (Table 12.4).

12.4.2   Thiazolidinediones (TZDs)

Thiazolidinediones (TZDs) act through intranuclear, peroxisome proliferator- activated receptors (PPARs) by regulating gene expression in several target organs (Table 12.5). TZDs improve insulin sensitivity at peripheral tissue by facilitating glucose transport activity, thereby increasing peripheral glucose utilization. TZDs also promote fatty acid uptake and storage in adipose tissue mass, and they regulate the release of adiponectin. In turn, adiponectin regulates adipose tissue differentiation and improves insulin sensitivity [37].

Table 12.5

Distribution of peroxisome proliferator activated receptors (PPARs) [37]

Receptors	Target organs	Function
PPAR-α	Liver, heart, vascular wall, muscle	Enhancing free fatty acid oxidation and regulation lipoprotein concentration
PPAR-γ	Adipose tissue, pancreatic beta cell, vascular endothelium, macrophage	Adipocyte differentiation, intravascular lipolysis, fatty acid uptake and storage, and glucose uptake
PPAR-δ	Skin, brain, adipose tissue	Mostly in lipid homeostasis

[a]Rosiglitazone is a pure PPAR-γ agonist; pioglitazone exerts PPAR-γ and PPAR-α effects

Two TZDs are currently available for treatment of T2DM in adults. Rosiglitazone (Avandia®) is a pure PPAR-γ agonist. Pioglitazone (Actos®) exerts both PPAR-γ and PPAR-α effects. As monotherapy, either agent can lower HbA_{1c} by 1–2% in adults with T2DM. They can also be used in combination with a sulfonylurea or metformin. Pioglitazone has also been approved for use in combination with insulin. Table 12.4 shows efficacy data, recommended dosage, and safety profiles of TZDs in adults with T2DM.

Strong evidence indicates that TZDs cause fluid retention and can contribute to heart failure [38–43], especially among those who use TZDs in combination with insulin therapy. The mechanism is thought to be PPAR-α-stimulated sodium reabsorption in the kidney [44]. TZDs should be avoided in patients with symptomatic heart failure and are contraindicated in patients with New York Heart Association (NYHA) classes III–IV heart failure [45]. Rosiglitazone can be associated with an increased risk of major cardiovascular events, myocardial infarction, and serious ischemic events in adults [46–49]. Pioglitazone does not appear to increase cardiovascular risk, or in some circumstances, may protect against myocardial infarction [50]. At the time of this writing, the risk–benefit ratio of each TZD on the cardiovascular system is not entirely clear. The FDA has added a black box warning about myocardial ischemia to rosiglitazone's label [51]. On September 23, 2010 FDA announced that it would significantly restrict the use of rosiglitazone-containing medicines to patients with T2DM who can not control their blood sugar on other medications. In addition, EMA has recommended the suspension of the marketing authorization for all rosiglitazone-containing medicines in Europe [52, 53].

Data on using TZDs in pediatric patients are very limited. Small studies have demonstrated the safety of TZDs in children with type 1 diabetes mellitus (T1DM) and in patients with polycystic ovarian syndrome (PCOS) [54, 55]. A study in pediatric patients with T2DM demonstrated that the efficacy of rosiglitazone was comparable to metformin. Participants were randomized to rosiglitazone (maximum dose of 4 mg orally twice daily) or metformin (maximum dose of 1,000 mg orally twice daily). By week 24, the proportion of subjects who achieved glycemic goals ($HbA_{1C} \leq 7\%$ and glucose ≤ 126 mg/dL) was comparable in both groups. Rosiglitazone appeared to be well tolerated except for one child who developed peripheral edema [56]. Further clinical trials are needed to determine the risks and benefits of using TZDs in pediatric patients. TZDs have not yet been FDA-approved for use in children.

12.5   AGENTS THAT MODIFY CARBOHYDRATE AND LIPID ABSORPTION

12.5.1   *Alpha-Glucosidase Inhibitors (Acarbose and Miglitol)*

These agents inhibit α-glucosidase activity in the intestinal brush border, where complex carbohydrates get converted into monosaccharides. By slowing this transition, these drugs delay glucose absorption and slow the postprandial rise of blood glucose. Studies have evaluated the use of acarbose in adults with T1DM and T2DM. Acarbose decreases the amplitude of postprandial glycemic excursions and improves HbA_{1C} [57–62]. Studies in pediatric patients with either T1DM or nondiabetic cystic fibrosis indicated that Acarbose can improve insulin sensitivity and glycemic control [63–68]. However, data on the effect of alpha-glucosidase inhibitors in children with T2DM remain unpublished. Table 12.4 provides data on the efficacy, adverse effects, and recommended dosage of acarbose in pediatric populations.

12.5.2   *Lipase Inhibitors (Orlistat®, Xenical®, Alli®)*

Orlistat inhibits fat absorption at the level of the small intestines and is mainly used in the treatment of obesity. Owing to the effect of weight reduction, studies in adults demonstrated its efficacy in improving glucose tolerance and delay progression of T2DM [69]. Orlistat® has been approved for treatment of obesity in children older than 12 years old.

12.6   GLUCAGON-LIKE PEPTIDE-1 (GLP-1) AGONISTS

The incretins – glucagon-like peptide-1 (GLP-1) and glucose-dependent insulinotropic polypeptide (GIP) – are gut hormones that increase glucose-induced insulin release. GLP-1 secretion is impaired in T2DM.

Table 12.6
Properties and biological actions of GLP-1 and GIP [37, 70]

	GLP-1	*GIP*
Properties	30/31-amino acid peptide	42-amino acid peptide
Site of synthesis	L-cell, distal small intestine and colon	K-cells, duodenum and stomach
Effect on pancreas	Stimulates insulin secretion	Stimulate insulin secretion
	Inhibits glucagon secretion	No effect on glucagon secretion
	Stimulate somatostatin secretion	No effect on somatostatin secretion
	Promotes beta-cell differentiation and expansion of beta-cell mass	Promotes beta-cell differentiation and expansion of beta-cell mass
	Inhibits beta-cell apoptosis	Inhibits beta-cell apoptosis
Effect on GI tract	Delays gastric emptying time	No effect on gastric emptying
Effect on CNS	Inhibits food intake, promotes satiety and weight loss, increases nausea	No regulation of appetite and body weight
Other effect	No effect on lipid metabolism	Increases lipolysis and free fatty acid synthesis
Deficiency in T2DM	Reduces GLP-1 secretion in T2DM	No defect in GIP secretion or GIP response in T2DM
	Preserve GLP-1 response in T2 DM	

By infusing GLP-1 in patients with T2DM, insulin secretion is amplified in a glucose-dependent manner, and blood glucose levels improve. Table 12.6 summarizes the role of GLP-1 and GIP hormones to support T2DM management.

GLP-1 improves blood glucose levels through several mechanisms [37, 70]. The glucose-dependent insulin stimulatory effect is enhanced, and both first-phase and second-phase insulin release are restored. GLP-1 also suppresses postprandial glucagon secretion, delays gastric emptying, and reduces food intake and body weight. GLP-1 also preserves pancreatic islet integrity, promoting beta-cell proliferation and decreasing beta cell apoptosis in animal models. The main barrier to use of native GLP-1 in diabetes treatment is its short half-life of 1.5–2 min [71]. GLP-1 is rapidly degraded by dipeptidyl peptidase IV (DPP-IV) and neural endopeptidase (NEP) enzymes. Given the potential role of GLP-1 in the treatment of T2DM, research has focused on developing therapeutic agents that resist DDP-IV degradation or inhibit DDP-IV, thus resulting in a longer half-life of endogenous GLP-1.

12.6.1   Incretin Mimetics

Exendin-4 (exenatide) is a GLP-1 agonist isolated from the saliva of the Gila monster, a lizard native to the Southwestern USA. This compound resists DPP-IV degradation. Exenatide was the first GLP-1 based therapy to be approved by the FDA and EMA for treatment of adult patients with T2DM who had not achieved adequate glycemic control with other oral hypoglycemic agents. Several studies have shown that exenatide, when used as an adjunctive therapy with other oral hypoglycemic agents (TZD, sulfonylurea, and/or metformin), effectively improves glycemic control [72–77], comparable with insulin glargine [78] but with less nocturnal hypoglycemia. The usual dose of exenatide is 5–10 mg by subcutaneous injection within 60 min prior to the morning and evening meals, or before the two main meals of the day (approximately 6 h or more apart). Exenatide is also approved for use as monotherapy, or in combination with oral hypoglycemic agents, with the precaution that the risk of hypoglycemia increases in combination with sulfonylureas.

Liraglutide is a modified, long-acting GLP-1 analog that binds to serum albumin, resulting in a slower degradation. Liraglutide resists degradation by DPP-IV and NEP. As a result, liraglutide has a half-life of 13 h and can be administered once daily, subcutaneously without regard to meals. Liraglutide has shown to be effective in lowering blood glucose in adult patients with T2DM, either as monotherapy [79, 80] or in combination with oral hypoglycemic agents (*i.e.*, sulfonylurea and TZD, with or without combination of metformin) [81–83]. Liraglutide is indicated as an adjunct to diet and exercise to improve glycemic control in adults with T2DM. However, it is not recommended as a first-line therapy for patients who have inadequate glycemic control after diet and exercise. Its side effects are similar to exenatide, including nausea, vomiting, and diarrhea. In animal models, liraglutide was associated with thyroid C-cell tumors [84, 85]. More data on its long-term clinical effects are still needed, and a phase I trial is ongoing in adolescents with T2DM.

12.6.2 DPP-IV Inhibitors

Unlike GLP-1 analogs, DPP-IV inhibitors can be administered more conveniently via the oral route. DPP-IV inhibitors are another option for combination therapy with oral hypoglycemic agents. Sitagliptin and saxagliptin are DPP-IV inhibitors approved by FDA for treatment of T2DM in adults, as an initial pharmacological treatment or as adjunct in combination with sulfonylurea, TZDs, or metformin [86–93].

Data using GLP-1 based therapy in pediatric patients are very limited. A small, randomized, placebo-controlled trial evaluating the pharmacology and tolerability of a single dose of exenatide in adolescent patients with T2DM (aged 10–16 years old) showed that administration of a single 2.5- or 5-mg dose resulted in dose-dependent increases in plasma exenatide concentrations and improved postprandial blood sugar levels [94]. Both doses were well tolerated. Further studies are still needed to determine the efficacy and safety of exenatide and other GLP-1 analogs in children and adolescents with T2DM.

12.6.3 Amylin Analogs

Amylin is a pancreatic islet amyloid polypeptide that is cosecreted from pancreatic beta-cells with insulin. Insulin and amylin complement each other's action on the regulation of glucose homeostasis. Amylin lowers circulating glucose by delaying gastric emptying, suppressing glucagon secretion, and decreasing appetite [95–98]. Pramlintide is a synthetic analog of amylin approved by FDA as adjunct therapy for the treatment of both T1DM and insulin-treated T2DM in adults. Results from randomized controlled trials in both T1DM and T2DM showed that pramlintide, when added to insulin therapy (with or without preexisting combination of sulfonylurea or metformin) could lower HbA_{1C} approximately 0.4–0.6% and resulted in modest weight reduction [97, 99–105]. The most common side effect is nausea. Hypoglycemia is also reported in patients with T1DM treated with amylin. Slow titration of pramlintide along with insulin dose adjustments is recommended.

Data using amylin in children and adolescents are still limited. Most studies of pramlintide in adolescents were conducted in patients with T1DM [100]. In these patients, pramlintide was shown to reduce postprandial glucagon and glucose excursions, similar to its effect in adults. Hypoglycemia was reported in the group of patients that neither titrated pramlintide nor adjusted insulin dose [100]. Information on pramlintide use in children with T2DM has *not* been reported. Further study is required to determine the efficacy, long-term effects, and safety profile of pramlintide in children and adolescents. Amylin does not yet have regulatory approval for use in children.

12.7   EXOGENOUS INSULIN

Insulin therapy is indicated in pediatric patients with T2DM whose glycemic control cannot be optimized with lifestyle modification, diet, and oral hypoglycemic agents. Four principal types of biosynthetic human insulin are currently available: (1) rapid-acting analogs (lispro, aspart, and glulisine), (2) short-acting regular, (3) intermediate-acting neutral protamine Hagedorn (NPH), and (4) long-acting analogs (primarily detemir and glargine). Table 12.7 summarizes these insulin formulations.

Children or adolescents who present with severe hyperglycemia or diabetic ketoacidosis (DKA) should be treated initially with insulin in an attempt to achieve glycemic control as soon as possible and prevent acute

Table 12.7
Insulin preparations and bioavailability characteristics [168–174]

Insulin formulations	Onset of action	Peak action	Effective duration
Rapid acting			
Lispro (Humalog®)	0–15 min	30–90 min	<5 h
Aspart (Novolog®)	10–20 min	40–50 min	3–5 h
Glulisine (Apidra®)	15–20 min	40–120 min	3–5 h
Short acting			
Regular insulin (Humulin® R or Novolin® R)	30 min	80–120 min	Up to 8 h
Intermediate acting			
NPH insulin (Humulin® N or Novolin® N)	1.8–2 h	4–12 h	12–24 h
Long acting			
Glargine (Lantus®)	1.5–2 h	Flat	Up to 24 h
Detemir (Levemir®)	1.6 h	Flat	Up to 24 h

Generally, 40–50% of the patient's total daily insulin dose should be given once daily as long-acting basal insulin (*e.g.*, detemir or glargine). Fast-acting insulin should be given with or immediately after each meal (breakfast, lunch, and dinner) to correct for any high blood glucose before the meal and to cover consumed carbohydrate (carb). One typical prescription for an adolescent with T2DM might start, for example, aspart insulin at meals as 1 unit for every 15 g carb + 1 unit for every 50 mg/dL above target of 110 mg/dL (within range of 80–140 mg/dL). Total daily insulin requirement usually ranges from 0.7 unit/kg/day (*e.g.*, adult with T1DM) to 1 unit/kg/day (*e.g.*, active prepubertal child with established T1DM), to >2.4 units/kg/day (*e.g.*, ill adolescent with T2DM receiving acute glucocorticoid). An otherwise well and active adolescent usually requires between 1.2 units/kg/day (for established T1DM) up to 2.0 units/kg/day (for established T2DM). Recent onset T1DM typically requires 10–20% less total daily insulin than established T1DM due to the honeymoon period, an effect seen less often in T2DM patients.

Table 12.8
Premixed insulin

Premixed insulin	Brands
70% NPH/30% regular insulin	Humulin 70/30® or Novolin 70/30®
Premixed insulin with rapid short acting	
70% insulin NPH/30% aspart	Novolog Mix 70/30®
75% insulin NPH/25% lispro	Humalog Mix 75/25®
50% insulin NPH/50% lispro	Humalog Mix 50/50®

hyperglycemic complications. Once the patient is stable, and the diagnosis of T2DM has been established, metformin therapy or lifestyle intervention should be offered, along with gradual weaning of the insulin therapy while maintaining optimal glycemic control. However, some patients present with a rapid deterioration of pancreatic beta-cell function. In these patients, early insulin treatment might be required to improve metabolic outcome and insulin sensitivity [106]. Glargine and determir are basal insulin analogs commonly used to provide up to 24 h of coverage. These long-acting analogs provide more consistent glycemic control by avoiding peaks of action and lowering blood glucose with less frequent incidence of hypoglycemia. Insulin glargine and insulin determir are approved by FDA for T1DM treatment in children ≥6 years old. Premixed insulin regimens (Table 12.8) also provide more flexibility and may improve compliance in children and adolescents with T2DM.

Continuous subcutaneous insulin infusion (CSII) via a pump is an additional treatment option for diabetes. An insulin pump replaces multiple dose injection regimens and typically improves glycemic control. Although most often used for T1DM, CSII has emerged as an option for T2DM patients who otherwise display difficulty in achieving glycemic control. Insulin aspart is FDA-approved for use in adults and children aged 2 years and older for subcutaneous daily injection and for subcutaneous continuous infusion by external insulin pump. This option requires close follow-up and education for both patients and clinicians. This approach is detailed by Dr. Gregory in Chap. 13.

12.8 LEPTIN

Leptin is a hormone produced by adipocytes that suppresses hunger. Large clinical trials in adults with T2DM conducted during the 1990s did not confirm a significant therapeutic benefit. However, leptin has been reported as successful monotherapy for patients with rare congenital or acquired lipodystrophic diabetes.

12.9   MANAGEMENT OF COMPLICATIONS OF T2DM

Evidence-based studies in adults suggest that T2DM and its comorbidities are strongly associated with cardiovascular disease [107–113]. It is crucial for children and adolescent with T2DM to be screened for comorbidities and to receive proper medical intervention if indicated. Pediatric patients with T2DM should be screened for dyslipidemia and hypertension (HTN), and treated if diagnosed [114]. Screening for microvascular complications should be done at least annually after the onset of puberty. Figures 12.3 and 12.4 suggests comprehensive review of screening and treatment of T2DM complications in children and adolescents [20, 115–117].

12.10   FUTURE DIRECTIONS FOR PHARMACOLOGIC MANAGEMENT OF PEDIATRIC T2DM AND OBESITY

The incidence of obesity and T2DM in children and adolescents is still increasing at an epidemic rate [118–128]. Studies evaluating the safety and efficacy of pharmacological treatment in this population are clearly needed. Since evidence-based research in adults indicates that T2DM and associated comorbidities are well-known risk factors for cardiovascular disease,

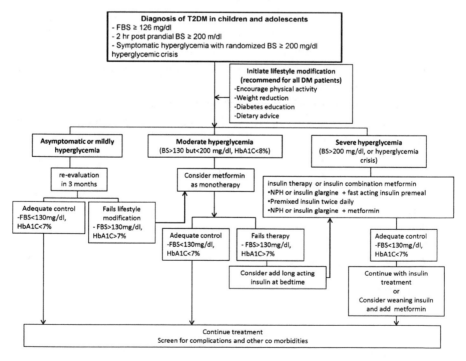

Fig. 12.3. Proposed algorithm for treatment of T2DM in children and adolescents [20, 116].

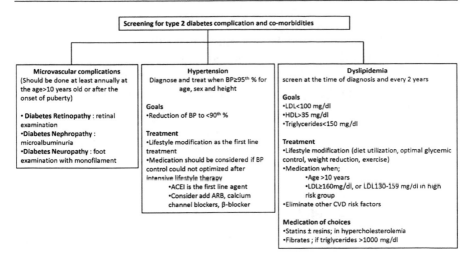

Fig. 12.4. Proposed algorithm for screening of T2DM complications in children and adolescents [116, 117].

it might be reasonable to approach and treat pediatric patients with T2DM with goals similar to those used in adults (Table 12.2), at least until more pediatric data become available. There are very limited data on the prevention of T2DM in children and adolescents. Most behavioral modification treatment is focused on weight control, which is considered to be the best strategy to prevent T2DM in children and adolescents at the greatest risk (overweight, strong family history of T2DM, and displaying signs or conditions related to insulin resistance such as Acanthosis nigricans or PCOS) [116]. More clinical trials are needed to determine the efficacy and safety profile on new therapeutic agents to optimize their roles in the treatment of pediatric T2DM and obesity.

The inhibition of glucose reabsorption at kidney is under intense study as a possible novel approach to treat diabetes. After plasma is filtered by the renal glomeruli, glucose is reabsorbed by renal sodium-glucose cotransporters (SGLTs) in the renal tubules, leaving <1% to be excreted in urine [129–131]. By inhibiting these symporters, the glucose renal threshold is lowered, allowing excess glucose in the plasma to be secreted in the urine, thus resulting in lower blood glucose levels. Several studies evaluating SGLT inhibitors have been conducted in animal models [132–137]. Phlorizin, a nonselective SGLT inhibitor, demonstrates ability as a potent glucosuric and antihyperglycemic agent in animal models [132, 133]. Studies with T-1095, another renal SGLT inhibitor, yielded similar results [138]. Recently, Han *et al.* have reported that dapagliflozin, a selective

SGLT2 inhibitor, lowered fasting and fed glucose levels in Zucker diabetic fatty rats [130]. Clinical studies in adults are underway.

The National Institute of Diabetes and Digestive and Kidney Diseases (NIDDK) of the National Institutes of Health has been sponsoring "Studies to Treat or Prevent Pediatric T2DM" (STOPP-T2D) to assess treatment options for T2DM in adolescents [139]. Another NIDDK-sponsored, multi-center trial called "Treatment Options for T2DM in Adolescent and Youth" (TODAY) is designed to compare the efficacy of metformin alone, or in combination with either rosiglitazone or lifestyle intervention in adolescents with T2DM [140].

12.11   CURRENT PRACTICE RECOMMENDATION

A team approach should be applied to manage pediatric T2DM, incorporating a diabetes nurse educator, licensed clinical dietitian, behavioral specialist, health-care provider (nurse practitioner or physician), and the patient's family. The most widely accepted therapeutic goals for pediatric T2DM are fasting glucose levels 80–130 mg/dL in the morning and $HbA_{1c} \leq 7\%$, with minimal hypoglycemic events in young patients who are vulnerable to hypoglycemia [114]. Lifestyle modification should be recommended as first-line therapy when possible and as an adjunctive treatment when pharmacological therapy is initiated. Family planning should be discussed in all pediatric patients of reproductive age, given the high risks of pregnancy in this population. Apart from medical interventions, surgical weight loss might be considered in selected adolescents with severe obesity and T2DM (see Chap. 9). Figure 12.3 summarizes a proposed algorithm for the management of pediatric T2DM.

12.11.1   Medication Treatment in Childhood Obesity (Table 12.9)

The primary goal of obesity treatment is to improve long-term health outcomes by establishing permanent, healthy lifestyle habits. Treatment of childhood obesity is based on age and underlying medical conditions. The goal of therapy in young healthy children (both overweight and obesity) is to maintain weight and BMI in a healthier range for age. Weight reduction is typically considered for older adolescents or patients with serious comorbidities (e.g., obstructive sleep apnea). The initial primary approach is usually lifestyle modification, specifically focusing on a healthy diet and on increasing physical activity while decreasing sedentary activities. However, under extreme circumstances, pharmacological treatment and/or weight loss surgery should be considered. The latest clinical practice guideline (CPG) from The Endocrine Society [141] suggests medical treatment (in combination with lifestyle modification) should be considered for: (1) obese children

Table 12.9
Medications available for treatment of pediatric obesity [141]

Mechanism of action	Name	Indication	Pediatric dosing	Route
Decreased fat digestion/absorption	Orlilstat (Xenical)	*FDA-approved* in patients older than 12 years in treatment of obesity (Xenical only) [175, 176]	120 mg, 3 times/day with meal	Oral
Antihyperglycemic medications (not FDA-approved)	Metformin	PCOS, impaired glucose tolerance, prediabetes [175, 177, 178]	500–2,000 mg, once or twice daily	Oral
	Exenatide, liraglutide, and amylin	Potentially promote weight loss in obese T2DM patients [72, 95]	5–10 μg SQ bid	Subcutaneous injection
Hormonal therapy	Growth hormone	*FDA-approved* for Prader–Willi syndrome [179]	1–3 mg/m², at bedtime daily	Subcutaneous injection
	Octreotide	Hypothalamic obesity, not FDA-approved for use in children [180, 181]	5–15 μg/kg/day, divided into 3 times/day	Subcutaneous injection
	Leptin	Congenital or acquired leptin deficiency, not FDA-approved [182, 183]	Titrate dose to serum levels	Subcutaneous injection
Antiepileptic drug	Topiramate	Potential weight loss and anorexia [184]; but not approved for treatment of obesity in children due to adverse event	96–256 mg/day	Oral

(BMI more than 95th percentile) only after a formal program of intensive lifestyle modification fails and (2) overweight children (BMI between 85–95th percentiles) only if severe comorbidities persist despite intensive lifestyle modification, especially in children with strong family history of T2DM or premature cardiovascular disease.

12.11.2 Sibutramine (Meridia®)

Sibutramine inhibits serotonin, norepinephrine, and (to a lesser degree) dopamine reuptake, thus suppressing appetite. Meta-analysis showed that sibutramine can decrease BMI by 2.4 kg/m^2 after 6 months and is considered to be the most effective medication [142]. Moreover, obese subjects treated with sibutramine had greater improvement in lipid parameter, when compared to placebo. However, adolescent patients receiving sibutramine had a greater increase in blood pressure and pulse rate [143–146]. Sibutramine is approved by the FDA for treatment of obesity in adolescents older than 16 years. Usual dosage is 5–15 mg orally once day.

The FDA is currently reviewing additional data that sibutramine-treated patients with a history of CVD are at risk of developing cardiovascular events, compared to placebo-treated patients [147, 148]. Current labeling recommends avoiding the use of sibutramine in patients with a history of coronary artery disease, congestive heart failure, cardiac arrhythmias, or stroke [148]. Because of these safety concerns, the EMA have recently decided to withdraw sibutramine from European markets [149]. In October 2010, Abbot laboratories announced that it is voluntary withdrawing sibutramine from the US market under the pressure of FDA, citing concerns over increased risk of cardiovascular events [150].

12.11.3 Orlistat (Xenical®, Alli®)

Orlistat acts by inhibiting gastric and pancreatic lipase, thus blocking fat absorption in the intestines. Treatment with orlistat was associated with a significant fall in BMI of 0.7 kg/m^2 in adults [142]; however, patients also experienced some gastrointestinal side effects, including abdominal discomfort, pain, and steatorrhea. The side effects are usually mild to moderate degree and generally improve over time. Orlistat must be taken with meals. At present, only Xenical® is approved by the FDA for treatment of obesity in adolescents older than 12 years old. Other medications, such as metformin, growth hormone, and octreotide, have been used to treat obesity in some clinical conditions other than common T2DM.

Obesity-related comorbidities include T2DM, metabolic syndrome, cardiovascular risk factors (HTN, dyslipidemia, and atherosclerosis), hyperandrogenism and infertility, precocious puberty, nonalcoholic fatty liver disease (NAFLD), pulmonary HTN, obstructive sleep apnea, and adverse psychosocial consequences [141]. Thus, it is reasonable to recommend that children and adolescent with BMI ≥85th percentile, apart from complete history and physical examination, undergo basic screening with fasting glucose, insulin, and lipid profile, as well as liver function testing and assessment for other obesity associated morbidities as clinically indicated [141]. Formal sleep study is often indicated to confirm/exclude obstructive sleep apnea. Surgical management of childhood obesity is discussed in Chap.9 by Dr. Al-Qahtani.

12.11.4 Current Recommendations

Figure 12.5 proposes an algorithm for management of childhood obesity. Pharmacological treatment, in combination with lifestyle modification, should be reserved only for patients who fail a formal intensive lifestyle modification, or in those who have severe comorbidities [141]. Pharmacotherapy should be offered only by experienced clinicians and only if the benefits of using medication clearly outweigh the risks [141]. Children and adolescents with BMI ≥85th percentile should be screened for obesity-associated morbidities, especially insulin resistance, T2DM, cardiovascular risk factors, and fatty liver disease [141].

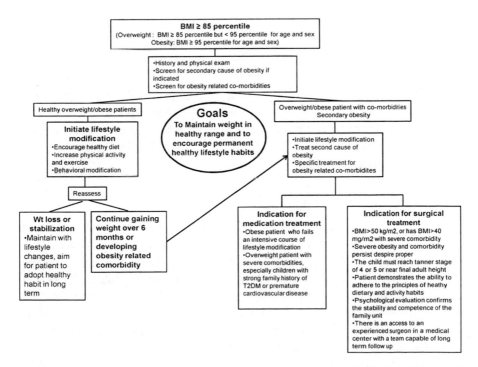

Fig. 12.5. Proposed algorithm for management of overweight and obesity in children and adolescents [141].

12.12   INSULIN RESISTANCE AND POLYCYSTIC OVARIAN SYNDROME

PCOS represents a heterogeneous group of disorders sharing insulin resistance and excess androgen action, leading to a higher risk of cardiovascular complications. PCOS is characterized by hyperandrogenism and insulin resistance. Patients can present with overt virilization: hirsutism, irregular menses, persistent acne, scalp hair loss, or hyperandrosis in adolescents and precocious adrenarche in children. Moreover, as insulin resistance is part of PCOS, these patients display risk of developing infertility, T2DM, and cardiovascular disease in the future.

Antiandrogen and estrogen–progestin therapies have been the predominant strategies for hyperandrogenism and irregular menses [151]. In PCOS patients with obesity, in addition to weight reduction, insulin sensitizing agents can also improve insulin sensitivity, promote ovulation, and lower androgen levels. Metformin has proven effective in both adults and adolescents for improving insulin sensitivity and lipid profiles [152, 153], regulating menses and inducing ovulation [154–156], and lowering androgen levels [157–160]. TZDs have also been shown to improve the metabolic profile and ovarian steroid biosynthesis in patients with PCOS [161, 162]. A small study conducted in obese adolescents with PCOS, aged 9–19 years, suggested a possible role for rosiglitazone treatment [55]. However, due to lack of long-term safety data, TZDs are not currently recommended in adolescents, especially in patients who do not have T2DM. Also, TZDs lack regulatory approval for treatment of pediatric T2DM. Given that treatment of PCOS increases fertility rates, contraceptive options should be discussed with all patients who are using metformin or TZDs for treatment of PCOS. Preconception care should be offered for those who desire to become pregnant, and screening for gestational diabetes should be done for those who are at risk [114] (Table 12.10).

12.13   CONCLUSION

Obesity and T2DM in children and adolescents continue to emerge with increasing prevalence and at earlier ages. Lack of data on long-term outcomes in pediatric populations has forced clinicians to treat pediatric T2DM, for now and judiciously, based on data from adult studies (Table 12.11). The risk–benefit ratio must be carefully considered before treating obese children and adolescents with medications given their uncertainty with respect to growth, development, and fertility. Behavioral modification still remains the first approach for treatment of both pediatric obesity and T2DM. Although metformin and insulin are the only two medications approved by

Table 12.10
Recommendation of screening and diagnosis of gestational diabetes (GDM)

Screening and diagnosis of gestational diabetes

High risk groups should be screened for GDM as soon as pregnancy is confirmed and again at 24–28 weeks if initial test is normal

Severe obesity

History of GDM

Presence of glycosuria

Diagnosis of PCOS

Low-risk groups do not require GDM screening

Age <25 years

Weight normal before pregnancy

Low risk ethnic group

No family history of diabetes (first degree relatives)

No history of abnormal OGTT

No history of poor obstetrical outcome

All patients who have greater risk than low-risk group but not at high risk, should undergo GDM screening test at the gestational age of 24–28 weeks

Diagnostic tests for GDM

Two-step approach

Initial screening with plasma glucose at 1 h after 50 g glucose loading test (positive screening test is in range of 130–140 mg/dL)

Perform a diagnostic 100 g oral glucose tolerance test (OGTT) on a separate day in patient who has positive result from step 1

or

One-step approach

Perform a diagnostic 100 g OGTT in all women to be tested at 24–28 weeks. The test should be done after an overnight fast of at least 8 h

Criteria of diagnosis GDM

At least two positive findings of:

- Fasting glucose $\geq$ 95 mg/dL
- 1-h glucose $\geq$ 180 mg/dL
- 2-h glucose $\geq$ 155 mg/dL
- 3-h glucose $\geq$ 140 mg/dL

Table 12.11
Management of dyslipidemia in pediatric T2DM [117]

Goals

LDL < 100 mg/dL

HDL > 35 mg/dL

TG < 150 mg/dL

Approaches

Initiate lifestyle modification

- Diet control with daily cholesterol intake <200 mg/day and saturated fat <7% of total daily calories
- Weight reduction
- Encourage physical activity

Optimize glycemic control

Modify other cardiovascular risks (smoking cessation; control blood pressure)

Consider medication when:

- Age > 10 years old
- LDL levels remain high despite intensive lifestyle modification, or if fasting TG > 1,000 mg/dL

Hypercholesterolemia

Consider medication when:

- Fasting LDL 160 mg/dL
- Fasting LDL 130–159 mg/dL in high-risk groups (strong family history of premature CAD, CVD, or peripheral vascular disease, HTN, smoking)
- Medications of choice: bile acid sequestrants[a] or statin drugs[b]

Hypertriglyceridemia (fasting TG > 150 mg/dL)

- Usually not directly managed with medication
- Consider intensive lifestyle modification, blood sugar control, and weight
- Reduction if indicated
- TG >1,000 mg/dL; consider fibric acid derivatives[c]

CAD coronary artery disease; *CVD* cerebrovascular disease; *HDL* high-density lipoprotein; *HTN* hypertension; *LDL* low-density lipoprotein; *TG* triglyceride

[a] Resins or bile acid sequestrants (cholestyramine powder; dose 240 mg/kg daily per oral, divided 3 times daily with maximum dose of 16 g daily, colesevalam – the second generation sequestrant; dose 625 mg/tablet, 3 or 6 times daily can also be used in a lower dose) are generally recommended as first choice therapy; however, due to side effects from medications, compliance rates are low in children and adolescents

[b] Statins (HMG-CoA reductase inhibitors) can also be considered as first-line treatment in hypercholesterolemia. Atorvastatin, lovastatin, pravastatin, and simvastatin given orally are approved by the FDA

(continued)

Table 12.11
(continued)

for use in adolescents with familial hypercholesterolemia [185]; however, data for statin use in pediatric T2DM and the very young remain limited. Treatment should be started with the lowest available dose (atorvastatin 10 mg daily, lovastatin 40 mg daily, pravastatin 40 mg daily, and simvastatin 20 mg daily [185]) and gradually adjusted, based on LDL levels and tolerance of side effects. Medication should be discontinued if liver function tests are greater than 3 times the upper normal limit

ᶜFibric acid derivatives (gemfibrozil, fenofibrate) have not been well investigated in pediatric population and should be used cautiously. The medication should be initiated with low dose and gradually adjusted. Common side effects of the medications include myalgia, myopathy, rhabdomyosis (especially using gemfibrozil in combination with statins), gall stone, and glucose intolerance. Liver functions should be monitored every 3 months when using medications

the FDA and EMA for treatment of pediatric T2DM, active studies hold promise for new approaches. Given the acute risks of DKA, sleep apnea, and other serious comorbidities, the prudent clinician should consider all aspects of available medical approaches to maximize their potential benefits.

REFERENCES

1. Ten S, Maclaren N (2004) Insulin resistance syndrome in children. J Clin Endocrinol Metab 89:2526–2539
2. Legido A, Sarria A, Bueno M *et al.* (1989) Relationship of body fat distribution to metabolic complications in obese prepubertal boys: gender related differences. Acta Paediatr Scand 78:440–446
3. Huang TT, Johnson MS, Gower BA, Goran MI (2002) Effect of changes in fat distribution on the rates of change of insulin response in children. Obes Res 10:978–984
4. Srinivasan SR, Myers L, Berenson GS (2002) Predictability of childhood adiposity and insulin for developing insulin resistance syndrome (syndrome X) in young adulthood: the Bogalusa Heart Study. Diabetes 51:204–209
5. Owens S, Gutin B, Barbeau P *et al.* (2000) Visceral adipose tissue and markers of the insulin resistance syndrome in obese black and white teenagers. Obes Res 8:287–293
6. Caprio S, Hyman LD, McCarthy S, Lange R, Bronson M, Tamborlane WV (1996) Fat distribution and cardiovascular risk factors in obese adolescent girls: importance of the intraabdominal fat depot. Am J Clin Nutr 64:12–17
7. Gutin B, Basch C, Shea S *et al.* (1990) Blood pressure, fitness, and fatness in 5- and 6-year-old children. JAMA 264:1123–1127
8. Berenson GS, Srinivasan SR, Wattigney WA, Harsha DW (1993) Obesity and cardiovascular risk in children. Ann N Y Acad Sci 699:93–103
9. Freedman DS, Mei Z, Srinivasan SR, Berenson GS, Dietz WH (2007) Cardiovascular risk factors and excess adiposity among overweight children and adolescents: the Bogalusa Heart Study. J Pediatr 150:12–17, e12
10. Mahoney LT, Burns TL, Stanford W *et al.* (1996) Coronary risk factors measured in childhood and young adult life are associated with coronary artery calcification in young adults: the Muscatine Study. J Am Coll Cardiol 27:277–284
11. McGill HC Jr, McMahan CA, Herderick EE *et al.* (2002) Obesity accelerates the progression of coronary atherosclerosis in young men. Circulation 105:2712–2718
12. Visser M (2001) Higher levels of inflammation in obese children. Nutrition 17:480–481

13. Daniels SR, Morrison JA, Sprecher DL, Khoury P, Kimball TR (1999) Association of body fat distribution and cardiovascular risk factors in children and adolescents. Circulation 99:541–545
14. Weyer C, Bogardus C, Mott DM, Pratley RE (1999) The natural history of insulin secretory dysfunction and insulin resistance in the pathogenesis of type 2 diabetes mellitus. J Clin Invest 104:787–794
15. Weyer C, Tataranni PA, Bogardus C, Pratley RE (2001) Insulin resistance and insulin secretory dysfunction are independent predictors of worsening of glucose tolerance during each stage of type 2 diabetes development. Diabetes Care 24:89–94
16. Gungor N, Bacha F, Saad R, Janosky J, Arslanian S (2005) Youth type 2 diabetes: insulin resistance, beta-cell failure, or both? Diabetes Care 28:638–644
17. Gungor N, Hannon T, Libman I, Bacha F, Arslanian S (2005) Type 2 diabetes mellitus in youth: the complete picture to date. Pediatr Clin North Am 52:1579–1609
18. Tripathy D, Carlsson M, Almgren P et al. (2000) Insulin secretion and insulin sensitivity in relation to glucose tolerance: lessons from the Botnia Study. Diabetes 49:975–980
19. Kobayashi K, Amemiya S, Higashida K et al. (2000) Pathogenic factors of glucose intolerance in obese Japanese adolescents with type 2 diabetes. Metabolism 49:186–191
20. Libman IM, Arslanian SA (2007) Prevention and treatment of type 2 diabetes in youth. Horm Res 67:22–34
21. Masharani U, German M (2007) Pancreatic hormones & diabetes mellitus. In: Gardner DG, Shoback D (eds) Greenspan's basic & clinical endocrinology, 8th edn. McGraw-Hill, Columbus, pp 661–747
22. DeFronzo RA (2000) Pharmacologic therapy for type 2 diabetes mellitus. Ann Intern Med 133:73–74
23. Bressler R, Johnson DG (1997) Pharmacological regulation of blood glucose levels in non-insulin-dependent diabetes mellitus. Arch Intern Med 157:836–848
24. Hermann LS, Schersten B, Bitzen PO, Kjellstrom T, Lindgarde F, Melander A (1994) Therapeutic comparison of metformin and sulfonylurea, alone and in various combinations. A double-blind controlled study. Diabetes Care 17:1100–1109
25. DeFronzo RA, Goodman AM (1995) Efficacy of metformin in patients with non-insulin-dependent diabetes mellitus. The Multicenter Metformin Study Group. N Engl J Med 333:541–549
26. Jeppesen J, Zhou MY, Chen YD, Reaven GM (1994) Effect of metformin on postprandial lipemia in patients with fairly to poorly controlled NIDDM. Diabetes Care 17:1093–1099
27. Culler FL, McKean LP, Buchanan CN, Caplan DB, Meacham LR (1994) Glipizide treatment of patients with cystic fibrosis and impaired glucose tolerance. J Pediatr Gastroenterol Nutr 18:375–378
28. Gottschalk M, Danne T, Vlajnic A, Cara JF (2007) Glimepiride versus metformin as monotherapy in pediatric patients with type 2 diabetes: a randomized, single-blind comparative study. Diabetes Care 30:790–794
29. United Kingdom Prospective Diabetes Study (UKPDS) (1995) 13: Relative efficacy of randomly allocated diet, sulphonylurea, insulin, or metformin in patients with newly diagnosed non-insulin dependent diabetes followed for three years. BMJ 310:83–88
30. Wu MS, Johnston P, Sheu WH et al. (1990) Effect of metformin on carbohydrate and lipoprotein metabolism in NIDDM patients. Diabetes Care 13:1–8
31. Bailey CJ, Wilcock C, Day C (1992) Effect of metformin on glucose metabolism in the splanchnic bed. Br J Pharmacol 105:1009–1013
32. Lutjens A, Smit JL (1977) Effect of biguanide treatment in obese children. Helv Paediatr Acta 31:473–480
33. Jones KL, Arslanian S, Peterokova VA, Park JS, Tomlinson MJ (2002) Effect of metformin in pediatric patients with type 2 diabetes: a randomized controlled trial. Diabetes Care 25:89–94

34. Zuhri-Yafi MI, Brosnan PG, Hardin DS (2002) Treatment of type 2 diabetes mellitus in children and adolescents. J Pediatr Endocrinol Metab 15(Suppl 1):541–546
35. Castells S (2002) Management of hyperglycemia in minority children with type 2 diabetes mellitus. J Pediatr Endocrinol Metab 15(Suppl 1):531–540
36. Srinivasan S, Ambler GR, Baur LA et al. (2006) Randomized, controlled trial of metformin for obesity and insulin resistance in children and adolescents: improvement in body composition and fasting insulin. J Clin Endocrinol Metab 91:2074–2080
37. Yki-Jarvinen H (2004) Thiazolidinediones. N Engl J Med 351:1106–1118
38. Home PD, Pocock SJ, Beck-Nielsen H et al. (2009) Rosiglitazone evaluated for cardiovascular outcomes in oral agent combination therapy for type 2 diabetes (RECORD): a multicentre, randomised, open-label trial. Lancet 373:2125–2135
39. Lago RM, Singh PP, Nesto RW (2007) Congestive heart failure and cardiovascular death in patients with prediabetes and type 2 diabetes given thiazolidinediones: a meta-analysis of randomised clinical trials. Lancet 370:1129–1136
40. Masoudi FA, Inzucchi SE, Wang Y, Havranek EP, Foody JM, Krumholz HM (2005) Thiazolidinediones, metformin, and outcomes in older patients with diabetes and heart failure: an observational study. Circulation 111:583–590
41. Dargie HJ, Hildebrandt PR, Riegger GA et al. (2007) A randomized, placebo-controlled trial assessing the effects of rosiglitazone on echocardiographic function and cardiac status in type 2 diabetic patients with New York Heart Association Functional Class I or II Heart Failure. J Am Coll Cardiol 49:1696–1704
42. Delea TE, Edelsberg JS, Hagiwara M, Oster G, Phillips LS (2003) Use of thiazolidinediones and risk of heart failure in people with type 2 diabetes: a retrospective cohort study. Diabetes Care 26:2983–2989
43. Singh S, Loke YK, Furberg CD (2007) Thiazolidinediones and heart failure: a teleoanalysis. Diabetes Care 30:2148–2153
44. Guan Y, Hao C, Cha DR et al. (2005) Thiazolidinediones expand body fluid volume through PPARgamma stimulation of ENaC-mediated renal salt absorption. Nat Med 11:861–866
45. Nesto RW, Bell D, Bonow RO et al. (2003) Thiazolidinedione use, fluid retention, and congestive heart failure: a consensus statement from the American Heart Association and American Diabetes Association. Circulation 108:2941–2948
46. Rosen CJ (2007) The rosiglitazone story – lessons from an FDA Advisory Committee meeting. N Engl J Med 357:844–846
47. Rosen CJ (2010) Revisiting the rosiglitazone story – lessons learned. N Engl J Med 363:803–806
48. Nissen SE, Wolski K (2010) Rosiglitazone revisited: an updated meta-analysis of risk for myocardial infarction and cardiovascular mortality. Arch Intern Med 170:1191–1201
49. Nissen SE, Wolski K (2007) Effect of rosiglitazone on the risk of myocardial infarction and death from cardiovascular causes. N Engl J Med 356:2457–2471
50. Graham DJ, Ouellet-Hellstrom R, MaCurdy TE et al. (2010) Risk of acute myocardial infarction, stroke, heart failure, and death in elderly medicare patients treated with rosiglitazone or pioglitazone. JAMA 304:411–418
51. http://www.accessdata.fda.gov/drugsatfda_docs/label/2008/021071s034lbl.pdf. Accessed 15 Sept 2010
52. http://www.fda.gov/Drugs/DrugSafety/PostmarketDrugSafetyInformationforPatients andProviders/ucm226956.htm. Accessed 15 Feb 2011
53. http://www.ema.europa.eu/docs/en_GB/document_library/Press_release/2010/09/ WC500096996.pdf. Accessed 15 Feb 2011
54. Zdravkovic V, Hamilton JK, Daneman D, Cummings EA (2006) Pioglitazone as adjunctive therapy in adolescents with type 1 diabetes. J Pediatr 149:845–849
55. Marcado-Asis L, Mercado A. Rosiglitazone is safe and effective in the treatment of insulin resistance syndrome in children and young adults. In: Proceedings of the 84th

annual meeting of the endocrine society, San Francisco, 19–21 June 2002 [abstract P2-720]

56. Dabiri G, Jones KL, Krebs J, Sun Y, Mudd P. Benefit of rosiglitazone in children with T2DM. Diabetes 2005 [abstract A457]

57. Hollander P, Pi-Sunyer X, Coniff RF (1997) Acarbose in the treatment of type I diabetes. Diabetes Care 20:248–253

58. McCulloch DK, Kurtz AB, Tattersall RB (1983) A new approach to the treatment of nocturnal hypoglycemia using alpha-glucosidase inhibition. Diabetes Care 6:483–487

59. Meneilly GS, Ryan EA, Radziuk J et al. (2000) Effect of acarbose on insulin sensitivity in elderly patients with diabetes. Diabetes Care 23:1162–1167

60. Hoffmann J, Spengler M (1994) Efficacy of 24-week monotherapy with acarbose, glibenclamide, or placebo in NIDDM patients. The Essen Study. Diabetes Care 17:561–566

61. Chiasson JL, Josse RG, Hunt JA et al. (1994) The efficacy of acarbose in the treatment of patients with non-insulin-dependent diabetes mellitus. A multicenter controlled clinical trial. Ann Intern Med 121:928–935

62. Holman RR, Cull CA, Turner RC (1999) A randomized double-blind trial of acarbose in type 2 diabetes shows improved glycemic control over 3 years (U.K. Prospective Diabetes Study 44). Diabetes Care 22:960–964

63. Kane MP, Abu-Baker A, Busch RS (2005) The utility of oral diabetes medications in type 2 diabetes of the young. Curr Diabetes Rev 1:83–92

64. Kentrup H, Bongers H, Spengler M, Kusenbach G, Skopnik H (1999) Efficacy and safety of acarbose in patients with cystic fibrosis and impaired glucose tolerance. Eur J Pediatr 158:455–459

65. Spengler M, Cagatay M. Assessment of efficacy and tolerability of acarbose in diabetic patients 5–16 years of age. In: Proceedings of the third international symposium on Acarbose, Berlin, 1992, pp 289–291

66. Henrichs I, Heinze E, Kohne E, Teller W. Improved management of juvenile diabetes by acarbose. In: Proceed 1; International symposium on Acarbose Berlin (West), 12–14 Nov 1987. Acarbose for the treatment of diabetes mellitus [abstract]

67. Bartsocas C, Papachristou C, Hillebrand I, Papadatos C. Acarbose as an adjunct in the management of juvenile-onset diabetes. In: International symposium on Acarbose. Effects on carbohydrate and fat metabolism, Montreux, Oct 1981 [abstract S27]

68. Damjanova M. Non randomized follow-up study with acarbose treatment and pre- and post-treatment with placebo in diabetes children (type 1). In: International symposium on Acarbose, Berline (West), 12–14 Nov 1987. Acarbose for the treatment of diabetes mellitus [abstract 74]

69. Heymsfield SB, Segal KR, Hauptman J et al. (2000) Effects of weight loss with orlistat on glucose tolerance and progression to type 2 diabetes in obese adults. Arch Intern Med 160:1321–1326

70. Drucker DJ (2007) The role of gut hormones in glucose homeostasis. J Clin Invest 117:24–32

71. Holst JJ, Vilsboll T, Deacon CF (2009) The incretin system and its role in type 2 diabetes mellitus. Mol Cell Endocrinol 297:127–136

72. DeFronzo RA, Ratner RE, Han J, Kim DD, Fineman MS, Baron AD (2005) Effects of exenatide (exendin-4) on glycemic control and weight over 30 weeks in metformin-treated patients with type 2 diabetes. Diabetes Care 28:1092–1100

73. Buse JB, Henry RR, Han J, Kim DD, Fineman MS, Baron AD (2004) Effects of exenatide (exendin-4) on glycemic control over 30 weeks in sulfonylurea-treated patients with type 2 diabetes. Diabetes Care 27:2628–2635

74. Kendall DM, Riddle MC, Rosenstock J et al. (2005) Effects of exenatide (exendin-4) on glycemic control over 30 weeks in patients with type 2 diabetes treated with metformin and a sulfonylurea. Diabetes Care 28:1083–1091

75. Zinman B, Hoogwerf BJ, Duran Garcia S *et al.* (2007) The effect of adding exenatide to a thiazolidinedione in suboptimally controlled type 2 diabetes: a randomized trial. Ann Intern Med 146:477–485
76. Riddle MC, Henry RR, Poon TH *et al.* (2006) Exenatide elicits sustained glycaemic control and progressive reduction of body weight in patients with type 2 diabetes inadequately controlled by sulphonylureas with or without metformin. Diabetes Metab Res Rev 22:483–491
77. Ratner RE, Maggs D, Nielsen LL *et al.* (2006) Long-term effects of exenatide therapy over 82 weeks on glycaemic control and weight in over-weight metformin-treated patients with type 2 diabetes mellitus. Diabetes Obes Metab 8:419–428
78. Heine RJ, Van Gaal LF, Johns D, Mihm MJ, Widel MH, Brodows RG (2005) Exenatide versus insulin glargine in patients with suboptimally controlled type 2 diabetes: a randomized trial. Ann Intern Med 143:559–569
79. Vilsboll T, Zdravkovic M, Le-Thi T *et al.* (2007) Liraglutide, a long-acting human glucagon-like peptide-1 analog, given as monotherapy significantly improves glycemic control and lowers body weight without risk of hypoglycemia in patients with type 2 diabetes. Diabetes Care 30:1608–1610
80. Garber A, Henry R, Ratner R *et al.* (2009) Liraglutide versus glimepiride monotherapy for type 2 diabetes (LEAD-3 Mono): a randomised, 52-week, phase III, double-blind, parallel-treatment trial. Lancet 373:473–481
81. Nauck M, Marre M (2009) Adding liraglutide to oral antidiabetic drug monotherapy: efficacy and weight benefits. Postgrad Med 121:5–15
82. Marre M, Shaw J, Brandle M *et al.* (2009) Liraglutide, a once-daily human GLP-1 analogue, added to a sulphonylurea over 26 weeks produces greater improvements in glycaemic and weight control compared with adding rosiglitazone or placebo in subjects with Type 2 diabetes (LEAD-1 SU). Diabet Med 26:268–278
83. Zinman B, Gerich J, Buse JB *et al.* (2009) Efficacy and safety of the human glucagon-like peptide-1 analog liraglutide in combination with metformin and thiazolidinedione in patients with type 2 diabetes (LEAD-4 Met+TZD). Diabetes Care 32:1224–1230
84. NDA 22-341 Victoza (Lariglutide {rDNA origin} injection). 2010. http://www.fda.gov/downloads/Drugs/DrugSafety/PostmarketDrugSafetyInformationforPatientsand Providers/UCM202063.pdf. Accessed 18 March 2010
85. Parks M, Rosebraugh C (2010) Weighing risks and benefits of liraglutide – the FDA's review of a new antidiabetic therapy. N Engl J Med 362:774–777
86. DeFronzo RA, Fleck PR, Wilson CA, Mekki Q (2008) Efficacy and safety of the dipeptidyl peptidase-4 inhibitor alogliptin in patients with type 2 diabetes and inadequate glycemic control: a randomized, double-blind, placebo-controlled study. Diabetes Care 31:2315–2317
87. Raz I, Hanefeld M, Xu L, Caria C, Williams-Herman D, Khatami H (2006) Efficacy and safety of the dipeptidyl peptidase-4 inhibitor sitagliptin as monotherapy in patients with type 2 diabetes mellitus. Diabetologia 49:2564–2571
88. Aschner P, Kipnes MS, Lunceford JK, Sanchez M, Mickel C, Williams-Herman DE (2006) Effect of the dipeptidyl peptidase-4 inhibitor sitagliptin as monotherapy on glycemic control in patients with type 2 diabetes. Diabetes Care 29:2632–2637
89. Charbonnel B, Karasik A, Liu J, Wu M, Meininger G (2006) Efficacy and safety of the dipeptidyl peptidase-4 inhibitor sitagliptin added to ongoing metformin therapy in patients with type 2 diabetes inadequately controlled with metformin alone. Diabetes Care 29:2638–2643
90. Goldstein BJ, Feinglos MN, Lunceford JK, Johnson J, Williams-Herman DE (2007) Effect of initial combination therapy with sitagliptin, a dipeptidyl peptidase-4 inhibitor, and metformin on glycemic control in patients with type 2 diabetes. Diabetes Care 30:1979–1987
91. Nauck MA, Meininger G, Sheng D, Terranella L, Stein PP (2007) Efficacy and safety of the dipeptidyl peptidase-4 inhibitor, sitagliptin, compared with the sulfonylurea,

glipizide, in patients with type 2 diabetes inadequately controlled on metformin alone: a randomized, double-blind, non-inferiority trial. Diabetes Obes Metab 9:194–205

92. Rosenstock J, Brazg R, Andryuk PJ, Lu K, Stein P (2006) Efficacy and safety of the dipeptidyl peptidase-4 inhibitor sitagliptin added to ongoing pioglitazone therapy in patients with type 2 diabetes: a 24-week, multicenter, randomized, double-blind, placebo-controlled, parallel-group study. Clin Ther 28:1556–1568

93. Hermansen K, Kipnes M, Luo E, Fanurik D, Khatami H, Stein P (2007) Efficacy and safety of the dipeptidyl peptidase-4 inhibitor, sitagliptin, in patients with type 2 diabetes mellitus inadequately controlled on glimepiride alone or on glimepiride and metformin. Diabetes Obes Metab 9:733–745

94. Malloy J, Capparelli E, Gottschalk M, Guan X, Kothare P, Fineman M (2009) Pharmacology and tolerability of a single dose of exenatide in adolescent patients with type 2 diabetes mellitus being treated with metformin: a randomized, placebo-controlled, single-blind, dose-escalation, crossover study. Clin Ther 31:806–815

95. Edelman SV, Darsow T, Frias JP (2006) Pramlintide in the treatment of diabetes. Int J Clin Pract 60:1647–1653

96. Chapman I, Parker B, Doran S et al. (2005) Effect of pramlintide on satiety and food intake in obese subjects and subjects with type 2 diabetes. Diabetologia 48:838–848

97. Whitehouse F, Kruger DF, Fineman M et al. (2002) A randomized study and open-label extension evaluating the long-term efficacy of pramlintide as an adjunct to insulin therapy in type 1 diabetes. Diabetes Care 25:724–730

98. Ratner RE, Dickey R, Fineman M et al. (2004) Amylin replacement with pramlintide as an adjunct to insulin therapy improves long-term glycaemic and weight control in Type 1 diabetes mellitus: a 1-year, randomized controlled trial. Diabet Med 21:1204–1212

99. Ratner RE, Want LL, Fineman MS et al. (2002) Adjunctive therapy with the amylin analogue pramlintide leads to a combined improvement in glycemic and weight control in insulin-treated subjects with type 2 diabetes. Diabetes Technol Ther 4:51–61

100. Chase HP, Lutz K, Pencek R, Zhang B, Porter L (2009) Pramlintide lowered glucose excursions and was well-tolerated in adolescents with type 1 diabetes: results from a randomized, single-blind, placebo-controlled, crossover study. J Pediatr 155:369–373

101. Edelman S, Garg S, Frias J et al. (2006) A double-blind, placebo-controlled trial assessing pramlintide treatment in the setting of intensive insulin therapy in type 1 diabetes. Diabetes Care 29:2189–2195

102. Levetan C, Want LL, Weyer C et al. (2003) Impact of pramlintide on glucose fluctuations and postprandial glucose, glucagon, and triglyceride excursions among patients with type 1 diabetes intensively treated with insulin pumps. Diabetes Care 26:1–8

103. Hollander P, Maggs DG, Ruggles JA et al. (2004) Effect of pramlintide on weight in overweight and obese insulin-treated type 2 diabetes patients. Obes Res 12:661–668

104. Weyer C, Gottlieb A, Kim DD et al. (2003) Pramlintide reduces postprandial glucose excursions when added to regular insulin or insulin lispro in subjects with type 1 diabetes: a dose-timing study. Diabetes Care 26:3074–3079

105. Hollander PA, Levy P, Fineman MS et al. (2003) Pramlintide as an adjunct to insulin therapy improves long-term glycemic and weight control in patients with type 2 diabetes: a 1-year randomized controlled trial. Diabetes Care 26:784–790

106. Sellers EA, Dean HJ (2004) Short-term insulin therapy in adolescents with type 2 diabetes mellitus. J Pediatr Endocrinol Metab 17:1561–1564

107. Booth GL, Kapral MK, Fung K, Tu JV (2006) Relation between age and cardiovascular disease in men and women with diabetes compared with non-diabetic people: a population-based retrospective cohort study. Lancet 368:29–36

108. Alexander CM, Landsman PB, Teutsch SM (2000) Diabetes mellitus, impaired fasting glucose, atherosclerotic risk factors, and prevalence of coronary heart disease. Am J Cardiol 86:897–902

109. National Cholesterol Education Program (NCEP) Expert Panel on Detection, Evaluation, and Treatment of High Blood Cholesterol in Adults (Adult Treatment Panel III) (2002) Third Report of the National Cholesterol Education Program (NCEP) Expert Panel on Detection, Evaluation, and Treatment of High Blood Cholesterol in Adults (Adult Treatment Panel III) final report. Circulation 106:3143–3421

110. De Backer G, Ambrosioni E, Borch-Johnsen K et al. (2003) European guidelines on cardiovascular disease prevention in clinical practice: third joint task force of European and other societies on cardiovascular disease prevention in clinical practice (constituted by representatives of eight societies and by invited experts). Eur J Cardiovasc Prev Rehabil 10:S1–S10

111. Haffner SM, Lehto S, Ronnemaa T, Pyorala K, Laakso M (1998) Mortality from coronary heart disease in subjects with type 2 diabetes and in nondiabetic subjects with and without prior myocardial infarction. N Engl J Med 339:229–234

112. Kannel WB, McGee DL (1979) Diabetes and cardiovascular disease. The Framingham Study. JAMA 241:2035–2038

113. Stamler J, Vaccaro O, Neaton JD, Wentworth D (1993) Diabetes, other risk factors, and 12-yr cardiovascular mortality for men screened in the Multiple Risk Factor Intervention Trial. Diabetes Care 16:434–444

114. American Diabetes Association (2010) Standards of medical care in diabetes – 2010. Diabetes Care 33(Suppl 1):S11–S61

115. American Diabetic Association (2010) Executive summary: standards of medical care in diabetes – 2010. Diabetes Care 33(Suppl 1):S4–S10

116. American Diabetes Association (2000) Type 2 diabetes in children and adolescents. Pediatrics 105(3 Pt 1):671–680

117. American Diabetes Association (2003) Management of dyslipidemia in children and adolescents with diabetes. Diabetes Care 26:2194–2197

118. Fagot-Campagna A, Pettitt DJ, Engelgau MM et al. (2000) Type 2 diabetes among North American children and adolescents: an epidemiologic review and a public health perspective. J Pediatr 136:664–672

119. Dabelea D, Hanson RL, Bennett PH, Roumain J, Knowler WC, Pettitt DJ (1998) Increasing prevalence of Type II diabetes in American Indian children. Diabetologia 41:904–910

120. Neufeld ND, Raffel LJ, Landon C, Chen YD, Vadheim CM (1998) Early presentation of type 2 diabetes in Mexican-American youth. Diabetes Care 21:80–86

121. Pihoker C, Scott CR, Lensing SY, Cradock MM, Smith J (1998) Non-insulin dependent diabetes mellitus in African-American youths of Arkansas. Clin Pediatr (Phila) 37:97–102

122. Pinhas-Hamiel O, Dolan LM, Daniels SR, Standiford D, Khoury PR, Zeitler P (1996) Increased incidence of non-insulin-dependent diabetes mellitus among adolescents. J Pediatr 128(5 Pt 1): 608–615

123. Dean HJ, Young TK, Flett B, Wood-Steiman P (1998) Screening for type-2 diabetes in aboriginal children in northern Canada. Lancet 352:1523–1524

124. Huen KF, Low LC, Wong GW et al. (2000) Epidemiology of diabetes mellitus in children in Hong Kong: the Hong Kong childhood diabetes register. J Pediatr Endocrinol Metab 13:297–302

125. Wei JN, Chuang LM, Lin CC, Chiang CC, Lin RS, Sung FC (2003) Childhood diabetes identified in mass urine screening program in Taiwan, 1993–1999. Diabetes Res Clin Pract 59:201–206

126. Kitagawa T, Owada M, Urakami T, Yamauchi K (1998) Increased incidence of non-insulin dependent diabetes mellitus among Japanese schoolchildren correlates with an increased intake of animal protein and fat. Clin Pediatr (Phila) 37:111–115

127. Likitmaskul S, Kiattisathavee P, Chaichanwatanakul K, Punnakanta L, Angsusingha K, Tuchinda C (2003) Increasing prevalence of type 2 diabetes mellitus in Thai children and adolescents associated with increasing prevalence of obesity. J Pediatr Endocrinol Metab 16:71–77

128. Braun B, Zimmermann MB, Kretchmer N, Spargo RM, Smith RM, Gracey M (1996) Risk factors for diabetes and cardiovascular disease in young Australian aborigines. A 5-year follow-up study. Diabetes Care 19:472–479

129. Moe O, Berry C, Rector FJ (1996) Renal transport of glucose, amino acids, sodium, chloride and water. In: Brenner B (ed) Brenner and rector's the kidney, 5th edn. WB Saunders, Philadelphiapp 375–415

130. Han S, Hagan DL, Taylor JR et al. (2008) Dapagliflozin, a selective SGLT2 inhibitor, improves glucose homeostasis in normal and diabetic rats. Diabetes 57:1723–1729

131. Deetjen P, Von Baeyer H, Drexel H (1992) Renal glucose transport. In: Seldin D, Giebisch G (eds) Seldin and Giebisch's the kidney, 2nd edn. Raven Press, New York, pp 2873–2888

132. Rossetti L, Smith D, Shulman GI, Papachristou D, DeFronzo RA (1987) Correction of hyperglycemia with phlorizin normalizes tissue sensitivity to insulin in diabetic rats. J Clin Invest 79:1510–1515

133. Kahn BB, Shulman GI, DeFronzo RA, Cushman SW, Rossetti L (1991) Normalization of blood glucose in diabetic rats with phlorizin treatment reverses insulin-resistant glucose transport in adipose cells without restoring glucose transporter gene expression. J Clin Invest 87:561–570

134. Dimitrakoudis D, Vranic M, Klip A (1992) Effects of hyperglycemia on glucose transporters of the muscle: use of the renal glucose reabsorption inhibitor phlorizin to control glycemia. J Am Soc Nephrol 3:1078–1091

135. Shi ZQ, Rastogi KS, Lekas M, Efendic S, Drucker DJ, Vranic M (1996) Glucagon response to hypoglycemia is improved by insulin-independent restoration of normoglycemia in diabetic rats. Endocrinology 137:3193–3199

136. Marette A, Dimitrakoudis D, Shi Q, Rodgers CD, Klip A, Vranic M (1999) Glucose rapidly decreases plasma membrane GLUT4 content in rat skeletal muscle. Endocrine 10:13–18

137. Kim JK, Zisman A, Fillmore JJ et al. (2001) Glucose toxicity and the development of diabetes in mice with muscle-specific inactivation of GLUT4. J Clin Invest 108:153–160

138. Oku A, Ueta K, Arakawa K et al. (2000) Antihyperglycemic effect of T-1095 via inhibition of renal Na+-glucose cotransporters in streptozotocin-induced diabetic rats. Biol Pharm Bull 23:1434–1437

139. Baranowski T, Cooper DM, Harrell J et al. (2006) Presence of diabetes risk factors in a large U.S. eighth-grade cohort. Diabetes Care 29:212–217

140. Zeitler P, Epstein L, Grey M et al. (2007) Treatment options for type 2 diabetes in adolescents and youth: a study of the comparative efficacy of metformin alone or in combination with rosiglitazone or lifestyle intervention in adolescents with type 2 diabetes. Pediatr Diabetes 8:74–87

141. August GP, Caprio S, Fennoy I et al. (2008) Prevention and treatment of pediatric obesity: an endocrine society clinical practice guideline based on expert opinion. J Clin Endocrinol Metab 93:4576–4599

142. McGovern L, Johnson JN, Paulo R et al. (2008) Clinical review: treatment of pediatric obesity: a systematic review and meta-analysis of randomized trials. J Clin Endocrinol Metab 93:4600–4605

143. Berkowitz RI, Wadden TA, Tershakovec AM, Cronquist JL (2003) Behavior therapy and sibutramine for the treatment of adolescent obesity: a randomized controlled trial. JAMA 289:1805–1812

144. McMahon FG, Weinstein SP, Rowe E, Ernst KR, Johnson F, Fujioka K (2002) Sibutramine is safe and effective for weight loss in obese patients whose hypertension is well controlled with angiotensin-converting enzyme inhibitors. J Hum Hypertens 16:5–11

145. Sramek JJ, Leibowitz MT, Weinstein SP et al. (2002) Efficacy and safety of sibutramine for weight loss in obese patients with hypertension well controlled by beta-adrenergic

blocking agents: a placebo-controlled, double-blind, randomised trial. J Hum Hypertens 16:13–19

146. Kim SH, Lee YM, Jee SH, Nam CM (2003) Effect of sibutramine on weight loss and blood pressure: a meta-analysis of controlled trials. Obes Res 11(9):1116–1123

147. James WP, Caterson ID, Coutinho W et al. (2010) Effect of sibutramine on cardiovascular outcomes in overweight and obese subjects. N Engl J Med 363:905–917

148. http://www.fda.gov/Drugs/DrugSafety/PostmarketDrugSafetyInformationforPatients andProviders/DrugSafetyInformationforHeathcareProfessionals/ucm198206.htm. Accessed 10 Sept 2010

149. Williams G (2010) Withdrawal of sibutramine in Europe. BMJ 340:c824

150. http://wwww.abbott.com/global/url/pressRelease/en_US/Press_Release_0908.htm. Accessed 15 Feb 2011.

151. Ehrmann DA (2005) Polycystic ovary syndrome. N Engl J Med 352:1223–1236

152. Nestler JE (2008) Metformin for the treatment of the polycystic ovary syndrome. N Engl J Med 358:47–54

153. Sharma ST, Wickham EP III, Nestler JE (2007) Changes in glucose tolerance with metformin treatment in polycystic ovary syndrome: a retrospective analysis. Endocr Pract 13:373–379

154. Glueck CJ, Goldenberg N, Pranikoff J, Loftspring M, Sieve L, Wang P (2004) Height, weight, and motor-social development during the first 18 months of life in 126 infants born to 109 mothers with polycystic ovary syndrome who conceived on and continued metformin through pregnancy. Hum Reprod 19:1323–1330

155. Glueck CJ, Bornovali S, Pranikoff J, Goldenberg N, Dharashivkar S, Wang P (2004) Metformin, pre-eclampsia, and pregnancy outcomes in women with polycystic ovary syndrome. Diabet Med 21:829–836

156. Nestler JE (2008) Metformin in the treatment of infertility in polycystic ovarian syndrome: an alternative perspective. Fertil Steril 90:14–16

157. Harborne L, Fleming R, Lyall H, Norman J, Sattar N (2003) Descriptive review of the evidence for the use of metformin in polycystic ovary syndrome. Lancet 361:1894–1901

158. Attia GR, Rainey WE, Carr BR (2001) Metformin directly inhibits androgen production in human thecal cells. Fertil Steril 76:517–524

159. Crave JC, Fimbel S, Lejeune H, Cugnardey N, Dechaud H, Pugeat M (1995) Effects of diet and metformin administration on sex hormone-binding globulin, androgens, and insulin in hirsute and obese women. J Clin Endocrinol Metab 80:2057–2062

160. Mansfield R, Galea R, Brincat M, Hole D, Mason H (2003) Metformin has direct effects on human ovarian steroidogenesis. Fertil Steril 79:956–962

161. Ehrmann DA, Schneider DJ, Sobel BE et al. (1997) Troglitazone improves defects in insulin action, insulin secretion, ovarian steroidogenesis, and fibrinolysis in women with polycystic ovary syndrome. J Clin Endocrinol Metab 82:2108–2116

162. Dunaif A, Scott D, Finegood D, Quintana B, Whitcomb R (1996) The insulin-sensitizing agent troglitazone improves metabolic and reproductive abnormalities in the polycystic ovary syndrome. J Clin Endocrinol Metab 81:3299–3306

163. Silverstein JH, Rosenbloom AL (2000) Treatment of type 2 diabetes mellitus in children and adolescents. J Pediatr Endocrinol Metab 13(Suppl 6):1403–1409

164. Byetta® package insert. San Diego: Amylin Pharmaceuticals Inc. and Eli Lilly & Co.; Sept 2010

165. Victoza® package insert. Princeton: Novo Nordisk Inc.; Jan 2010

166. Januvia® package insert. Whitehouse Station: Merk & Co. Inc.; June 2009

167. Onglyza® package insert. Princeton: Bristo-Myers Squibb Inc.; July 2009

168. Levemir® package insert. Princeton: Novo Nordisk Inc.; July 2009

169. Novolog® package insert. Princeton: Novo Nordisk Inc.; March 2010

170. Novolin R® package insert. Princeton: Novo Nordisk Inc.; June 2009

171. Novolin N® package insert. Princeton: Novo Nordisk Inc.; June 2009

172. Plank J, Bodenlenz M, Sinner F *et al.* (2005) A double-blind, randomized, dose-response study investigating the pharmacodynamic and pharmacokinetic properties of the long-acting insulin analog detemir. Diabetes Care 28:1107–1112

173. Apidra® package insert. Bridgewater: Sanofi-Aventis Inc.; Feb 2009

174. Humalog® package insert. Indianapolis: Eli Lilly & Co.; Sept 2009

175. Freemark M (2007) Pharmacotherapy of childhood obesity: an evidence-based, conceptual approach. Diabetes Care 30:395–402

176. Chanoine JP, Hampl S, Jensen C, Boldrin M, Hauptman J (2005) Effect of orlistat on weight and body composition in obese adolescents: a randomized controlled trial. JAMA 293:2873–2883

177. Freemark M, Bursey D (2001) The effects of metformin on body mass index and glucose tolerance in obese adolescents with fasting hyperinsulinemia and a family history of type 2 diabetes. Pediatrics 107:E55

178. Kay JP, Alemzadeh R, Langley G, D'Angelo L, Smith P, Holshouser S (2001) Beneficial effects of metformin in normoglycemic morbidly obese adolescents. Metabolism 50:1457–1461

179. Stafler P, Wallis C (2008) Prader–Willi syndrome: who can have growth hormone? Arch Dis Child 93:341–345

180. Lustig RH, Hinds PS, Ringwald-Smith K *et al.* (2003) Octreotide therapy of pediatric hypothalamic obesity: a double-blind, placebo-controlled trial. J Clin Endocrinol Metab 88:2586–2592

181. Lustig RH, Rose SR, Burghen GA *et al.* (1999) Hypothalamic obesity caused by cranial insult in children: altered glucose and insulin dynamics and reversal by a somatostatin agonist. J Pediatr 135(2 Pt 1):162–168

182. Farooqi IS, Matarese G, Lord GM *et al.* (2002) Beneficial effects of leptin on obesity, T cell hyporesponsiveness, and neuroendocrine/metabolic dysfunction of human congenital leptin deficiency. J Clin Invest 110:1093–1103

183. Farooqi IS, Jebb SA, Langmack G *et al.* (1999) Effects of recombinant leptin therapy in a child with congenital leptin deficiency. N Engl J Med 341:879–884

184. Wilding J, Van Gaal L, Rissanen A, Vercruysse F, Fitchet M (2004) A randomized double-blind placebo-controlled study of the long-term efficacy and safety of topiramate in the treatment of obese subjects. Int J Obes Relat Metab Disord 28:1399–1410

185. Kwiterovich PO Jr (2008) Recognition and management of dyslipidemia in children and adolescents. J Clin Endocrinol Metab 93:4200–4209

186. Robertson RP. Antagonist: diabetes and insulin resistance – philosophy, science, and the multiplier hypothesis. J Lab Clin Med 1995;125:560–564; discussion 565

187. Beck-Nielsen H, Groop LC (1994) Metabolic and genetic characterization of prediabetic states. Sequence of events leading to non-insulin-dependent diabetes mellitus. J Clin Invest 94:1714–1721

13 Insulin Pump Management

Justin M. Gregory

Key Points

- Insulin remains among the few FDA-approved therapies for pediatric T2DM to date.
- Although traditionally used for management of type 1 diabetes, pump-delivered insulin therapy can improve glycemic control for pediatric T2DM in a cost-effective manner.

Keywords: Insulin pump, Diabetes, Continuous subcutaneous insulin infusion, Continuous glucose monitoring, Multiple daily injections

13.1 INTRODUCTION

The pump has gained increasing popularity as an insulin delivery system in recent years. Many users find that, in addition to decreasing the number of injections they take each day, the device allows for increased flexibility in their daily insulin regimen and mealtimes.

13.2 HISTORY

The notion of an insulin pump first arose in the early 1960s, when Dr. Arnold Kadish designed a backpack-sized pump. Although novel, it was too large to be clinically practical. Researchers explored ways to make the delivery of insulin more physiologic and to miniaturize the technology, leading to the introduction of a brick-sized pump by the late 1970s. These

From: *Nutrition and Health: Management of Pediatric Obesity and Diabetes*,
Edited by: R.J. Ferry, Jr., DOI 10.1007/978-1-60327-256-8_13,
© Springer Science+Business Media, LLC 2011

early sets offered little flexibility for basal infusion rates, required frequent battery changes, and employed infusion sets with metal needles, necessitating diluted insulin suspensions. The injection sites frequently became infected or clogged and often dislodged. Thus, pumps were not widely used until the 1990s [1].

The paradigm shift from intermittent subcutaneous injections to continuous subcutaneous insulin infusion (CSII) via insulin pumps resulted from major innovations in diabetes care during the 1990s. First, the landmark Diabetes Control and Complication Trial (DCCT) and the United Kingdom Prospective Diabetes Study (UKPDS) highlighted that tight blood glucose control –albeit at the expense of frequent injections of insulin and risk of more frequent hypoglycemia – significantly decreases major adverse complications (*i.e.*, diabetic retinopathy, nephropathy, and neuropathy). After the DCCT's publication in 1993, the number of patients using CSII exploded from 15,000 to over 162,000 by 2001 [2]. Second, technological advancements reduced the pump to a pocket size. Third, new synthetic insulin formulations (lispro, aspart, etc.) hastened the development of flexible dosing protocols taking advantage of the newer pumps. Fortunately, other patients with nondiabetic conditions benefited from these advances in drug delivery systems.

13.3   HOW A PUMP WORKS

13.3.1   *Parts, Components, and Models*

The commercially available insulin pumps share their essential components and design. Most pump models are about the size and shape of a deck of cards. They can be worn by a clip on a belt or carried in a pocket (Fig. 13.1).

A display screen allows the user to control dosing, set alarms, and follow the pump's status. Within the pump's housing, a disposable cartridge holds the insulin. It resembles the cylinder section of a syringe and is approximately 200 units in volume (Fig. 13.2).

Typically, the cartridge is changed and replaced every 2–3 days. A small, battery-powered piston ejects insulin from the cartridge, usually into a plastic tube which is connected to an infusion set. The subcutaneous portion of the infusion set is introduced using a needle sheathed inside a plastic tube (Figs. 13.3 and 13.4).

Once inserted subcutaneously, the needle is removed leaving the plastic tube under the skin. The infusion set is designed such that the tube can be disconnected for a short amount of time, leaving the set under the skin. Disconnection allows the user to bathe, swim, or pursue other desired

Fig. 13.1. A generic insulin pump.

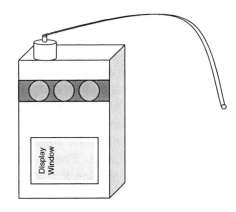

Fig. 13.2. Generic insulin cartridge.

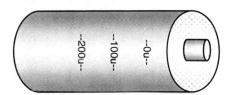

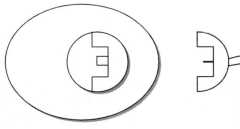

Fig. 13.3. Catheter and tube insert.

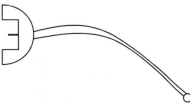

Fig. 13.4. Tube inserted into catheter.

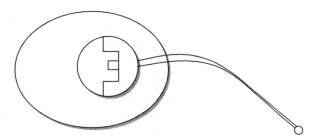

activities. Nevertheless, most pumps today can be worn while swimming or exercising.

Several models are available in the U.S. market, including the OneTouch Ping (Animas Corporation, West Chester, PA), the Accu-Chek Spirit (Roche Diagnostics, Basel, Switzerland), Paradigm 522 and 722 (Medtronic, Inc., Minneapolis, MN), and the OmniPod (Insulet Corporation, Bedford, MA). With the exception of the Omnipod, which employs a tubeless delivery system, insulin pumps are similar in size and most companies guarantee their pumps for 4 years. They tend to have a 1–2 month battery life (with lithium batteries), similar programming interfaces, and are water resistant.

13.3.2   Insulin Delivery

The major advantage of a pump is enabling the use of rapidly acting insulin in two ways. First, a pump provides immediate, bolus doses of insulin. The patient can self-deliver a single dose, either to cover a meal or to correct an elevated blood glucose level. Second, a pump delivers a continuous, basal infusion. The basal dose provides insulin between meals and overnight (to prevent excessive glucose release from the liver). Basal dosing is expressed as a rate, most commonly as units of insulin per hour (*i.e.*, units/hour).

Once the patient and clinician plan to begin pump therapy, the initial consideration is the insulin regimen. Either short-acting or rapid-acting insulin analogs may be administered as continuous subcutaneous infusions. The short-acting formulation is regular insulin (R), manufactured since the mid-1920s and available from several commercial sources. Action of regular insulin displays onset within 30–60 min, peaks at 2 h, and effectively lasts 6–8 h. Rapid-acting insulin analogs are lispro, aspart, and glulisine – each produced by recombinant DNA technology with minimal changes in the molecule designed to reduce aggregation. These rapid analogs display onset within 5–15 min, peak at 1–1.5 h, and effectively last 3–4 h [2]. Several studies suggest the rapid analogs exert equal or improved efficacy toward reducing postprandial glucose excursions, hemoglobin A1c values, and hypoglycemic episodes while preventing weight gain [3, 4]. Generally, most clinicians prefer to recommend a rapid analog for use with a pump to aid prompt diabetic control upon pump activation and to reduce the chance of delayed recognition when the pump is not functioning properly.

The previous insulin requirement and target for glycemic control are useful starting points to design the dosing regimen for CSII. Patients with previously well-controlled blood glucose values (hemoglobin A$_{1c}$ less than 7.0%) usually will require 10–20% less total daily insulin by CSII compared to their multiple daily injection (MDI) regimen. Patients with suboptimal blood glucose control may be started on the same amount of total daily insulin [5]. Divide the total daily insulin dose, and give half as bolus and half as basal. Most prepubertal children with type 1 diabetes beyond the "honeymoon" period require between 0.6 and 0.7 insulin units per kilogram body weight daily. Increased adiposity or normal puberty (increased steroid and growth hormone levels) can increase this requirement by up to 20%. The basal rate is usually between 0.01 and 0.015 units per kilogram body weight per hour [5]. The rate can then be adjusted as indicated on the patient's home blood glucose monitoring. Preprandial bolus dosing is proportionately dosed based on the carbohydrate content of what is being consumed. A frequently used starting ratio is one unit of insulin for every 15 g of carbohydrate. This dose should also be adjusted based on a truthful home blood glucose log. Bolus dosing is also generated to correct glycemic excursions from the target range. One unit of rapid-acting insulin can reduce blood glucose levels by as much as 100 mg/dL [6], and this value is often called the correction factor, or sensitivity factor. A widely accepted formula used to calculate the correction factor is:

$$\text{correction factor} = \frac{\text{TDD}_{\text{insulin}}}{C_{\text{insulin}}} \tag{13.1}$$

where $\text{TDD}_{\text{insulin}}$ is the total daily insulin dose and C_{insulin} is equal to 1,800 for rapid-acting insulin and 1,500 for short-acting insulin [7]. Using a number in this range as a correction factor, a correcting dose may be calculated using the formula:

$$\text{correction dose} = \frac{\text{BG} - \text{BG}_{\text{ideal}}}{\text{correction factor}} \tag{13.2}$$

Where BG is the current high blood glucose needing correction and BG_{ideal} is the desired blood glucose, usually between 100 and 120 mg/dL, unless there is increased concern for hypoglycemia, in which case BG_{ideal} should be set higher.

A major feature of the insulin pump is its ability to fine-tune and automate the delivery of basal and bolus insulin dosages. The basal insulin regimen can be tailored to fit the individual's changing insulin needs throughout the day. For instance, many patients experience a "dawn phenomenon," where a circadian overnight rise in two of insulin's counterregulatory hormones, growth hormone and cortisol, lead to an elevated waking blood glucose value after being normoglycemic at bedtime. The insulin pump allows the clinician to program the hourly infusion rate. Thus, the basal insulin rate can be raised in the hours leading up to the anticipated rise in blood glucose, maintaining normoglycemia throughout the night (Table 13.1).

Table 13.1
Sample basal-rate profile

Start	End	Rate (U/h)
12:00 AM	1:00 AM	0.500
1:00 AM	3:00 AM	0.525
3:00 AM	10:00 AM	0.800
10:00 AM	11:00 PM	0.325

Most pumps have programs that let the user devise different daily basal-rate profiles, such as a weekday profile, when he is at work or school, and a weekend profile, when one might sleep in or have a reduced amount of stress – requiring less total daily insulin. Some pumps allow the user to create sick-day profiles, when higher total daily insulin doses are needed. Another feature is that the user can program one-time temporary basal rates before periods when insulin needs will change. Exercising is one example where a temporary basal rate can be dropped by a certain percentage for the duration of the exercise. The key to fine-tuning is frequent monitoring and recording of the blood glucose. Changes in the basal rates should be guided by excursions from normoglycemia 4 or more hours after eating [1]. Ideally, the clinician works closely with the patient and/or family to direct these changes as the blood glucose log indicates. The physician should then strive to teach the patient and family to interpret and adjust their basal rates incrementally to achieve normoglycemia throughout the week. With their doctor's guidance, the patient and family can become their own best diabetes expert.

Delivery of bolus insulin can also be adapted to meet the patient's needs. Most pumps have multiple programs for delivering insulin. The "normal" bolus program allows the user to simply dose and deliver insulin. Most pumps allow for doses as precise as one-twentieth of a unit. Before eating, the patient may calculate the needed insulin dose using the insulin to carbohydrate ratio mentioned earlier. To correct hyperglycemia, he may use the correction dose Eq. (13.1) above (Fig. 13.5).

Bolus doses can be shaped to fit certain meals with the "extended" bolus. For instance, meals with high-fat, high-protein content tend to slow gastric peristalsis and gastrointestinal digestion, leading to increased blood glucose levels hours after the meal is eaten. To counteract this effect, the user may program an extended bolus dose, where the bolus insulin is slowly infused over a designated amount of time. This way, the insulin enters the circulation steadily over a longer period of time, avoiding hypoglycemia in the period immediately after a meal and also avoiding hyperglycemia several hours later (Fig. 13.6).

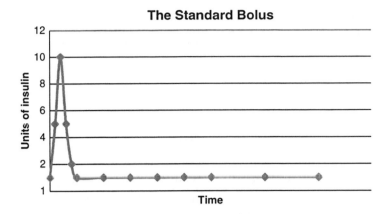

Fig. 13.5. The standard bolus.

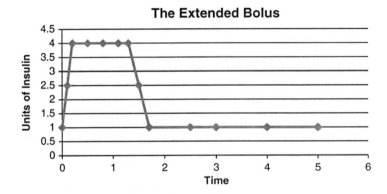

Fig. 13.6. The extended bolus.

Insulin pumps also allow for automated correction of hyperglycemia. Most have a "correction bolus program" where the user simply enters in his current blood glucose level and the pump calculates a correcting dose that he can accept or alter. This correcting dose is calculated by the pump with several factors, largely using Eq. (13.2). First, the clinician can set a target blood glucose (BG_{ideal}) to achieve in correcting the high blood glucose. The correction factor, which can be programmed for different values at various points during the day based on times of increased or decreased insulin sensitivity, is also designated and used by the program in calculating the correcting dose. Most pumps also calculate the "insulin on board" in the patient and factor this into the correcting dose. Assuming the pharmacokinetic parameters of the rapid-acting insulin analogs, the insulin on board function uses a curvilinear algorithm to account for the decay of previous bolus doses in the bloodstream. The effective duration of the rapid-acting

Table 13.2
Insulin to carbohydrate ratios (units insulin: grams carbs)

Start time	End time	I:C ratio
12:00 AM	6:00 AM	1:15
6:00 AM	11:00 AM	1:12
11:00 AM	8:00 PM	1:18
8:00 PM	12:00 AM	1:15

insulins is 3–4 h. The clinician can input this value into the program that calculates the insulin on board and alter this value if necessary. Subtracting the insulin on board from the correcting dose prevents "stacking" of insulin doses that might lead to overcorrection of the hyperglycemia.

Before eating, a meal dose can also be calculated. The clinician can designate the insulin to carbohydrate (I:C) ratio into a pump's "meal dose program," which he may choose to vary for different times of day as insulin sensitivity varies (Table 13.2).

The user enters the number of grams of carbohydrates to be eaten and the program uses the I:C ratio to make an initial dose calculation. The patient next enters his current blood glucose level and a correcting dose is added. Then the insulin on board is subtracted, outputting a meal dose which the user can accept or alter.

Some patients find that eating certain foods with high fat and starch content lead to a late rise in blood glucose level, even when dosing their usually effective I:C ratio of insulin. For example, a 9-year-old boy with diabetes eats a slice of pizza with 40 g of carbs and 12 g of fat. Usually, 2.70 units of insulin works well, but his parents find that while his blood glucose was 110 2 h after the meal, 4 h after the meal it is 275. High-fat foods have a tendency to slow the stomach's emptying of food into the small intestine and this effect is worse in individuals with gastroparesis. To counteract this effect, many pumps have a "combination bolus" program designed to allow the user to deliver a percentage of the total dose immediately and the remainder over an extended amount of time. A clinician might recommend that the parents give 50% of the bolus immediately and 50% over the next 4 h to cover the late rise in blood glucose but increasing the total dose might also be necessary (Fig. 13.7).

13.4 ADVANTAGES AND DISADVANTAGES

Physicians, nurses, diabetes educators, and nutritionists are frequently called upon to help their patients and families consider the advantages and disadvantages of initiating pump therapy. The list of considerations is long and varies from individual to individual.

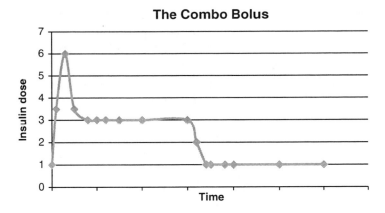

Fig. 13.7. The combo bolus.

13.4.1   Advantages

As alluded to earlier, a significant advantage of CSII comes from its ability to fine-tune a basal insulin profile for each patient. Because the basal insulin can be tailored to maintain normoglycemia between meals, a patient is allowed more flexibility to delay or skip meals and vary the size and composition of the serving [2]. Periods of increased insulin sensitivity, such as exercise, or decreased insulin sensitivity, such as sick days, can be adjusted for by altering the basal rate.

Another advantage is consistency in pharmacokinetics. As opposed to MDI, CSII uses a single, rapid-acting insulin compared to at least two in MDI: a long acting insulin analog and a short- or rapid-acting insulin. Rapid- and short-acting insulin analogs have significantly more reproducibility in their pharmacokinetic profiles compared to longer acting insulin in absorption from the subcutaneous tissue to the bloodstream [1]. A group of studies showed that absorption of intermediate-acting insulin varies anywhere between 10% and 52% compared to 2.8% absorption of regular acting insulin over a 24-h period [1, 8, 9]. Infusing insulin in the same site for 2–3 days lends itself to predictability and consistency in blood glucose profiles after insulin is infused [5]. Insulin uptake is variable from injection site to injection site, with factors such as skin temperature and thickness of subcutaneous fat contributing to the variability with each MDI [10]. Because CSII infusions are continuous and short-acting insulin is used exclusively, there is a minimal subcutaneous depot of insulin at any one time, decreasing the probability of excessive mobilization of insulin from the subcutaneous tissue into the bloodstream during exercise.

The automated programs included with the pump simplify calculation of appropriate doses for the patient. A patient can input a blood glucose value and the pump calculates a dose to correct hyperglycemia. Before a meal, he may simply input the carbs he is about to eat plus his current blood glucose value to calculate a dose that has taken into account the insulin he should already have on board, his insulin to carb ratio for that particular time of day, and the degree of low or high blood glucose that needs to be corrected to normoglycemia. If these programs are used consistently, trends can be observed more readily to allow for empirical adjustment of correction factors and I:C ratios. A pump is also able to use combination bolusing for foods that are digested more slowly, such as pizza, as mentioned in the example earlier. Finally, pumps have a lockout feature where the clinician may set a maximal dose of insulin to help prevent an accidental – and potentially life threatening – insulin overdose.

Many patients find the pump more convenient. Instead of seven or more daily injections, the infusion set is changed every 2–3 days. Users often find delivering insulin with the pump is more discreet and less time consuming than injecting a dose with a syringe or insulin pen. Correction doses are as simple as a few button pushes. Before meals a patient no longer has to prep an injection site, draw up insulin, prepare an insulin pen needle, or keep up with as many insulin supplies. One longitudinal study showed that in a cohort of 161 youth with type 1 diabetes who initiated pump therapy between 1998 and 2001, greater than 80% continued to use their insulin pumps. In addition, the study noted that patients who returned to daily injection therapy checked their blood glucose levels significantly less frequently than those who stayed on the pump [11].

Several studies have compared the efficacy of CSII to MDI. In general, these trials tend to show slight, but statistically significant improvement in glycosylated hemoglobin (HbA_{1c}) with initiation of CSII compared to MDI. HbA_{1c} is a lab value frequently used to extrapolate the average blood glucose over the previous 3 months. A meta-analysis by Pickup et al. in 2002 showed somewhat better control when using CSII. Twelve randomized control trials from 1982 to 2000 followed 600 type 1 diabetes patients, 301 allocated to CSII and 299 allocated to MDI for anywhere from 2.5 to 24 months. The CSII group had a 0.51% lower HbA_{1c} than MDI; however, most of the CSII used short-acting insulins that are not as effective as the rapid-acting insulin analogs currently available [8]. The studies in this meta-analysis also used insulin NPH, an intermediate-acting insulin, in the MDI groups as the basal insulin instead of insulin glargine or detemir, the long-acting insulins available today. Another meta-analysis by Weissberg-Benchell in 2003 evaluated 52 studies and also found improved glycemic control in CSII compared to conventional therapies and MDI [12]. This analysis, however, has been criticized for including nonrandomized trials

[13]. A randomized, prospective, short-term study by Doyle *et al.* used newer analogs to compare MDI versus CSII in 2004. Thirty two youth with type 1 diabetes were randomized to either receive MDI with once daily insulin glargine (a long acting analog with an effective duration of approximately 24 h) and premeal insulin aspart or CSII with aspart. The two groups had no statistically significant difference in HbA_{1c} at baseline and levels were checked again at 16 weeks. While the MDI group did not have a statistically significant decrease in HbA_{1c} from its baseline, the CSII group had a significantly lower HbA_{1c} from its baseline as compared to the MDI group. The MDI cohort had an HbA_{1c} of 8.2% at baseline compared to 8.1% 16 weeks later. The HbA_{1c} of the CSII group changed from 8.1% at baseline to 7.2% 16 weeks later [14]. Other studies suggest that hypoglycemic events are fewer in CSII regimens compared to MDI [15]. A randomized open crossover trail by Weintrob *et al.* took 23 children with type 1 diabetes and placed half on a CSII regimen and half on a MDI regimen for 3.5 months, then switched the groups onto the opposite regimen for another 3.5 months. HbA_{1c} was similar between CSII and MDI and no clinically significant difference was observed in hyperglycemic or hypoglycemic events.

13.4.2 Disadvantages

A regimen using an insulin pump is much more expensive than one using syringes or insulin pens. Depending on the manufacturer, the upfront cost of a pump is approximately \$5,000–6,000 [16, 17]. The largest cost associated with insulin pumps is that of replacing consumable components such as the insulin cartridges and infusion sets. In 2002, Conrad *et al.* calculated the annual cost of CSII is approximately \$3,400 compared to \$1,800 for MDI [17]. While conceptually the improvement in HbA_{1c} noted with CSII over MDI would seemingly lead to fewer long-term complications associated with insufficient glycemic control, a satisfactory method has not been devised to convert these observed benefits into a cost per quality-adjusted life-year [18]. Thus, the savings benefit of improved glycemic control with CSII at the expense of increased annual cost over MDI has not been fully elucidated. It is critical that parents and patients know that Federal law allows them to appeal denials of durable medical equipment (DME) and medical therapies (such as novel but more costly insulin analogs) when the prescribing physician has deemed it medically necessary. Plan language often excludes insulin pumps and glucose sensors as DME, requiring the patient or practitioner to request an independent, third-party review of the denial.

Because an insulin pump uses a relatively low depot of subcutaneous insulin, an interruption in the insulin flow can lead to hypoinsulinemia, hyperglycemia, and possibly diabetic ketoacidosis [5]. For the same reason, a malfunction in the pump must be quickly addressed. Pump therapy can be prone to occlusions in tubing, dead batteries, poor upkeep, and being misplaced. The clinical team should advise their patients to always have a back-up supply of insulin available for injection should delivery via the pump be interrupted.

Patients often complain of being attached or tethered to the pump. Although it can be attached to clothing, it is often bothersome to wear during vigorous exercise. Some also find it problematic during times of intimacy, although it can be detached from the infusion site for short periods of time.

While current models of pumps claim to be swimming and bathing compatible, they are still prone to small nicks in and around the display screen, allowing water to enter and break the display.

Often overlooked is that a considerable amount of technical expertise is required to effectively operate an insulin pump. A patient or parent must be able to work through the pump's program menus, understand how to count carbohydrates, and properly change out insulin cartridges and infusion sets. In order to start pump therapy, a significant amount of time and money must be spent in training to ensure safe and effective use of the pump.

Another disadvantage is the potential for weight gain with pump use. During the DCCT, weight gain was reported when patients switched to intensive insulin therapy, either with MDI or CSII [19]. Tamborlane *et al.* however, make the case that an increase in body mass index (BMI) was only seen in one of the seven studies completed since the DCCT where patients switched from injections to CSII [20].

13.5   THE IDEAL CANDIDATE FOR AN INSULIN PUMP

Physicians are often put in the position of deciding who is and who is not a good candidate for insulin pump therapy. Complicating the decision is that there is little in the way of evidenced based guidelines indicating what kind of patient will be successful on CSII, as opposed to MDI. Usually, financial means are the first consideration as the high cost of insulin pump therapy is prohibitive in a great many patients. Successful pump therapy requires frequent blood glucose checking and logging, carbohydrate counting, medication compliance, and a minimal level of recognizing trends in blood glucose control over time. Some argue that if a patient and family are unable to achieve these basic requirements when using MDI, it is unlikely CSII will work well. For this reason, many experts recommend that patients first demonstrate mastery of MDI before progressing on to CSII [21]. Other experts, however, have seen success in patients with poor control on MDI who switched to pump therapy, particularly patients who had frustration achieving their goals with MDI [1].

Often considered is the age of the patient at initiation of pump therapy. One randomized control trial analyzed pump therapy in patients between the ages of 1 and 6 [22]. After 6 months, no difference was seen in mean HbA$_{1c}$ and mean blood glucose between a CSII group and a group receiving current therapy of NPH and a rapid-acting analog. The frequency of severe hypoglycemia, ketoacidosis, and hospitalization was similar between the two groups throughout the trial. Patients in the CSII had more fasting and predinner mild/moderate hypoglycemia at the 1 and 6 month time points. Quality of life improved in CSII users' fathers from baseline to 6 months while psychological distress increased in mothers in the current therapy group. A position paper by Euster *et al.* in 2006 proposed that all patients with T1D be considered for pump therapy regardless of age. Suggested baseline eligibility criteria included motivated parents with good compliance with diabetes care and demonstrated mastery of carbohydrate counting [17].

Perhaps the patients who benefit most from pump therapy are those individuals whose variable lifestyles require increased flexibility in their insulin regimen.

13.6 ONGOING MANAGEMENT WITH PUMP THERAPY

Once a patient starts pump therapy, close follow-up is necessary to achieve success in management, particularly in the first few months. Adjustments are usually needed in basal and bolus dosing. Experts recommend adjusting the basal rate only if significant blood glucose excursions are seen more than 4 h after a meal bolus or during the occasional skipped meal while monitoring blood glucose every 2 h in the fasted state [1]. Small, incremental changes should be made with consideration of the context in which the excursions occurred, such as times when sedentary or physically active. When adjusting the meal bolus dose, measurements taken 2 h after each dose should be recorded. Small, incremental changes in the I:C ratio should then be made to counteract blood glucose values outside an acceptable range determined by the clinician. The key to successful follow-up is good record keeping by the patient and/or family. A reasonable follow-up plan would be to return to the physician 2–4 weeks after starting pump therapy and then on a quarterly basis once blood glucose values become stable. Many doctors ask their patients to e-mail them their blood glucose log at least once each week during the first few weeks of pump therapy so incremental changes can be made, as necessary.

During follow-up visits, HbA$_{1c}$ values should be checked. If control is not optimal, reviewing the pump's memory function may be helpful in addition to reviewing the patient's blood glucose and insulin log. Thought should be given to whether the patient is remembering to bolus with small snacks, if meal doses are being skipped, and if the patient understands how to correct high blood glucose values. Physical exam should include checking the skin where infusion sets are placed to look for atropy, hypertrophy, or inflammation [1].

13.7 FUTURE ADVANCEMENTS

Several advancements are on the horizon that will further improve pump therapy in the next decade. One promising development is the advent of the continuous glucose monitor (CGM). The CGM is a device with several components. A subcutaneous sensor is placed under the skin and replaced every 3–7 days, comparable to the infusion set of an insulin pump. The sensor uses technology similar to the standard blood glucose monitor in measuring the level of glucose in the surrounding interstitial fluid. Throughout the day and night, the interstitial glucose values are measured and the sensor telemetrically "talks" to an electronic receiver or insulin pump. Newer monitors are able to sound alarms when it predicts trends toward hypo- or hyperglycemia. They also provide the clinician with insight into the patient's blood glucose dynamics, especially during times when blood glucose values are not checked, such as when sleeping or in the period following a meal. These data allow for optimizing the basal and bolus insulin regimens.

There are currently several limitations associated with CGM. CGM measures interstitial glucose rather than blood glucose, as does standard blood glucose monitoring. Because of this, the measurements seen in real time from the CGM are lagging behind the blood glucose concentration in well-mixed blood, usually by 5–15 min. While the lag is not significant when blood glucose levels are not changing with time, it presents a problem when blood glucose levels are acutely falling or rising. If the patient relies solely on CGM, an imminent hypoglycemic event might be detected too late. Another limitation is the cost associated with CGM. The sensors cost hundreds of dollars and must be changed every 3–7 days.

A recent study evaluating the efficacy of CGM found a statistically significant improvement in HbA_{1c} of type 1 diabetes patients, age 25 and older who use CGM compared to regular blood glucose monitoring. The study did not find improvement in subjects in age groups 8–14 or 15–24 [22]. The authors concluded that further work is needed to understand barriers to effective blood glucose control in younger patients using CGM.

While much work on continuous glucose monitoring remains, it represents the next step toward developing the long-awaited artificial pancreas, a device that would both sense glycemic excursions and secrete the appropriate correcting dose of insulin to maintain normoglycemia.

13.8   CONCLUSION

While the advantages and disadvantages of CSII must be weighed on a case by case basis by the clinical team, patient, and family, for many it represents an exceptionally useful device for managing diabetes. A pump's benefits for increasing flexibility and improving glycemic control have made it an increasingly popular tool for millions of diabetic individuals.

REFERENCES

1. Bode BW, Tamborlane WV, Davidson PC (2002) Insulin pump therapy in the 21st century. Strategies for successful use in adults, adolescents, and children with diabetes. Postgrad Med 111(5):69–77, quiz 27
2. Gardner DG, Shoback D (eds) (2007) Greenspan's basic and clinical endocrinology, 8th edn. McGraw-Hill, New York, pp 661–747
3. Zinman B et al. (1997) Insulin lispro in CSII: results of a double-blind crossover study. Diabetes 46(3):440–443
4. Bode B et al. (2002) Comparison of insulin aspart with buffered regular insulin and insulin lispro in continuous subcutaneous insulin infusion: a randomized study in type 1 diabetes. Diabetes Care 25(3):439–444
5. McCulloch D (2008) Insulin therapy in type 1 diabetes mellitus, vol. 6. In: Basow DS (ed). UpToDate: Waltham, MA
6. Havas S, Donner T (2006) Tight control of type 1 diabetes: recommendations for patients. Am Fam Physician 74(6):971–978
7. Delahanty L, McCulloch D (2008) Nutritional considerations in type 1 diabetes, vol. 6. Basow DS (ed). UpToDate: Waltham, MA
8. Pickup J, Mattock M, Kerry S (2002) Glycaemic control with continuous subcutaneous insulin infusion compared with intensive insulin injections in patients with type 1 diabetes: meta-analysis of randomised controlled trials. BMJ 324(7339):705
9. Lauritzen T et al. (1982) Absorption of isophane (NPH) insulin and its clinical implications. Br Med J (Clin Res Ed) 285(6336):159–162
10. Sindelka G et al. (1994) Effect of insulin concentration, subcutaneous fat thickness and skin temperature on subcutaneous insulin absorption in healthy subjects. Diabetologia 37(4):377–380
11. Wood JR et al. (2006) Durability of insulin pump use in pediatric patients with type 1 diabetes. Diabetes Care 29(11):2355–2360
12. Weissberg-Benchell J, Antisdel-Lomaglio J, Seshadri R (2003) Insulin pump therapy: a meta-analysis. Diabetes Care 26(4):1079–1087
13. DeVries JH, Heine RJ (2003) Insulin pump therapy: a meta-analysis: response to Weissberg-Benchell et al. Diabetes Care 26:2485; author reply 2485–2486
14. Doyle EA et al. (2004) A randomized, prospective trial comparing the efficacy of continuous subcutaneous insulin infusion with multiple daily injections using insulin glargine. Diabetes Care 27:1554–1558
15. Bode BW, Steed RD, Davidson PC (1996) Reduction in severe hypoglycemia with long-term continuous subcutaneous insulin infusion in type I diabetes. Diabetes Care 19:324–327
16. Schade DS, Valentine V (2002) To pump or not to pump. Diabetes Care 25:2100–2102
17. Eugster EA, Francis G (2006) Position statement: continuous subcutaneous insulin infusion in very young children with type 1 diabetes. Pediatrics 118:e1244–e1249
18. Colquitt JL et al. (2004) Clinical and cost-effectiveness of continuous subcutaneous insulin infusion for diabetes. Health Technol Assess 8(43):iii, 1–171

19. Anonymous (1993) The effect of intensive treatment of diabetes on the development and progression of long-term complications in insulin-dependent diabetes mellitus. The Diabetes Control and Complications Trial Research Group. N Engl J Med 329:977–986

20. Tamborlane WV *et al.* (2006) Continuous subcutaneous insulin infusion (CSII) in children with type 1 diabetes. Diabetes Res Clin Pract 74(Suppl 2):S112–S115

21. Schade DS, Valentine V (2006) Are insulin pumps underutilized in type 1 diabetes? No. Diabetes Care 29:1453–1455

22. Tamborlane WV *et al.* (2008) Continuous glucose monitoring and intensive treatment of type 1 diabetes. N Engl J Med 359:1464–1476

14 Hyperglycemic Crises in Diabetes Mellitus: Diabetic Ketoacidosis and Hyperglycemic Hyperosmolar State

Dwain E. Woode and
Abbas E. Kitabchi

Key Points

- Although preventable in many cases, DKA and HHS remain among the most morbid of the acute sequelae of diabetes mellitus in children and adolescents.
- Recent innovations reduce cost and resource utilization during stabilization, transport, and definitive care of pediatric patients with DKA.
- The two-bag approach for initial resuscitation and stabilization of DKA has become the standard of care for pediatric DKA.

Keywords: Pediatric diabetes, Diabetic ketoacidosis, Two-bag system, Hyperglycemic hyperosmolar state

14.1 INTRODUCTION

Among the many complications of diabetes, diabetic ketoacidosis (DKA) and hyperglycemic hyperosmolar state (HHS) remain the most serious in the acute setting [1–5]. Estimates put the number or hospitalizations for DKA at greater than 135,000/year with a total cost of $17,559 per episode. Less than 1% of all diabetes-related hospital admissions are due to HHS placing it lower than that of DKA [3]. DKA has a reported annual medical

From: *Nutrition and Health: Management of Pediatric Obesity and Diabetes*,
Edited by: R.J. Ferry, Jr., DOI 10.1007/978-1-60327-256-8_14,
© Springer Science+Business Media, LLC 2011

expense of 2.4 billion [6, 7]. Data from The National Center for Health Statistics indicate that the rate of increase in DKA was faster than the rate of newly diagnosed cases of diabetes from 1996 to 2006.

It has been estimated that 15–67% of patients with new onset type 1 diabetes mellitus (T1DM) present in DKA [8]. DKA and HHS can be seen as points along a continuum of hyperglycemic emergencies. They are characterized by relative insulinopenia. The clinical presentation is determined mostly by the degree of dehydration and the severity of metabolic acidosis [1, 3, 9]. Although DKA is most commonly seen in patients with T1DM, it can occur in T2DM patients. The terms "type 1½ diabetes mellitus" or "ketosis-prone diabetes" have been used to describe the phenomenon of DKA in patients with T2DM [10–12]. T2DM was once thought to be solely a disease of the adult population. However, as the pediatric population follows the national trend in obesity, an increasing number of pediatric patients are diagnosed with T2DM [13].

Table 14.1

Diagnostic criteria and classification

| | DKA | | | |
	Mild	Moderate	Severe	HHS
Plasma glucose (mg/dL)	>250	>250	>250	>600
Arterial pH	7.25–7.30	7.00 to <7.24	<7.00	>7.30
Serum bicarbonate (mEq/L)	15–18	10 to <15	<10	>15
Urine ketone*	Positive	Positive	Positive	Small
Serum ketone*	Positive	Positive	Positive	Small
Anion gap	>12	>12	>12	Variable
Effective serum osmolality (mOsm/kg)**	Variable	Variable	Variable	>320
Alteration in sensorium or mental obtundation	Alert	Alert/drowsy	Stupor/coma	Stupor/coma
Water deficit (% total body water)	<5	5	10	>10

*Nitroprusside reaction method

**Effective serum osmolality: 2[measured Na (mEq/L)] + glucose (mg/dL)/18 = mOsm/kg H_2O. Total serum osmolality: Serum Na (mEq/L) × 2 + Serum glucose (mg/dL)/18 + BUN (mg/dL)/2.8 = mOsm/kg H_2O.

Although HHS occurs most commonly in patients with T2DM, it can also occur with T1DM during episodes of DKA. Table 14.1 lists the typical biochemical criteria for diagnosing DKA and HHS.

14.2 PATHOGENESIS

As a consequence of the relative insulin deficiency existing in DKA or HHS, glucose cannot be utilized by insulin-sensitive tissues (*e.g.*, muscle, liver, adipose tissue), resulting in hyperglycemia and dehydration which is further exacerbated by elevation of catecholamines, glucagon, growth hormone [GH], and cortisol [3, 9, 14–16]. In the evaluation of patients with suspected DKA, it is useful to remember that although the metabolic derangement found can all be independently caused by other pathologies, in combination they should cause a high index of suspicion.

14.2.1 Diabetic Ketoacidosis

DKA results in metabolic derangements causing severe alterations of carbohydrate, protein, and lipid metabolism. These are due to the ineffectiveness, or deficiency of insulin and concomitant elevations of catecholamines, glucagon, GH, and cortisol. Hyperglycemia and lipolysis are central to the development of the metabolic decompensation in DKA [14, 16].

In DKA, stress hormones are increased while blood concentration of insulin is minimal. Since the brain uses glucose as its major fuel and does not require insulin for glucose metabolism, this process ensures a ready supply of fuel. Hyperglycemia in DKA, then, is due to: (1) increased gluconeogenesis, (2) accelerated glycogenolysis, and (3) impaired glucose utilization by peripheral tissues (*e.g.*, liver, muscle, and fat) [2, 15] (Fig. 14.1). Decreased insulin and increased cortisol levels lead to inhibition of protein synthesis and increased proteolysis. The resulting amino acids are then substrates for gluconeogenesis [14].

The imbalance between cortisol and glucagon, on the one hand, and insulin, on the other, augments gluconeogenesis through stimulation of the rate-limiting enzymes of the gluconeogenic pathway [2, 3, 14, 16, 17]. Hyperglycemia results from increased gluconeogenesis and, to a lesser degree, increased glycogenolysis and decreased glucose utilization. Additionally, poor glucose utilization is further exaggerated by increased levels of circulating catecholamines and free fatty acids (FFA) [18]. Glycosuria, polyuria, polydipsia, and polyphagia are the direct result of hyperglycemia [3]. If not corrected promptly, these symptoms can lead to weight loss, dehydration, severe electrolyte imbalances, and death. In DKA, excess catecholamines combined with the absence of effective insulin concentration, promote the breakdown of triglycerides to FFA and glycerol, providing additional substrates for gluconeogenesis [14, 16, 17].

Pathogenesis of DKA and HHS
Stress, Infection and / or insufficient insulin intake

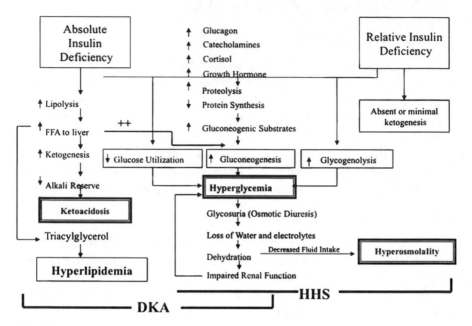

Fig. 14.1. Pathogenesis of DKA and HHS stress, infection, and/or insufficient insulin intake.

This and other alterations in lipid metabolism are the result of major hormonal changes. Facilitated by increased lipolysis, there is a resultant increase in β-oxidation of FFA, ketone body formation, and conversion of FFA to very-low-density lipoprotein (VLDL) by the liver. Decreased concentrations of malonyl co-enzyme A (CoA) further enhances ketogenesis because of increased glucagon. Increased concentration of glucagon, relative to insulin, blocks the conversion of pyruvate to acetyl-CoA by inhibiting acetyl-CoA carboxylase, the first rate-limiting enzyme in *de novo* fatty acid synthesis [16, 18]. Malonyl CoA inhibits carnitine palmitoyl acyl transferase (CPT1), the rate-limiting enzyme of ketogenesis; therefore, reduction in malonyl CoA leads to stimulation of CPT1 and effective increase in ketogenesis [16].

The insulin-sensitive tissues, therefore, change from their usual carbo-hydrate metabolism to metabolizing fat. Increased ketone production and a concomitant decrease in the metabolism of ketone bodies [acetoacetate (AcAc), and β-hydroxybutyrate (BOHB)] leads to ketonemia [18, 19]. Osmotic diuresis, due to hyperglycemia, results in shifts of water along with potassium and phosphate from the intracellular to the extracellular space and leads to elevations in serum levels of both ions despite a total body deficit. Three mechanisms contribute to these electrolyte abnormalities.

First, insulin stimulates salt and water reabsorption in the proximal and distal nephron and phosphate reabsorption in the proximal tubules. In DKA, the deficiency of insulin interrupts this normal process and allows potassium and phosphate to be lost in the urine. Second, urinary loss of ketoions causes an obligatory loss of cations in the form of sodium, potassium, and ammonium salts. Third, osmotic diuresis promotes the net loss of electrolytes.

There is growing evidence that hyperglycemia induces proinflammatory cytokines and chemokines, such as tumor necrosis factor alpha, interleukins, and reactive oxygen species among others [20]. After appropriate treatment (with insulin and hydration), all are seen to return to near normal values [21].

14.2.2 Hyperglycemic Hyperosmolar State

DKA and HHS can be viewed as points along a spectrum and therefore share a very similar pathogenesis (Fig. 14.1). There are, however, some major differences [3–5, 22] (Table 14.2). In HHS, there is some residual insulin production, which is enough to prevent major lipolysis. Additionally, there is a greater degree of dehydration and smaller increases in counter-regulatory hormones in HHS.

14.2.3 DKA in Type 2 Diabetes

Just as T2DM was once thought to be exclusively an adult disease, so too was DKA once thought to be exclusive to T1DM. However, in recent years there has been a new classification added to the list of type of diabetes – so-called "type 1 ½" diabetes [23], also called ketosis prone diabetes. These patients are typically Hispanic or African-American, older, and more obese than those with T1DM. They often present with DKA but require insulin only acutely and can subsequently be treated with oral hypoglycemic agents. They do not typically require life-long insulin therapy. When meas-ured several weeks after the presentation of DKA, the beta-cell function in these patient is robust, and 40% of these patients remain insulin-independent after 10 years out from initial presentation [13].

14.3 PRECIPITATING FACTORS

Infection is a common precipitating factor in both DKA and HHS [3, 22]. In older populations, DKA can be precipitated by cerebrovascular accident (CVA), myocardial infarction (MI), pancreatitis, inadequate insulin therapy, and inadvertent omission of basal insulin. The use of insulin pumps was previously associated with increased episodes of DKA. However, it appears that the incidence of DKA was only elevated in the adolescent population

Table 14.2

Admission biochemical data in patients with hyperglycemic hyperosmolar
state (HHS) or diabetic ketoacidosis (DKA)[a]

	Mean ± SEM	
Parameters measured	HHS (n = 12)	DKA (n = 22)
Glucose (mg/dL)	930 ± 83	616 ± 36
Na$^+$ (mEq/L)	149 ± 3.2	134 ± 1.0
K$^+$ (mEq/L)	3.9 ± 0.2	4.5 ± 0.13
BUN (mg/dL)	61 ± 11	32 ± 3
Creatinine (mg/dL)	1.4 ± 0.1	1.1 ± 0.1
pH	7.3 ± 0.03	7.12 ± 0.04
Bicarbonate (mEq/L)	18 ± 1.1	9.4 ± 1.4
3-β-hydroxybutyrate (mM)	1.0 ± 0.2	9.1 ± 0.85
Total osmolality[b]	380 ± 5.7	323 ± 2.5
IRI (nM)	0.08 ± 0.01	0.07 ± 0.01
C-peptide (nM)	1.14 ± 0.1	0.21 ± 0.03
FFA (mM)	1.5 ± 0.19	1.6 ± 0.16
Human growth hormone (ng/mL)	1.9 ± 0.2	6.1 ± 1.2
Cortisol (ng/mL)	570 ± 49	500 ± 61
IRI (nM)[c]	0.27 ± 0.05	0.09 ± 0.01
C-peptide (nM)[c]	1.75 ± 0.23	0.25 ± 0.05
Catecholamines (ng/mL)	28 ± 0.09	1.78 ± 0.4
Growth hormone (ng/mL)	1.1	7.9
DGap: anion gap – 12 (mEq/L)	11	17

[a]Data are from Chupin et al. [19]. *IRI* immunoreactive insulin

[b]According to the formula: $2(Na + K) + urea (mM)/2.8 + glucose (mM)/18$

[c]Values following intravenous administration of tolbutamide

[3, 11, 24, 25]. In younger patients, omission of insulin may be a consequence
of fear of weight gain, fear of hypoglycemia, immaturity (disorganization),
or rebellion against authority. One study found that more than one–half of
all newly diagnosed diabetic patients (age <20 years old) presented with
DKA. Of these patients, 29.4% had T1DM and 9.7% had T2DM [24]. In
adolescents, DKA may be precipitated by psychological issues or eating
disorders. This group is responsible for as much as 20% of recurrent DKA.
The use of risperidone has also been associated with an increased prevalence
of DKA in schizophrenic patients [26, 27].

At diagnosis, DKA is more common in children younger than 5 years of age and in children within families at low socio-economic status. Poor control or previous episodes of DKA are additional risk factors for recurrent DKA. Peripubertal and adolescent girls, children with clinical depression or other psychiatric disorders, and children with difficult or unstable family circumstances are also at risk for DKA [28].

14.4   DIAGNOSIS

14.4.1   History and Physical Examination

A concise history is very important in the diagnosis and management of DKA and HHS. The younger the child, the more difficult it is to obtain a history of polydipsia, polyuria, and weight loss. Many other diagnoses, which explain the symptoms, may be made in a child prior to the diagnosis of DKA. In T1DM, the symptoms of DKA begin within a few hours of the precipitating event(s). Several studies have demonstrated that insulin levels begin decreasing immediately at interruption of CSII, but glucose levels are maintained in the normal range for approximately 1–2 h. Ketosis can be seen within 4–6 h of insulin interruption. HHS usually develops over the course of days or weeks and may include clouding of sensorium, which can progresses to mental obtundation and coma. Patients in both DKA and HHS can present with polyuria, polyphagia, polydipsia, weight loss, weakness, dehydration, and poor skin turgor. In addition, patients with DKA may have abdominal pain, emesis, and Kussmaul breathing [3, 4, 22]. Patients may also be normothermic or mildly hypothermic, despite harboring some infection.

With DKA, abdominal pain which does not resolve with hydration and correction of acidosis should prompt a judicious search for other causes of the clinical presentation. The majority of patients with an effective osmolality above 330 mOsm/kg are severely obtunded, but mental obtundation rarely exists in patients with osmolality below 320 mOsm/kg. Severe obtundation with an effective osmolality under 320 mOsm/kg requires evaluation for other precipitating events [29].

14.4.2   Laboratory Evaluation

Although findings from a prompt physical examination and a high blood glucose level (by finger stick) in association with ketonuria can strongly suggest the presence of DKA, a definitive diagnosis must be verified by laboratory tests including blood pH and serum bicarbonate. The initial laboratory evaluation for DKA and HHS should consist of a metabolic profile, including blood glucose, blood urea nitrogen (BUN), serum ketones, electrolytes, creatinine, capillary blood gases, complete blood count with differential, and a urinalysis. DKA can be classified as mild, moderate, or severe based on the degree of acidemia and change in mental status [17] (Table 14.1).

The anion gap (AG) is a reflection of unbalanced anion and cations in the body. It is calculated as the difference between the major measured anions ($[Cl^- + HCO_3^-]$) and the major measured cations ($[Na^+ + K^+]$). Adding an acid to the body increases the hydrogen ion concentration with a concurrent decrease in bicarbonate concentration. An associated increase in the anion concentration is reflected as increased AG. Because of fluctuating levels of potassium during DKA and its subsequent treatment, the potassium level is not routinely used to calculate the AG.

Leukocytosis is a typical finding in hyperglycemic crises, with white blood cell counts up to $25,000/mm^3$, but seldom higher unless there is a concomitant bacterial infection [30]. In DKA, the serum sodium level in DKA is usually decreased because of osmotic flux of water from the intracellular to extracellular space due to hyperglycemia. Moreover, modern laboratory assays based on electrical impedance falsely lower the measured sodium in hyperosmolar specimens (*i.e.*, from DKA patients), often referred to as pseudohyponatremia. The *corrected* serum sodium is calculated adding 1.6 mM to the measured serum sodium for every 100 mg/dL of glucose above 200 mg/dL. The corrected serum sodium level should be stable or rise (but not fall) during the initial 12–16 h of resuscitation.

Serum potassium concentration can be normal or high, depending on the shift of potassium between the intracellular to the extracellular space because of acidemia, insulin deficiency, and hypertonicity [3]. In HHS, serum sodium level is usually normal or elevated, with elevated BUN and serum creatinine due to dehydration.

The insulinopenia that exists in DKA leads to increased ketogenesis and a ketone body ratio (BOHB: AcAc) disproportionately in favor of BOHB. The higher BOHB reflects the redox state of hepatic mitochondria. As treatment progresses, the reduced state is improved, and the ketone body ratio becomes more balanced.

14.5 DIFFERENTIAL DIAGNOSIS

Since most patients in DKA present with abdominal pain, nausea, or vomiting, the differential diagnosis of pancreatitis should be considered. Unfortunately, increased serum amylase, which may be released from extrapancreatic tissues [3], is not definitive for the diagnosis of pancreatitis in DKA.

Patients may present with metabolic conditions resembling DKA or HHS, which emphasizes the need for laboratory and physical evaluation. Patients may present in mild ketoacidosis, if they have had decreased oral intake (starvation ketosis). However, it is rare for these patients to present with a serum bicarbonate concentration below 18 mEq/L and hyperglycemia. Other entities in the differential diagnosis of DKA are the high AG acidosis (including lactic acidosis), advanced chronic renal failure, and ingestion of drugs such as salicylate, methanol, and ethylene glycol. "MUDPILES" is a classic mnemonic for causes of high ion gap acidosis such as: Methanol, Uremia, DKA, Paraldehyde, Isoniazid, Lactic Acidosis, Ethylene glycol, and Salicylates. Additionally, patients can present with multiple acid base disorders that may confound the presentation of DKA. This is especially true in patients with chronic respiratory illnesses, where there is a high bicarbonate concentration at baseline, or with metabolic acidosis seen in chronic renal disease. Dehydration due to vomiting can cause a metabolic alkalosis from loss of hydrogen ions. In lactic acidosis, a decrease in circulating bicarbonate level may falsely suggest a more severe case of DKA than the one that actually exists [31]. Table 14.3 shows a partial differential diagnosis.

14.6 TREATMENT

The goals of DKA therapy should be fourfold: (1) to improve tissue perfusion by increasing circulatory volume; (2) to correct hyperglycemia and improve plasma osmolality; (3) to correct electrolyte imbalance and to reduce serum and urine ketone bodies to normal; and (4) to identify and treat precipitating events. Successful treatment of DKA and HHS requires frequent reassessment of the above goals to ensure appropriate improvements [3]. A suggested flow sheet for recording results is presented in Table 14.4 [1], and Fig. 14.2a summarizes a protocol for managing DKA and HHS.

14.6.1 Fluids

Both DKA and HHS are volume-depleted states [5, 17, 22]. Therefore, initial fluid therapy attempts to expand the interstitial (ISC), intravascular (IVC), and intracellular (ICS) compartments along with restoring renal perfusion. Paradoxically, despite being dehydrated, most patients continue to produce considerable urine output due to osmotic diuresis. A patient presenting with a diagnosis of DKA who is not producing large amounts of urine is likely to be severely dehydrated. Children with mild DKA are likely to be 5–7% total body water fluid deficient and those with severe DKA can be assumed to be fluid deficient by at least 10% [28]. Corrected serum sodium level can be used as a marker during volume repletion. As serum glucose levels fall, the corrected serum sodium should increase. Assuming no contraindication, the initial fluid should be isotonic saline. This expands

Table 14.3
Laboratory evaluation of metabolic causes of acidosis and coma

	Starvation or high fat intake	DKA	Lactic acidosis	Uremic acidosis	Alcoholic ketosis (starvation)	Salicylate intoxication	Methanol or ethylene glycol intoxication	Hyperosmolar coma	Hypoglycemic coma	Rhabdomyolysis
pH	Normal	↓	↓	Mild ↓	↓↑	↓↑	↓	Normal	Normal	Mild ↓ maybe ↓↓
Plasma glucose	Normal	↑	Normal	Normal	↓ or normal	Normal or ↓	Normal	↑↑ >500 mg/dL	↓↓ <30 mg/dL	Normal
Glycosuria	Negative	++	Negative	Negative	Negative	Negative	Negative	++	Negative	Negative
Total plasma ketones	Slight ↑	↑↑	Normal	Normal	Slight to moderate ↑	Normal	Normal	Normal or slight ↑	Normal or slight ↑	Normal
Anion gap	Slight ↑	↑	↑	Slight ↑	↑	↑	↑	Normal	Normal or slight	↑↑
Osmolality	Normal	↑	Normal	↑	Normal	Normal	↑↑	↑↑ >330 mOsm/kg	Normal	Normal or slight ↑
Uric acid	Mild ↑ (starvation)	↑	Normal	Normal	↑	Normal	Normal	Normal	Normal	↑
Miscellaneous		May give false-positive for ethylene glycol	Serum lactate >7 mmol/L	BUN >200 mg/dL		Serum salicylate positive	Serum levels positive			Myoglobinuria hemoglobinuria

Table 14.4
DKA/HHS management flow sheet

	SUGGESTED
	DKA / HHS FLOWSHEET

Height: _____
Weight:
Initially: _____
After 24hr: _____

DATE: HOUR:															
MENTAL STATUS*															
TEMPERATURE															
PULSE															
RESPIRATION/DEPTH**															
BLOOD PRESSURE															
SERUM GLUCOSE (MG/DL)															
SERUM KETONES															
URINE KETONES															
ELECTROLYTES — SERUM Na$^+$ (mEq/L)															
SERUM K$^+$ (mEq/L)															
SERUM CL$^-$ (mEq/L)															
SERUM HCO$_3^-$ (mEq/L)															
SERUM BUN (mg/dl)															
EFFECTIVE OSMOLALITY 2 [measured Na (mEq/L)] + Glucose (mg/dl)/18															
ANION GAP															
ARTERIAL/VENOUS BLOOD GASES — pH VENOUS(V) ARTERIAL (A)															
pO$_2$															
pCO$_2$															
O$_2$ SAT															
INSULIN — UNITS in PAST HOUR															
ROUTE															
INTAKE FLUID/METABOLITES — 0.45% NaCl (ml) PAST HOUR															
0.9% NaCl (ml) PAST HOUR															
5% DEXTROSE (ml) PAST HOUR															
KCL (mEq) PAST HOUR															
PO$_4$ (mMOLES) PAST HOUR															
OTHER															
OUTPUT — URINE (ml)															
OTHER															

```
* A-ALERT      D-DROWSY      S-STUPOROUS      C-COMATOSE
** D-DEEP            S-SHALLOW                  N-NORMAL
```

a

MANAGEMENT OF PATIENTS WITH DKA

Algorithm assumes that patient is not in shock. If shock exists, resuscitate patient as would normally be done with intravenous fluids and support.

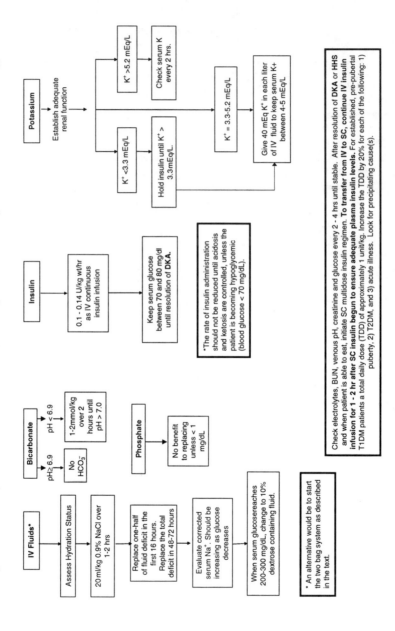

IV Fluids*

Assess Hydration Status

20ml/kg 0.9% NaCl over 1-2 hrs

Replace one-half of fluid deficit in the first 16 hours. Replace the total deficit in 48-72 hours

Evaluate corrected serum Na⁺. Should be increasing as glucose decreases

When serum glucose reaches 200-300 mg/dL, change to 10% dextrose containing fluid.

* An alternative would be to start the two bag system as described in the text.

Bicarbonate

pH≥6.9 → No HCO₃⁻

pH < 6.9 → 1-2mmol/kg over 2 hours until pH > 7.0

Phosphate

No benefit to replacing unless < 1 mg/dL

Insulin

0.1 - 0.14 U/kg wt/hr as IV continuous insulin infusion

Keep serum glucose between 70 and 80 mg/dl until resolution of **DKA**.

*The rate of insulin administration should not be reduced until acidosis and ketosis are controlled, unless the patient is becoming hypoglycemic (blood glucose < 70 mg/dL).

Potassium

Establish adequate renal function

K⁺ <3.3 mEq/L → Hold insulin until K⁺ > 3.3mEq/L.

K⁺ >5.2 mEq/L → Check serum K every 2 hrs.

K⁺ = 3.3-5.2 mEq/L

Give 40 mEq K⁺ in each liter of IV fluid to keep serum K+ between 4-5 mEq/L

Check electrolytes, BUN, venous pH, creatinine and glucose every 2 - 4 hrs until stable. After resolution of **DKA** or **HHS** and when patient is able to eat, initiate SC multidose insulin regimen. **To transfer from IV to SC, continue IV insulin infusion for 1 - 2 hr after SC insulin begun to ensure adequate plasma insulin levels.** For established, pre-pubertal T1DM patients a total daily dose (TDD) of approximately 1 unit/kg. Increase the TDD by 20% for each of the following: 1) puberty, 2) T2DM, and 3) acute illness. Look for precipitating cause(s).

Fig. 14.2.   (a) Management of patients with DKA (b) Two bag system.

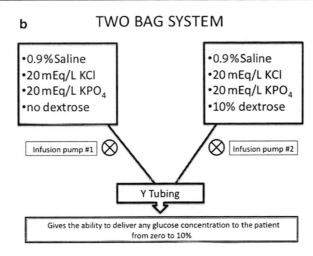

b   **TWO BAG SYSTEM**

- •0.9 % Saline
- •20 mEq/L KCl
- •20 mEq/L KPO$_4$
- •no dextrose

- •0.9 % Saline
- •20 mEq/L KCl
- •20 mEq/L KPO$_4$
- •10% dextrose

Infusion pump #1   Infusion pump #2

Y Tubing

Gives the ability to deliver any glucose concentration to the patient
from zero to 10%

Fig. 14.2. (continued).

the ISC and IVC volumes. Subsequent use of half-normal saline (which is similar in osmolarity to fluid loss in DKA) will expand the intracellular volume [32] but can increase the 1Jk of cerebral edema; thus, it should be avoided during the initial 24 h of resuscitation. The choice and rate of subsequent fluids will be based on the patient's sodium concentration and hydration status. The fluid replacement goal is to correct the estimated water deficit over a 48-h period or longer by replacing one-half the water deficit in the first 16 h and the remainder over the next ≥32 h. Iatrogenic fluid overload can be avoided by frequent patient monitoring. An effective serum osmolality above 320 mOsm/kg indicates severe dehydration.

In hemodynamically compromised patients, aggressive isotonic saline use should continue until stable. Providing a bolus of 20 mL/kg over 1 h and repeating if hemodynamically unstable. Nevertheless, most providers are overly aggressive with initial fluid resuscitation, which can increase the risk of cerebral edema. The use of insulin without adequate fluid replacement may aggravate hypotension, and insulin effectiveness is lessened in the hyperosmolar state [33, 34]. Therefore, expanding intravascular and intracellular compartments with hydration renders the body more sensitive to low dose insulin therapy. Hydration may also reduce the level of counterregulatory hormones and hyperglycemia [35], reduce serum blood glucose, BUN, hematocrit, and potassium levels without significant changes in pH or HCO$_3$ [29].

DKA patients require calories for proper metabolism of ketone bodies. Therefore, once the blood glucose level is approximately 200–300 mg/dL, the sodium chloride solution should be replaced with a dextrose-containing solution. The rate of insulin administration should not be reduced until acidosis and ketosis are controlled, unless the patient becomes hypoglycemic (blood glucose <70 mg/dL).

14.6.2 Insulin Therapy

The cornerstone of DKA and HHS therapy is the administration of insulin by continuous intravenous infusion [9, 36]. It is vital to determine the serum potassium level before insulin is given. Hypokalemia can be exacerbated if insulin is infused without correcting potassium deficiency [37]. It is recommended that no insulin be given to patients unless the potassium value is available and potassium is >3.3 mEq/L. However, it is also prudent to administer insulin promptly and continuously upon confirmation of DKA and renal function. Bolus insulin therapy is generally unwise in the setting of DKA.

Continuous intravenous insulin infusion is preferred to subcutaneous administration due to ease of control by intravenous drip and rapid onset of action [29]. Algorithms have, in the past, recommended the use of an initial bolus of regular insulin followed by a continuous infusion. A randomized prospective study has demonstrated that in the treatment of DKA, an initial bolus of insulin is *not* necessary, provided insulin is infused at an hourly rate of 0.1–0.14 units/kg body weight (Table 14.5). Additionally, when the potassium level is in the normal range, a bolus may precipitate hypokalemia. After the initial volume expansion and improved renal perfusion associated with 20 mL/kg of 0.9% saline, the blood glucose level may fall abruptly, but thereafter should fall hourly by 50–100 mg/dL. The rate of dextrose infusion can be adjusted to maintain blood glucose above 70–80 mg/dL until DKA is resolved. In HHS, this goal can be 250–300 mg/dL until mental obtundation and hyperosmolar state are corrected. The resolution of DKA is indicated by a blood glucose level below 200 mg/dL and the presence of any two of the following: serum bicarbonate ≥18 mEq/L, or pH>7.3, or AG ≤12 mEq/L. HHS is resolved when total osmolality is below 320 mOsm/kg with a gradual recovery to mental alertness.

Studies using rapid-acting insulin analogs suggest that for mild cases of DKA, the use of subcutaneous lispro or aspart given every 1–2 h [38, 39] is as effective as the use of regular insulin given intravenously in the intensive care unit (ICU). This requires that adequately informed personnel are available for frequent measuring of blood glucose by fingersticks every 2 h, for frequent monitoring of electrolytes and venous pH (every 4–6 h), and for adequate administration of fluid.

Table 14.5
Outline for treatment of DKA

Laboratory evaluation	After history and physical examination, initial laboratory evaluation should include determination of complete blood count, blood glucose, serum electrolytes, blood urea nitrogen (BUN), creatinine, serum ketones, osmolality, arterial blood gases, and urinalysis. Admission ECG, chest radiograph, and cultures of blood, urine, and sputum may be ordered if clinically indicated. During therapy, capillary blood glucose should be determined every 1–2 h at the bedside using a glucose oxidase reagent strip; and blood should be drawn every 2–4 h for determination of serum electrolytes, glucose, BUN, creatinine, phosphorus, and venous pH.
Fluids	10–20 mL/kg normal saline (0.9% sodium chloride) over first hour. Then, 0.9% saline at a rate depending on fluid status and serum sodium concentration, with a goal of correcting 50% of the fluid deficit in the first 16 h. When plasma glucose reaches 200–300 mg/dL, change to dextrose-containing fluid to support continued insulin administration until ketonemia is controlled, while avoiding hypoglycemia.
Insulin	Start regular insulin infusion at 0.1 unit/kg hourly as a continuous infusion. Alternatively, an infusion rate of at least 0.14 unit/kg/h can be used. After initial diuresis, the goal is to achieve a rate of decline of glucose of 50–100 mg/dL hourly. Maintain glucose levels between 80–150 mg/dL until ketoacidosis is resolved.
Potassium	Serum K^+ ≥5.2 mEq/L; no supplementation is required.
	Serum K^+=4–5 mEq/L; add 20 mEq/L to each liter of replacement fluid.
	Serum K^+=3–4 mEq/L; add 40 mEq/L to each liter of replacement fluid.
	Serum K^+≤3.3 mEq/L; hold insulin and give 10–20 mEq/h until K^+ >3, then add 40 mEq/L to each liter of replacement fluid.

(continued)

Table 14.5
(continued)

Bicarbonate	Usually reserved for cardiac arrest. When arterial pH <6.9 or bicarbonate <5 mM, carefully consider 100 mM of bicarbonate in 400 mL of H_2O with 20 mEq of potassium chloride over 2 h until pH increases to ≥7.0. Do *not* give bicarbonate if pH ≥7.0.
Phosphate	If indicated (serum levels <1 mg/dL), 20–30 mM potassium phosphate over 24 h. Monitor serum calcium level.
Transition to subcutaneous insulin	Insulin infusion should be continued until resolution of ketoacidosis (glucose ≤200 mg/dL, bicarbonate ≥15 mEq/L, pH>7.30, or patient ready to eat). When this occurs, start subcutaneous insulin regimen.
	To prevent recurrence of DKA during the transition period to subcutaneous insulin, consider continuation of intravenous insulin for 1 h after subcutaneous insulin is given.

Similar protocol should be used for HHS, except that no bicarbonate is needed for HHS and switching to glucose-containing fluid is done when blood glucose reaches 300 mg/dL. Adapted from Kitabchi [44].

No prospective, randomized studies have been conducted or reported to compare rapid-acting insulin analog infusion to intravenous regular insulin infusion in the ICU. Therefore, the use of rapid-acting insulin analogs is not recommended for patients with severe DKA or HHS.

14.6.3   The Two Bag System

Another method of fluid administration is the "two bag" system. This method was introduced in the 1990s and has gained wide acceptance in most pediatric hospitals. The main benefit of the system is the ease of titrating to any glucose infusion rate from 0 to 10%. Additionally, this approach significantly reduces cost if implemented correctly. The basic idea is to hang two identical bags of 0.9% sodium chloride, each with the appropriate electrolyte concentration for a desired patient. To the second bag is added 10% dextrose. These two bags (on separate infusion pumps) are then connected by Y-shaped tubing to the final common catheter for infusion (Fig. 14.2b). Since each bag can titrate independently, it is both easy and fast to administer and adjust various concentrations of dextrose-containing fluid to the patient. Shutting off Bag #1 (which lacks dextrose) will provide 10% dextrose; alternatively, shutting off Bag #2 (which contains dextrose) will provide no dextrose. As the electrolytes in each bag are the same, there should be no concern about mixing the electrolytes in each bag. A case-controlled retrospective analysis from a busy children's hospital compared this "two bag system" to the traditional "one bag" system for the management of DKA. The authors concluded that the two bag system provided "...more cost-effective intravenous dextrose and fluid delivery and enhance[d] quality of care by improving the efficiency, timeliness, and flexibility of overall control" [33].

14.6.4 Potassium

DKA and HHS patients can have total-body depletion of potassium despite elevated serum levels. This increase is secondary to the acidosis, which causes kaliuresis as well as transport of potassium from the intracellular to the extracellular compartment. Potassium should be carefully monitored during therapy, and no insulin shoud be given unless serum potassium is >3.3 mEq/L. Previous sections discussed several mechanisms that contribute to the total body depletion of potassium and phosphate. During treatment, insulin causes a shift of potassium into the intracellular space. Once serum potassium levels are within the normal range, and good renal function is established, 20–30 mEq of potassium added to the hydrating solution should suffice [2, 9]. Serum potassium levels should be maintained between 4 and 5 mEq/L. In cases of significant hypokalemia, potassium replacement should be initiated concurrently with fluid therapy. Insulin administration should be delayed until potassium levels are >3.3 mEq/L [15].

14.6.5 Bicarbonate

The use of bicarbonate in DKA is highly controversial, but a prospective randomized study suggests that use of bicarbonate in DKA is unnecessary when pH is above 6.9 [2, 3, 5, 39]. As ketone bodies decrease during treatment, there will be an adequate supply of bicarbonate except in severe cases of acidosis [15]. However, there are no comparative prospective randomized studies for pH below 6.9. Having said this, DKA in children is not usually treated with bicarbonate, even with lower pH [17]. There is no indication for treatment with bicarbonate in patients with HHS.

14.6.6 Phosphate

Along with sodium and potassium depletion, there is also a deficit of phosphate in DKA and HHS at presentation. As with potassium, the serum phosphate level is usually normal or increased, but decreases after insulin therapy is started. Prospective randomized studies [34] show that phosphate therapy offers little benefit in the clinical outcome of patients with DKA. In cases with complications of hypophosphatemia, judicious replacement of phosphate may be justified. The typical resuscitation includes 20–30 mEq/L of phosphate (as potassium phosphate). The use of phosphate in higher doses may cause hypocalcemia [34, 40]. The maximal rate of phosphate replacement should not exceed 4.5 mmol/h.

14.7   IMMEDIATE POSTHYPERGLYCEMIC CRISIS FOLLOW-UP CARE

Intravenous insulin therapy should continue until there is resolution of the hyperglycemic crisis and acidosis (criteria described previously). The half-life of regular insulin administered intravenously is very short (5–7 min). If there is sudden interruption of insulin infusion, blood insulin concentrations can plummet to undetectable levels, leading to a relapse of hyperglycemic crises. Therefore, the recommendation is that intravenous insulin infusion can continue for up to 2 h after subcutaneous regular insulin has been started. However, the insulin infusion can be stopped as soon as a fast-acting insulin (*e.g.*, lispro or aspart) has been given. While on an insulin infusion, blood sugar should be checked hourly. During recovery off the insulin infusion, serum glucose can be checked every 4 h until the patient eats. Once eating, the patient should monitor blood glucose before each meal, at bedtime, and once overnight (between midnight and 0300 h).

For established, prepubertal T1DM patients a total daily dose (TDD) of approximately 1 unit/kg is a good starting point for transition to subcutaneous insulin. From this starting point, increase the TDD by 20% for each of the following: (1) puberty, (2) T2DM, and (3) acute illness. For example, a newly diagnosed, pubertal, T2DM patient would start at TDD of 1.4–1.6 units/kg. Patients with cystic fibrosis-related diabetes on steroids may require more than 2–3 units/kg daily. Insulin should be administered in divided doses provided there is adequate glycemic control [15]. The choice of insulin regimen after resolution of the hyperglycemic crisis will be determined by the capabilities of the patient/family. A prospective randomized trial—comparing treatment with basal–bolus versus split-mixed regimen with NPH plus regular insulin—determined that there was similar glycemic control following the resolution of DKA. One advantage of the basal–bolus regimen was fewer hypoglycemic episodes [41].

The basal dose typically starts at 45–55% of the TDD as a long-acting insulin (*e.g.*, detemir or glargine) given once daily, typically at bedtime to improve convenience for busy families. Bolus dosing of fast-acting insulin (*e.g.*, lispro or aspart or glulisine) – based on a combination of correction factor and insulin:carbohydrate ratio (ICR) – comprises the remainder of the TDD. The typical range for the correction factor before meals (>20 g carbohydrate at breakfast, lunch, or dinner) is 1 unit for every 50 mg/dL above target of 120 mg/dL (*e.g.*, an insulin-resistant adolescent with T2DM) to 1 unit for every 100 mg/dL above target of 120 mg/dL (*e.g.*, an insulin-sensitive, pre-pubertal T1DM). The typical range for the ICR with meals is 1 unit for every 10 g of carbohydrate (*e.g.*, an insulin-resistant adolescent with T2DM) to 1 unit for every 30 g of carbohydrate (*e.g.*, an insulin-sensitive, pre-pubertal T1DM).

14.8 COMPLICATIONS OF THERAPY

In the past when higher doses of insulin were used, the most common complications of insulin therapy were hypokalemia and hypoglycemia [1]. These complications have been reduced with the use of lower-dose insulin infusions [9].

Cerebral edema is a complication that is relatively rare in adults and most often strikes children with hyperosmolar states, including DKA [28, 42]. Cerebral edema occurs in 0.5–1% of all DKA cases and remains the most common cause of mortality in children with DKA [43]. Cerebral edema is associated with 21–24% mortality and contributes to 57–87% of all DKA-associated deaths in children. Approximately 15–26% of survivors sustain permanent neurological injury. Signs and symptoms of cerebral edema include headache, decreased heart rate, and increasing blood pressure. Additionally, patients may be restless, irritable, drowsy, or have nonspecific neurological symptoms. Although clinical symptoms usually manifest 4–12 h after initiation of therapy, there are reported cases of cerebral edema even before therapy is started [28]. The pathophysiology of cerebral edema is poorly understood, but there is some evidence that over–hydration and possibly the use of bicarbonate may lead to cerebral edema [46]. Risk factors for the development of cerebral edema include: elevated BUN, hypocapnea, patients age five years and younger, sluggish improvement of hyponatremia as treatment for DKA ensues, and profound acidosis. The treatments include intravenous mannitol, reduction in rate of fluid administration, and mechanical ventilation.

14.9 PREVENTION

Most cases of DKA and HHS can be prevented by more ready access to medical care, improved effective communication between healthcare providers and patients, more engaged caretakers, and more robust patient education. One helpful feature of patient education is the "sick day rules." First, communicate to families that insulin therapy should never be discontinued.

Second, any diabetic patient who vomits more than once during a 24-h period should seek prompt medical attention with a licensed healthcare provider, regardless of circumstances. Third, promptly monitor urinary ketones whenever a diabetic patient appears ill. Fourth, promptly rehydrate and administer insulin when ketones are detected, following the advice of the assigned provider [15, 44, 45]. A rule of thumb in children over age 2 years and adolescents is that ketosis will require resuscitation with 1 oz/year of age hourly, avoiding drinks with caffeine, high fat content, or concentrated sweets. Minor ketosis in pediatic patients can be treated with fast- or short- acting insulin as 10% TDD given every 2 h subcutaneously.

Economic factors play a big part in access to care and comprise a major reason for discontinued insulin therapy. More than 50% of DKA admissions in some inner-city hospitals can be attributed to discontinuation of medication and noncompliance [11]. This underscores the need of a healthcare delivery system that is robust and innovative.

REFERENCES

1. Alberti KGMM (2001) Diabetic acidosis, hyperosmolar coma, and lactic acidosis. In: Becker KL (ed) *Principles and Practice of Endocrinology and Metabolism*, 3rd edn. Lippincott Williams and Wilkins, Philadelphia
2. Kitabchi AE, Fisher JN, Murphy MB, Rumbak MJ (1994) Diabetic ketoacidosis and the hyperglycemic hyperosmolar nonketotic state. *Joslin's Diabetes Mellitus*. In: Joslin EP, Kahn CR, Weir GC (eds) *Joslin's Diabetes Mellitus*, 13th edn. Lea & Febiger, Philadelphia, pp 738–770
3. Kitabchi AE, Umpierrez GE, Murphy MB (2001) Management of hyperglycemic crises in patients with diabetes. Diabetes Care 24:131–153
4. Matz R (1999) Management of the hyperosmolar hyperglycemic syndrome. Am Fam Physician 60:1468–1476
5. Kitabchi AE, Murphy MB (2002) Hyperglycemic crises in adult patients with diabetes mellitus. In: Wass JAH, Shalet SM, Gale EAM (eds) *Oxford Textbook of Endocrinology and Diabetes*. Oxford University Press, New York, pp 1734–1747
6. Johnson DD, Palumbo PJ, Chu CP (1980) Diabetic ketoacidosis in a community-based population. Mayo Clin Proc 55:83–88
7. Kim S (2007) Burden of hospitalizations primarily due to uncontrolled diabetes: implications of inadequate primary health care in the United States. Diabetes Care 30:1281–1282
8. Lawrence SE, Cummings EA, Gaboury I *et al.* (2005) Population-based study of incidence and risk factors for cerebral edema in pediatric diabetic ketoacidosis. J Pediatr 146:688–692
9. Alberti KG, Hockaday TD, Turner RC (1973) Small doses of intramuscular insulin in the treatment of diabetic "coma". Lancet 2:515–522
10. Kitabchi AE (2003) Ketosis-prone diabetes – a new subgroup of patients with atypical type 1 and type 2 diabetes? J Clin Endocrinol Metab 88:5087–5089
11. Umpierrez GE, Kelly JP, Navarrete JE *et al.* (1997) Hyperglycemic crises in urban blacks. Arch Intern Med 157:669–675
12. Umpierrez GE, Woo W, Hagopian WA *et al.* (1999) Immunogenetic analysis suggests different pathogenesis for obese and lean African-Americans with diabetic ketoacidosis. Diabetes Care 22:1517–1523

13. Mauvais-Jarvis F, Sobngwi E, Porcher R et al. (2004) Ketosis-prone type 2 diabetes in patients of sub-Saharan African origin: clinical pathophysiology and natural history of beta-cell dysfunction and insulin resistance. Diabetes 53:645–653

14. Exton JH (1987) Mechanisms of hormonal regulation of hepatic glucose metabolism. Diabetes Metab Rev 3:163–183

15. Kitabchi AE, Umpierrez GE, Miles JM et al. (2009) Hyperglycemic crises in adult patients with diabetes. Diabetes Care 32:1335–1343

16. McGarry JD, Woeltje KF, Kuwajima M et al. (1989) Regulation of ketogenesis and the renaissance of carnitine palmitoyltransferase. Diabetes Metab Rev 5:271–284

17. Kitabchi AE, Umpierrez GE, Murphy MB et al. (2004) Hyperglycemic crises in diabetes. Diabetes Care 27(suppl 1):S94–S102

18. Reichard GA Jr, Skutches CL, Hoeldtke RD et al. (1986) Acetone metabolism in humans during diabetic ketoacidosis. Diabetes 35:668–674

19. Balasse EO, Fery F (1989) Ketone body production and disposal: effects of fasting, diabetes, and exercise. Diabetes Metab Rev 5:247–270

20. Stentz FB, Umpierrez GE, Cuervo R et al. (2004) Proinflammatory cytokines, markers of cardiovascular risks, oxidative stress, and lipid peroxidation in patients with hyperglycemic crises. Diabetes 53:2079–2086

21. Buyukasik Y, Ileri NS, Haznedaroglu IC et al. (1998) Enhanced subclinical coagulation activation during diabetic ketoacidosis. Diabetes Care 21:868–870

22. Wachtel TJ, Silliman RA, Lamberton P (1987) Predisposing factors for the diabetic hyperosmolar state. Arch Intern Med 147:499–501

23. Maldonado M, Hampe CS, Gaur LK et al. (2003) Ketosis-prone diabetes: dissection of a heterogeneous syndrome using an immunogenetic and beta-cell functional classification, prospective analysis, and clinical outcomes. J Clin Endocrinol Metab 88:5090–5098

24. Kitabchi AE, Umpierrez GE, Fisher JN et al. (2008) Thirty years of personal experience in hyperglycemic crises: diabetic ketoacidosis and hyperglycemic hyperosmolar state. J Clin Endocrinol Metab 93:1541–1552

25. Nyenwe EA, Loganathan RS, Blum S et al. (2007) Active use of cocaine: an independent risk factor for recurrent diabetic ketoacidosis in a city hospital. Endocr Pract 13:22–29

26. Haupt DW, Newcomer JW (2001) Risperidone-associated diabetic ketoacidosis. Psychosomatics 42:279–280

27. Rydall AC, Rodin GM, Olmsted MP et al. (1997) Disordered eating behavior and microvascular complications in young women with insulin-dependent diabetes mellitus. N Engl J Med 336:1849–1854

28. Wolfsdorf J, Glaser N, Sperling MA (2006) Diabetic ketoacidosis in infants, children, and adolescents: a consensus statement from the American Diabetes Association. Diabetes Care 29:1150–1159

29. Kitabchi AE, Fisher JN (1981) Insulin therapy of diabetic ketoacidosis: physiologic versus pharmacologic doses of insulin and their routes of administration. In: Brownlee M (ed) Handbook of diabetes mellitus. Garland STPM Press, New York, pp 95–149

30. Slovis CM, Mork VG, Slovis RJ et al. (1987) Diabetic ketoacidosis and infection: leukocyte count and differential as early predictors of serious infection. Am J Emerg Med 5:1–5

31. Bjellerup P, Kallner A, Kollind M (1994) GLC determination of serum-ethylene glycol, interferences in ketotic patients. J Toxicol Clin Toxicol 32:85–87

32. Hillman K (1987) Fluid resuscitation in diabetic emergencies – a reappraisal. Intensive Care Med 13:4–8

33. Grimberg A, Cerri RW, Satin-Smith M et al. (1999) The "two bag system" for variable intravenous dextrose and fluid administration: benefits in diabetic ketoacidosis management. J Pediatr 134:376–378

34. Fisher JN, Kitabchi AE (1983) A randomized study of phosphate therapy in the treatment of diabetic ketoacidosis. J Clin Endocrinol Metab 57:177–180

35. Waldhausl W, Kleinberger G, Korn A *et al.* (1979) Severe hyperglycemia: effects of rehydration on endocrine derangements and blood glucose concentration. Diabetes 28:577–584
36. Kitabchi AE, Ayyagari V, Guerra SM (1976) The efficacy of low-dose versus conventional therapy of insulin for treatment of diabetic ketoacidosis. Ann Intern Med 84:633–638
37. Abramson E, Arky R (1966) Diabetic acidosis with initial hypokalemia. Therapeutic implications. JAMA 196:401–403
38. Umpierrez GE, Cuervo R, Karabell A *et al.* (2004) Treatment of diabetic ketoacidosis with subcutaneous insulin aspart. Diabetes Care 27:1873–1878
39. Umpierrez GE, Latif K, Stoever J *et al.* (2004) Efficacy of subcutaneous insulin lispro versus continuous intravenous regular insulin for the treatment of patients with diabetic ketoacidosis. Am J Med 117:291–296
40. Umpierrez GE, Jones S, Smiley D *et al.* (2009) Insulin analogs versus human insulin in the treatment of patients with diabetic ketoacidosis: a randomized controlled trial. Diabetes Care 32:1164–1169
41. Kreisberg RA (1977) Phosphorus deficiency and hypophosphatemia. Hosp Pract 12:121–128
42. Rosenbloom AL (1990) Intracerebral crises during treatment of diabetic ketoacidosis. Diabetes Care 13:22–33
43. Glaser N, Kuppermann N (2004) The evaluation and management of children with diabetic ketoacidosis in the emergency department. Pediatr Emerg Care 20:477–481, quiz 482–484
44. Kitabchi AE (2005) Hyperglycemic crises: improving prevention and management. Am Fam Physician 71:1659–1660
45. Laffel LM, Brackett J, Ho J *et al.* (1998) Changing the process of diabetes care improves metabolic outcomes and reduces hospitalizations. Qual Manag Health Care 6:53–62
46. Glaser N, Barnett P, McCaslin I *et al.* (2001) Risk factors for cerebral edema in children with diabetic ketoacidosis. The Pediatric Emergency Medicine Collaborative Research Committee of the American Academy of Pediatrics. N Engl J Med. 344:264–269

15 Monogenic Diabetes

Rabia Rehman, Hooman Oktaei, Dale Childress, and Solomon S. Solomon

Key Points

- MODY forms of diabetes are underdiagnosed, especially in very young and elderly populations.
- MODY should be suspected when a patient with "T2DM" presents before age 25 in the absence of obesity or clinical signs of insulin resistance, particularly when other family members share a history of such clinical features.
- Oral sulfonylurea therapy is preferred to injected insulin therapy for most patients with the commonest form of MODY.
- It is critical to confirm the specific form of MODY to individualize therapy.

Keywords: Maturity onset diabetes of youth, MODY, Monogenic diabetes, Glucokinase

15.1 INTRODUCTION

Monogenic but heterogeneous forms of diabetes mellitus comprise a group of disorders formerly classified as maturity onset diabetes of youth (MODY). These disorders typically manifest before age 25 years as non-ketotic diabetes mellitus. The clinical manifestations of monogenic diabetes result from a partial or total compromise of insulin secretion by the pancreatic beta-cells. These secretory defects are most often responsive to

From: *Nutrition and Health: Management of Pediatric Obesity and Diabetes*,
Edited by: R.J. Ferry, Jr., DOI 10.1007/978-1-60327-256-8_15,
© Springer Science+Business Media, LLC 2011

sulfonylureas or insulin secretagogues. While relatively rare, the management differs from other common forms of diabetes. Moreover, this area remains an active field of investigation.

Tattersall and Fajans (1975) coined the acronym MODY and defined these disorders as "fasting hyperglycemia diagnosed under the age of 25 which could be treated without insulin for more than two years" [1]. Monogenic forms of diabetes mellitus are often misdiagnosed as type 1 diabetes (T1DM) or type 2 DM (T2DM). Over the past 15 years, rapid discoveries have revealed novel, underlying molecular mechanisms for this group and prompted a novel classification of this spectrum. The defining clinical features for the majority of these patients remain nonketotic diabetes mellitus, early age of onset (usually before 25 years and most often during childhood or adolescence), and lack of obesity or overt insulin resistance (*e.g.*, lack of acanthosis nigricans). Monogenic diabetes can arise from any of several genetic defects which impair insulin secretion or development of adequate beta-cell mass (Table 15.1) [2].

Neonatal diabetes mellitus (NDM) is a rare cause of hyperglycemia, defined as persistent hyperglycemia occurring in the first months of life that lasts for more than 2 weeks and requires insulin for management [3]. NDM may be transient or permanent.

Transient NDM can result from unipaternal disomy of chromosome 6 or unbalanced duplication of paternal chromosome 6. The most common mutation occurs in a transcriptional regulator of pituitary adenylate cyclase-activating polypeptide [4]. No doubt, other gene candidates will be identified.

Permanent NDM is most often caused by mutation of the ATP-sensitive potassium channel which regulates the majority of glucose-stimulated insulin release. The most common cause is due to activating mutations in the *KCNJ11* gene that encodes Kir6.2 [5]. The K_{ATP} channel is composed of a small subunit Kir6.2 that creates a central pore for potassium egress surrounded by four regulatory sulfonylurea receptor (SUR1) subunits. Activating Kir6.2 mutations can prevent insulin release by increasing the number of open K_{ATP} channels at plasma membranes which results in hyperpolarization of the β-cells, resulting in hyperglycemia. Sulfonylurea therapy has been shown to be safe in the short term for these patients and probably more effective than insulin [6]. NDM can also result from other gene mutations, including insulin promoter factor 1 (*IPF-1*), *EIF2AK3*, glucokinase (*GCK*), *FOXP3*, *PTF1A*, *GLIS3*, and insulin (*INS2*).

With the exception of MODY2 (caused by a heterozygous *GCK* mutation affecting an enzyme [7]), all other identified forms of MODY result from heterozygous mutations in transcription factors. Hepatocyte nuclear factor 4α (HNF4α) defects are associated with MODY1 [2], and HNF1α defects

Table 15.1

MODY forms

Type	Gene	Chromosome	Affected protein	Average age of onset	Presentation	Severity	Treatment
1	HNF4α	CR 20	Hepatocyte nuclear factor 4α	26.3 (18.5–37.8) [27]	Early adult years. Significantly higher plasma glucose 2 h after glucose load in the face of mild fasting hyperglycemia	Mild elevations in fasting plasma glucose severity tends to increase over time [2]	Sulfonylureas; some may need insulin
2	GCK	CR 7	Glucokinase	20.9 (10.2–41.7) [27]	Heterogeneous mutation results in mild fasting hyperglycemia (complete deficiency of glucokinase results in permanent neonatal diabetes)	Mild stable, asymptomatic hyperglycemia present from birth [32] that does not increase substantially over the course of many years [2]	Diet and physical activity

(continued)

Table 15.1
(continued)

Type	Gene	Chromosome	Affected protein	Average age of onset	Presentation	Severity	Treatment
3	*TCF1*	CR 12	Hepatocyte nuclear factor 1α	20.4 (12.2–33.5) [27]	Age at onset of diabetes varies widely, influenced by type and position of mutations (ADA), familial factors, and parent of origin. 65% develop diabetes by 25 years and 100% by 50 years [52]. Diabetic retinopathy and nephropathy frequently occur.	Mild hyperglycemia that tends to worsen over time [2] usually develop severe hyperglycemia after puberty [32]	Initially, treat with dietary modification; can be treated with sulfonylureas, 30–40% may need insulin after 15 years of diabetes
4	*IPF1*	CR 13	Insulin promoter factor 1	42.7 (27.5–66.1) [27]	Expression of diabetes in this pedigree may occur at later ages than in families with other types of MODY [2]		Sulfonylureas, some may need insulin

#	Gene		Full name		Clinical features	Treatment
5	TCF2	CR17	Hepatocyte nuclear factor 1β	24.2 (17.9–32.7) [34]	Early onset of diabetes, renal cysts, genital abnormalities, elevated liver enzymes	Insulin and treatment of related conditions such as renal cysts and renal failure
6	NEUROD1	CR 2	Neurogenic differentiation factor 1			Insulin
7	KLF11		Krupple-like factor 11			
8	CEL (carboxyl ester lipase)		Bile salt dependent lipase			
9	PAX4					

with MODY3 [8, 9]. HNF1b mutants cause MODY5 [10]. Mutations in IPF1 cause MODY4 [11]. Neurogenic differentiation factor 1 (Neuro D1), also known as beta-cell E-box transactivator 2, associates with MODY6 [12]. MODY7 is caused by Krupple-like factor 11 (*KLF11*) mutations [13, 14]. Research is underway on newly recognized forms of MODY. Acinar Carboxyl Esterase Lipase deficiency can cause MODY8 [15]. Also known as diabetes-pancreatic exocrine dysfunction syndrome, MODY9 results from mutations in the paired box gene 4 (*PAX4*) genes [16].

MODY patients are estimated to comprise 1–5% of the diabetes population in the United States and other industrialized countries. The various genetic mutations which lead to MODY result in pancreatic β-cell dysfunction and consequent failure of insulin secretion. Nongenetic factors, like those leading to insulin resistance, may trigger the onset of diabetes mellitus and increase the severity of hyperglycemia. While these factors are involved in the development of the clinical manifestations of diabetes, they have little direct role in the development of the MODY component (failure of insulin secretion) of these disorders [2]. The different MODY types differ by their age of onset, severity of disease and progression of hyperglycemia, and the risk of microvascular complications, as well as the coexistence of other abnormalities.

15.1.1 Typical Case Presentation of Monogenic Diabetes

A 5-year-old boy was brought to the clinic by his mother who reported that he was lethargic and "not being himself" for the past few weeks. Fasting hyperglycemia was noted at 7.2 mM (normal <6.1 mM). A full evaluation for suspected T1DM revealed hemoglobin A_{1C} (HbA_{1C}) 6.2% (reference 4.1–5.7%), no glucosuria, and no ketonuria. No diabetes-related antibodies were detected in the circulation, including those against insulin, glutamic acid decarboxylase (GAD65), or protein tyrosine phosphatase-like molecule (IA-2). Basal serum C-peptide level was normal, 1.3 ng/mL (normal 1.1–5.0). Past history included birth after 37 weeks of gestation and normal birth weight (3,100 g). The pregnancy had been complicated by gestational diabetes (GDM), diagnosed by oral glucose tolerance test (OGTT) during second trimester. Mother had been maintained on glyburide during the pregnancy with "good" blood sugar control. The mother's glucose readings remained stable throughout life on diet alone. She did not develop any diabetic microvascular complications. She remained on diet alone, without any medication well into adulthood. OGTT performed on the child showed a small increment at the 2-h value (plasma glucose <3 mM). Further analysis of the family history revealed several members with mild hyperglycemia in successive generations. The child was initially maintained on insulin, and repeat testing after 5–6 months did not show any change in HbA_{1C}. Monogenic diabetes was suspected from the early age of presentation, mild hyperglycemia, no response to insulin therapy, and a strong family history of mild diabetes. Genetic testing confirmed MODY2 by demonstrating a shared, genomic, and heterozygous *GCK* mutation in both the child and mother.

15.2   MODY1 (HNF4A)

15.2.1   Genetics of MODY1

MODY1 is caused by mutations in the HNF4α gene. It constitutes about 2–4% of MODY types in a study conducted on 53 Caucasian families in the United States [12]. The mechanism by which this mutation results in diabetes is similar to the HNF1α gene mutation, which produces MODY3. As the name suggests, hepatocyte nuclear factor 4α is a liver-enriched transcription factor, but is found in other tissues including the pancreas, kidneys, and genital tissues [2, 17]. HNF4α interacts with multiple transcription factors, including HNF1α (HNF1α) and IPF1 [18, 19]; variants in each of which cause specific subtypes of MODY1. In liver, HNF4α plays a role in gluconeogenesis [20]. In pancreatic β-cells, it regulates expression of genes involved in glucose metabolism and insulin secretion [21, 22] and directly activates insulin gene expression [23, 24].

Raeder *et al.* reported MODY1 as the third most prevalent MODY form in a Norwegian registry. An HNF4α P2 promoter haplotype was also linked with the incidence of late-onset diabetes mellitus, further supporting the role of a region of the HNF4α gene in type 2 diabetes [25].

15.2.2   Clinical Features of MODY1

Mutations in HNF4α result in progressive deterioration of beta-cell function and loss of glycemic control. This eventually progresses to the need for treatment with oral hypoglycemic drugs or insulin in about 30–40% of these patients [2] (Table 15.1).

15.2.3   Complications of MODY1

Microvascular complications including retinopathy and nephropathy are common in MODY1 similar to patients with type 1 or type 2 diabetes mellitus [2].

15.2.4   Diagnosis of MODY1

Diagnosis can be made based on clinical suspicion with incidental detection of hyperglycemia and a positive family history of mild diabetes in multiple family members. A markedly impaired 2-h value on OGTT is frequently seen. Genetic testing is necessary in these patients to make a definitive diagnosis.

15.3 MODY2 (GCK)

15.3.1 Genetics of MODY2

Heterozygous mutations in the *GCK* gene located on chromosome 6 were first identified in 1992 [26]. Homozygous mutations in *GCK* result in permanent neonatal diabetes. *GCK*-related MODY2, together with MODY3, comprises the majority of the cases of MODY-related diabetes. A UK-based study reported MODY2 as the second most common form of MODY, constituting almost 20% of affected families [27]. Data from French families suggest *GCK* mutations can be the most common cause of MODY, accounting for >60% of studied pedigrees carrying the mutation [28].

The enzyme GCK phosphorylates glucose to glucose-6-phosphate, most abundantly in the pancreas and liver. Glucose phosphorylation represents the rate-limiting step for glycolysis [29]; therefore, GCK is the critical regulatory enzyme for ATP-mediated insulin secretion. Loss-of-function *GCK* mutations result in decreased sensing of glucose by the beta-cells. This increases the threshold of beta-cell responsiveness to trigger insulin secretion from a blood glucose level of 5 mM to about 6–7 mM. This shifts the dose–response curve, relating insulin secretion to blood glucose levels, rightward [30]. Consequently, heterozygous *GCK* mutations result clinically in mild hyperglycemia.

Mutations in *GCK* coding regions are also associated with decreased net accumulation of hepatic glycogen and augmented hepatic gluconeogenesis after meals. The former abnormality probably results from impaired glucose phosphorylation in hepatocytes, due to decreased enzymatic activity of mutant *GCK*. Both abnormalities contribute to postprandial hyperglycemia. Hence, hyperglycemia in MODY2 results from both altered beta-cell function and abnormalities in liver glycogen metabolism [31].

15.3.2 Clinical Features of MODY2

MODY2 results in stable, mild fasting hyperglycemia, present throughout life. In contrast to other forms of diabetes, hyperglycemia in MODY2 can be managed with dietary modification alone and rarely requires pharmacological treatment (Table 15.2). There is very little risk of developing microvascular (<5%) as well as macrovascular complications and the severity of hyperglycemia does not worsen with advancing age. Follow-up visits are recommended yearly only with measurement of glycosylated HbA_{1C} [32].

Table 15.2
MODY-specific requirements for treatment

MODY/mutant	% Requiring treatment[a]		
	Diet	Oral hypoglycemic	Insulin
1/HNF1α	27	43	31
2/GCK	84	14	2
3/HNF4α	25	75	0
4/IPF1	13	47	40
5/HNF1β	0	33	67
6/NDF1	32	42	26

[a]Adapted from data presented in ref. [27]

15.3.3 Who Should Be Tested?

Young children presenting with mild fasting hyperglycemia, and/or mild to moderate abnormalities on OGTT and a strong family history of diabetes, should receive genetic testing for MODY2. Although not inexpensive, confirmation of the diagnosis exerts a great impact on the quality of life of the children. Additionally, in women with GDM and a strong family history of diabetes (or continued impaired fasting blood glucose after an episode of GDM), establishing the exact diagnosis (*i.e.*, MODY) may be helpful to manage GDM and ultimately then the child [32].

15.4 MODY3

Mutations in the HNF-1α gene appear to be the most common cause of MODY among patients seen in adult diabetes clinics. Over 120 different HNF-1α mutations have been reported [2]. This group of mutation(s) in the gene encoding hepatocyte nuclear factor-1α (HNF-1α) was first identified in late 1996 in subjects with the MODY3 form of NIDDM. MODY3 was found to be the most common and constituted almost 63% of MODY families in a study conducted in the United Kingdom [27].

15.4.1 Genetics of MODY3

HNF-1α is a transcription factor which is encoded by the gene *TCF1*, located on chromosome 12q, which is a regulator of the tissue-specific expression of several liver genes [9]. High levels of HNF-1α expression are seen in the liver, pancreas, kidney, and gut [33]. Approximately 30% of HNF-1α mutations are nonsense frameshift sequences, which result in the production of premature termination codons [34]. Mutant RNAs formed as a result of this are subject to degradation by the "nonsense mediated decay (NMD)" pathway. Mutations are also likely to result in haplo-insufficiency as a consequence of a reduction in mRNA levels due to NMD, which can cause MODY from such a dominant negative effect *in vivo* [35].

15.4.2   Clinical Features of MODY3

MODY3 is the most common monogenic form of diabetes mellitus. MODY3 patients, like MODY2, also present with mild fasting hyperglycemia; however, the hyperglycemia worsens over time due to a progressive decrease in insulin secretion. A total of 30–40% of these patients eventually will require insulin therapy [2].

15.4.3   Complications of MODY3

Microvascular complications frequently occur in patients with MODY3. After 16 years of diabetes, the prevalance of retinopathy is about 50%, with severe forms of retinopathy affecting 15–20% of the patients. Incipient nephropathy (microalbuminuria) is present in about 20% of these cases. Thus, when considering the duration of diabetes and the level of glycemic control, the prevalence of microangiopathic complications is similar to that seen in type 1 and type 2 diabetes. However, the frequency of metabolic syndrome including hypertension, abnormal lipid levels, and macroangiopathy (coronary heart disease) is much lower than in type 2 diabetes [32].

15.4.4   Diagnosis of MODY3

The increment in blood glucose levels after a 2-h ODTT in MODY3 is >3.0 mM. By contrast, MODY2 patients show only a slight increase during the 2-h OGTT [36]. Genetic testing can be done for a confirmatory diagnosis, if the patient has no anti-islet autoantibodies, and there are no clinical features of type 2 diabetes and/or insulin resistance. In a study conducted among 28 Japanese patients thought to have type 1 diabetes, but who had no anti-islet cell autoantibodies, two (14%) were found to have a mutation in HNF1α [37].

15.5   LESS COMMON MODY FORMS

15.5.1   MODY4

MODY4, 5, and 6 are rare forms of MODY, respectively, representing 0, 1, and 0% of a cohort of 90 UK families [27]. MODY4 is caused by mutation in *IPF1*, which not only plays a role in regulation of genes in pancreatic islet cells, but also in the development of pancreas. Mutations in this gene result in impaired insulin secretion [2].

15.5.2 MODY5

Caused by HNF1β mutations, MODY5 is known to be frequently associated with nephropathy and kidney malformations, such as renal cyst formation and dysplastic kidneys [38]. Some reported cases also had co-existing genital malformations and liver test abnormalities. Therefore, in nonobese patients with diabetes and progressive nondiabetic nephropathy, along with coexisting renal malformations, genital abnormalities, and deranged liver tests, testing for HNF1β may be warranted [32]. Treatment of these less common forms of MODY is essentially similar to the other more common types, with diet and oral sulphonylureas in mild disease and insulin only in the more severe forms.

15.5.3 MODY6

Caused by mutations in neurogenic differentiation factor 1, MODY6 results in mild insulinopenia.

15.6 MAKING THE DIAGNOSIS

Physicians should pursue the diagnosis of MODY based on clinical suspicion in patients with mild nonketotic diabetes (especially if detected before age 25), with a positive family history of hyperglycemia, and in the absence of physical findings of insulin resistance. Making the correct diagnosis is always crucial. First, definitive diagnosis allows more accurate prediction of disease-related complications and treatment options for families. Complications are rare in some subgroups of these diabetes patients. Second, due to the known mode of inheritance and high penetrance, this would allow genetic counseling for families affected by MODY and these mutations. Accurate diagnosis of the specific MODY type will result in a significant reduction of costs of treatment as well as decrease in side effects from potential insulin therapy. As stated earlier, insulin therapy is seldom required for treatment of MODY. Early diagnosis and treatment then will also help to prevent complications that are known to occur in these diabetics. Studies on the genetics of MODY have been extremely successful in facilitating an increased understanding of the genes and pathways that are crucial for normal beta-cell function and improving all criteria for diagnosing/treating all forms of diabetes [39].

15.7 TESTING FOR MODY

Studies have shown striking differences in the response to an oral glucose load in patients with MODY2 and MODY3. After a standard OGTT, HNF-1α mutation carriers have a greatly elevated 2-h postprandial glucose (>3 mM) and increment in OGTT as compared with *GCK* patients. *GCK* patients also display lower fasting blood glucose, and they handle the glucose load of an OGTT better, *i.e.*, <3 mmol/L glucose increase during an OGTT. The difference is seen despite their having quantitatively similar beta-cell defects and less insulin resistance as measured by HOMA. However, differences in OGTT cannot be used for diagnosis as they are not sufficiently sensitive or specific, especially in young children (below the age of 10) [36]. Rather, insulin and C-peptide values are measured by RIA or ELISA after arginine infusion at 0 and 45 min [40, 41].

15.7.1 Genetic Testing

Original techniques involved separation by high-performance liquid chromatography and direct sequencing for routine detection of mutations [42]. These methods have largely been replaced by techniques outlined in these references: MODY1 [8], MODY2 [37, 43], MODY3 [9, 44], MODY4 [11], MODY5 [10, 45], and MODY6 [12].

The gold standard for diagnosis of MODY remains DNA sequencing. DNA is obtained from leukocytes present in a small blood or saliva sample. The coding sequences of HNF4a, GCK, TCF1, IPF1, or TCF2 are amplified in a highly specific manner through a polymerase chain reaction (PCR), and all PCR products are then fully sequenced. Hence, by the combination of genomic DNA extraction, PCR, and DNA sequence analysis, various MODY gene mutations can be readily identified.

Commercially available genetic tests to detect various types of monogenic diabetes include DNA sequencing, multiplex ligation-dependent probe amplification, and targeted mutation analysis with the test turnaround of 2–8 weeks. The high cost of these assays precludes genetic screening. Genetic tests should be selectively performed based upon the clinical presentation (Fig. 15.1).

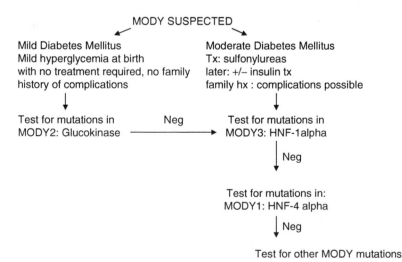

Fig. 15.1. A flow diagram for the clinical protocol (adapted from Athena Diagnostics).

15.7.2 Future of Diagnostic Technology for MODY

In the future, the availability of gene chip technology may allow rapid screening of mitochondrial and MODY mutations [46]. This might include a gene chip coding for DNA which identifies mutations specific for each different type of MODY.

15.8 TREATING MONOGENIC DIABETES

15.8.1 Treating MODY1

Due to the progressive decrease in beta–cell function in this MODY type, hyperglycemia also tends to increase over time. This results in the need for treatment with oral hypoglycemic drugs like sulfonylureas or insulin in a substantial proportion of these patients to maintain normoglycemia (30–40% require insulin) [2]. Monitoring of blood glucose and HbA_{1C} therefore is necessary in these patients to prevent or minimize complications.

15.8.2 Treating MODY2

Patients with *GCK* mutations have mild hyperglycemia and rarely have hyperosmolar syndrome (HHS) or diabetic ketoacidosis (DKA). The vast majority will therefore be detected during routine medical screening, during pregnancy, or during family screening when MODY is suspected. In most patients, the age of diagnosis is therefore the age at which they are first tested. Patients with *GCK* mutations rarely need any pharmacological treatment and the majority are managed on diet alone [47].

Mutations in HNF-1α result in progressive β-cell dysfunction as in MODY1 with increasing treatment requirements and greater risk of complications with aging [48, 49]. Hyperglycemia is treated with either oral hypoglycemic agents (sulfonylurea) or insulin. A recent case report shows that use of sitagliptin, an inhibitor of the enzyme dipeptidyl peptidase-4 (DPP-4), could improve the glycemic control of a 57-year-old woman with MODY3 who had a heterozygous R54X nonsense mutation in the HNF1-α gene [50]. Further study should be done to discover the potential role of using DPP-4 inhibitors in the treatment of MODY.

15.8.3 Treating MODY5

The coexisting pancreatic atrophy and associated insulin resistance means that diabetic HNF1β carriers are not sensitive to sulfonylurea medication, and early insulin therapy is required. Multiple organ abnormalities may require several different individualized treatments.

15.9   DETECTING MODY IN ELDERLY POPULATIONS

Older patients are usually diagnosed with type 2 diabetes by default, mostly based on age at clinical presentation. Insulin resistance is a key component of T2DM. Most of these patients have already been placed on insulin sensitizers (biguanides and thiazolidinediones) along with insulin secretagogues (sulfonylureas) or insulin itself. The underlying pathophysiologic defect in MODY is insulin secretion, requiring the use of insulin secretagogues or rarely insulin itself. MODY patients may not need insulin sensitizers. These patients can be identified with OGTT or arginine-stimulated insulin and C-peptide release. This will screen out 80%. The final diagnosis can then be made by PCR of leukocyte DNA, using specific primers to amplify genomic regions encoding MODY genes.

By correctly identifying MODY patients among those with T2DM, we can use appropriate therapy, decrease risk of microvascular and macrovascular complications, significantly decrease the cost of treatment (as sensitizers remain much more expensive than sulfonylureas or insulin), and also reduce the risk of serious side effects of individual drugs, such as hypoglycemia and lactic acidosis. Can an adult patient have both insulin resistance and MODY? Yes, one could start out with MODY, then become progressively more obese, and end up with a hard-to-diagnosis combination of both diseases. This could be deciphered by the use of a "euglycemic clamp" [51]. Then, individual therapy reflecting the specific pathophysiology could be designed and instituted. We estimate 2–3% undiagnosed MODY in elderly populations.

REFERENCES

1. Tattersall RB, Fajans SS (1975) A difference between the inheritance of classical juvenile-onset and maturity-onset type diabetes of young people. Diabetes 24:44–53
2. Fajans SS, Bell GI, Polonsky KS (2001) Molecular mechanisms and clinical pathophysiology of maturity-onset diabetes of the young. New Engl J Med 345:971–980
3. Kalhan SC, Parimi PS (2002) Disorders of carbohydrate metabolism. In: Fanaroff AA, Martin RJ (eds) Neonatal-perinatal medicine: diseases of the fetus and infant, 7th edn. Mosby, St. Louis, p 1351
4. Shield JP (2000) Neonatal diabetes: new insights into aetiology and implications. Horm Res 53(Suppl 1):7–11
5. Gloyn AL, Pearson ER, Antcliff JF, Proks P, Bruining GJ, Slingerland AS, Howard N, Srinivasan S, Silva JM, Molnes J, Edghill EL, Frayling TM, Temple IK, Mackay D, Shield JP, Sumnik Z, van Rhijn A, Wales JK, Clark P, Gorman S, Aisenberg J, Ellard S, Njolstad PR, Ashcroft FM, Hattersley AT (2004) Activating mutations in the gene encoding the ATP-sensitive potassium-channel subunit Kir6.2 and permanent neonatal diabetes. N Engl J Med 350:1838–1849
6. Pearson ER, Flechtner I, Njølstad PR, Malecki MT, Flanagan SE, Larkin B, Ashcroft FM, Klimes I, Codner E, Iotova V, Slingerland AS, Shield J, Robert JJ, Holst JJ, Clark PM, Ellard S, Søvik O, Polak M, Hattersley AT (2006) Switching from insulin to oral

sulfonylureas in patients with diabetes due to Kir6.2 mutations. N Engl J Med 355:467–477

7. Froguel P, Zouali H, Vionnet N, Velho G, Vaxillaire M, Sun F, Lesage S, Stoffel M, Takeda J, Passa P, Permutt MA, Beckmann JS, Bell GI, Cohen D (1993) Familial hyperglycemia due to mutations in glucokinase: definition of a subtype of diabetes mellitus. New Engl J Med 328:697–702

8. Yamagata K, Furuta H, Oda N et al. (1996) Mutations in the hepatocyte nuclear factor 4 alpha gene in maturity-onset diabetes of the young (MODY1). Nature 384:458–460

9. Yamagata K, Oda N, Kaisaki PJ et al. (1996) Mutations in the hepatic nuclear factor 1 alpha gene in maturity-onset diabetes of the young (MODY3). Nature 3:455–458

10. Horikawa Y, Iwasaki N, Hara M et al. (1997) Mutation in hepatocyte nuclear factor-1 β gene (TCF2) associated with MODY. Nat Genet 17:384–385

11. Stoffers DA, Ferrer J, Clarke WL, Habener JF (1997) Early-onset type-II diabetes mellitus (MODY4) linked to IPF1. Nat Genet 17:138–139

12. Malecki MT, Jhala US, Antonellis A et al. (1999) Mutations in NeurD1 are associated with the development of type 2 diabetes mellitus. Nat Genet 23:323–8

13. Neve B, Fernandez-Zapico ME, Ashkenazi-Katalan V et al. (2005) Role of transcription factor KLF11 and its diabetes-associated gene variants in pancreatic beta cell function. Proc Natl Acad Sci USA 102:4807–4812

14. Online Mendelian Inheritance in Man (OMIM) (2010) Maturity-onset diabetes of the young, type VII, 610508. Accessed 3 June 2010

15. Raeder H, Johansson S, Holm PI, Haldorsen IS, Mas E, Sbarra V, Nermoen I, Eide SA, Grevle L, Bjorkhaug L, Sagen JV, Aksnes L, Sovik O, Lombardo D, Molven A, Njolstad PR (2006) Mutations in the *CEL* VNTR cause a syndrome of diabetes and pancreatic exocrine dysfunction. Nat Genet 38:54–62

16. Plengvidhya N, Kooptiwut S, Songtawee N, Doi A, Furuta H, Nishi M, Nanjo K, Tantibhedhyangkul W, Boonyasrisawat W, Yenchitsomanus P, Doria A, Banchuin N (2007) PAX4 mutations in Thais with maturity onset diabetes of the young. J Clin Endocrinol Metab 92:2821–2826

17. Cereghini S (1996) Liver-enriched transcription factors and hepatocyte differentiation. FASEB J 10:267–282

18. Eeckhoute J, Moerman E, Bouckenooghe T, Lukoviak B, Pattou F, Formstecher P, Kerr-Conte J, Vandewalle B, Laine B (2003) Hepatocyte nuclear factor 4 alpha isoforms originated from the P1 promoter are expressed in human pancreatic beta-cells and exhibit stronger transcriptional potentials than P2 promoter-driven isoforms. Endocrinology 144:1686–1694

19. Boj SF, Parrizas M, Maestro MA, Ferrer J (2001) A transcription factor regulatory circuit in differentiated pancreatic cells. Proc Natl Acad Sci U S A 98:14481–14486

20. Rhee J, Inoue Y, Yoon JC, Puigserver P, Fan M, Gonzalez FJ, Spiegelman BM (2003) Regulation of hepatic fasting response by PPARgamma coactivator-1alpha (PGC-1): requirement for hepatocyte nuclear factor 4alpha in gluconeogenesis. Proc Natl Acad Sci USA 100:4012–4017

21. Stoffel M, Duncan SA (1997) The maturity-onset diabetes of the young (MODY1) transcription factor HNF4alpha regulates expression of genes required for glucose transport and metabolism. Proc Natl Acad Sci U S A 94:13209–13214

22. Wang H, Maechler P, Antinozzi PA, Hagenfeldt KA, Wollheim CB (2000) Hepatocyte nuclear factor 4alpha regulates the expression of pancreatic beta-cell genes implicated in glucose metabolism and nutrient-induced insulin secretion. J Biol Chem 275:35953–35959

23. Bartoov-Shifman R, Hertz R, Wang H, Wollheim CB, Bar-Tana J, Walker MD (2002) Activation of the insulin gene promoter through a direct effect of hepatocyte nuclear factor 4 alpha. J Biol Chem 277:25914–25919

24. Silander K, Mohlke KL, Scott LJ, Peck EC, Hollstein P, Skol AD, Jackson AU, Deloukas P, Hunt S, Stavrides G, Chines PS, Erdos MR, Narisu N, Conneely KN, Li C, Fingerlin TE, Dhanjal SK, Valle TT, Bergman RN, Tuomilehto J, Watanabe RM, Boehnke M, Collins FS

(2004) Genetic variation near the hepatocyte nuclear factor-4 gene predicts susceptibility to type2 diabetes. Diabetes 53:1141–1149

25. Raeder H, Bjorkhaug L, Johansson S, Mangseth K, Sagen JV, Hunting A *et al.* (2006) A hepatocyte nuclear factor-4{alpha} gene (HNF4A) P2 promoter haplotype linked with late-onset diabetes: studies of HNF4A variants in the Norwegian MODY registry. Diabetes 55:1899–1903

26. Hattersley AT, Turner RC, Permutt MA *et al.* (1992) Linkage of type 2 diabetes to the glucokinase gene. Lancet 339:1307–1310

27. Frayling TM, Evans JC, Bulman MP, Pearson E, Allen L, Owen K, Bingham C, Hannemann M, Shepherd M, Ellard S, Hattersley AT (2001) β-Cell genes and diabetes molecular and clinical characterization of mutations in transcription factors. Diabetes 50(Suppl 1):S94–100

28. Barrio R, Chantelot CB, Moreno JC, Morel V, Calle H, Alonso M, Mustieles C (2002) Nine novel mutations in maturity-onset diabetes of the young (MODY) candidate genes in 22 Spanish families. J Clin Endocrinol Metab 87:2532–2539

29. Randle PJ (1993) Glucokinase and candidate genes for type 2 (non-insulin dependent) diabetes mellitus. Diabetologia 36:269–275

30. Byrne MM, Sturis J, Clément K *et al.* (1994) Insulin secretory abnormalities in subjects with hyperglycemia due to glucokinase mutations. J Clin Invest 93:1120–1130

31. Velho G, Petersen KF, Perseghin G, Hwang JH, Rothman DL, Pueyo ME, Cline GW, Froguel P, Shulman GI (1996) Impaired hepatic glycogen synthesis in glucokinase-deficient (MODY-2) subjects. J Clin Invest 98:1755–1761

32. Timsit J, Bellanné-Chantelot C, Dubois-Laforgue D, Velho G (2005) Diagnosis and management of maturity-onset diabetes of the young. Treat Endocrinol 4:9–18

33. Pontoglio M, Barra J, Hadchouel M, Doyen A, Kress C, Poggi Bach J, Babinet C, Yaniv M (1996) Hepatocyte nuclear factor 1 inactivation results in hepatic dysfunction, phenylketonuria, and renal Fanconi syndrome. Cell 84:575–585

34. Ellard S (2000) Hepatocyte nuclear factor 1alpha (HNF-1alpha) mutations in maturity-onset diabetes of the young. Hum Mutat 16:377–385

35. Harries LW, Hattersley AT, Ellard S (2004) Messenger RNA transcripts of the hepatocyte nuclear factor-1α gene containing premature terminating codons are subject to nonsense mediated decay. Diabetes 53:500–504

36. Stride A, Vaxillaire M, Tuomi T, Barbetti F, Njolstad PR, Hansen T *et al.* (2002) The genetic abnormality in the beta cell determines the response to an oral glucose load. Diabetologia 45:427–435

37. Kawasaki E, Sera Y, Yamakawa K *et al.* (2000) Identification and functional analysis of mutations in the hepatocyte nuclear factor-1α gene in anti-islet auto-antibody-negative Japanese patients with type 1 diabetes. J Clin Endocrinol Metab 85:331–335

38. Kolatsi-Joannou M, Bingham C, Ellard S *et al.* (2001) Hepatocyte nuclear factor 1-beta: a new kindred with renal cysts and diabetes and gene expression in normal human development. J Am Soc Nephrol 12:2175–2180

39. Mitchell SM, Frayling TM (2002) The role of transcription factors in maturity-onset diabetes of the young. Mol Genet Metab 77:35–43

40. Duckworth WC, Solomon S, Kitabchi A (1972) Effect of chronic sulfonylurea therapy on plasma insulin and proinsulin levels. J Clin Endocrinol Metab 35:585–591

41. Solomon SS, Duckworth WC, Jallepalli P, Bobal MA, Iyer R (1980) The glucose intolerance of acute pancreatitis: hormonal response to arginine. Diabetes 29:22–26

42. Boutin P, Vasseur F, Samson C, Wahl C, Froguel P (2001) Routine mutation screening of HNF-1α and GCK genes in MODY diagnosis: how effective are the techniques of DHPLC and direct sequencing used in combination. Diabetologia 44:775–778

43. Ellard S, Beards F, Allen LI *et al.* (2000) A high prevalence of glucokinase mutations in gestational diabetic subjects selected by clinical criteria. Diabetologia 43:250–253

44. Bjorkhaug L, Sagen JV, Thorsby P, Sovik O, Molven A, Njolstad PR (2003) J Clin Endocrinol Metab 88:920–931

45. Iwasaki N, Okabe I, Momoi MY, Ohashi H, Ogata M, Iwamoto Y (2001) Splice site mutation in hepatocyte nuclear factor-1 β gene, IVS2nt+1G>A, associated with maturity onset diabetes of the young, renal dysphagia and bicornuate uterus. Diabetologia 44:387–388

46. Winter WE, Nakamura M, House DV (1999) Monogenic diabetes mellitus in youth. The MODY syndromes. Endocrinol Metab Clin North Am 28:765–785

47. Gloyn AL (2003) Glucokinase (*GCK*) mutations in hyper- and hypoglycemia: maturity-onset diabetes of the young, permanent neonatal diabetes, and hyperinsulinemia of infancy. Hum Mutat 22:353–362

48. Velho G, Vaxillaire M, Boccio V, Charpentier G, Froguel P (1996) Diabetes complications in NIDDM kindreds linked to the MODY3 locus on chromosome 12q. Diabetes Care 19:915–919

49. Lehto M, Tuomi T, Mahtani MM, Widen E, Forsblom C, Sarelin L, Gullstrom M, Isomaa B, Lehtovirta M, Hyrkko A, Kanninen T, Orho M, Manley S, Turner RC, Brettin T, Kirby A, Thomas J, Duyk G, Lander E, Taskinen M-R, Groop L (1997) Characterization of the MODY3 phenotype: early-onset diabetes caused by an insulin secretion defect. J Clin Invest 99:582–591

50. Lumb A, Gallan I (2009) Treatment of HNF1-alpha MODY with the DPP-4 inhibitor Sitagliptin. Diabet Med 26:189–190

51. Shankar T, Solomon SS, Duckworth WC, Jenkins T, Iyer RS, Bobal MA (1988) Growth hormone and carbohydrate metabolism in cirrhosis. Horm Metab Res 20:579–583

52. Klupa T, Warram JH, Antonellis A *et al.* (2002) Determinants of the development of diabetes (maturity-onset diabetes of the young-3) in carriers of HNF-1alpha mutations: evidence for parent-of-origin effect. Diabetes Care 25:2292–2301

16 Secondary Causes of Obesity in Childhood

Paula M. Hale, Tulay T. Cushman,
Edward S. Kimball, Aji Nair,
and Rebecca Gusic Shaffer

Key Points

- Secondary causes of obesity are frequent and must be diagnosed to assure optimal clinical care.

Keywords: Secondary causes of obesity, Syndromes, Endocrine disorders, Hypothalamic obesity, Iatrogenic causes

16.1 INTRODUCTION

Exogenous obesity, also referred to as idiopathic or primary obesity, is the most common form of obesity in childhood, and its etiology, as the name suggests, is mostly related to exogenous factors. It is important to differentiate between idiopathic obesity and secondary obesity, which occurs much less frequently. Secondary obesity in childhood is associated with diverse disorders, including genetic syndromes, endocrine diseases, central nervous system insults (hypothalamic obesity), and various other causes, such as iatrogenic obesity. The primary presentation of all of these disorders can be obesity in childhood [1] (see Table 16.1) [2].

From: *Nutrition and Health: Management of Pediatric Obesity and Diabetes*,
Edited by: R.J. Ferry, Jr., DOI 10.1007/978-1-60327-256-8_16,
© Springer Science+Business Media, LLC 2011

Table 16.1
Disorders associated with secondary obesity in childhood [2]

Genetic syndromes
- Prader–Willi syndrome
- Laurence–Moon–Biedl syndrome
- Alström syndrome
- Cohen syndrome
- Carpenter syndrome
- Klinefelter syndrome
- Turner syndrome

Endocrine disorders
- Insulinoma
- Diabetes mellitus
- Mauriac syndrome
- Pseudohypoparathyroidism (Albright's hereditary osteodystrophy)
- Pituitary dwarfism
- Growth hormone deficiency
- Hypercortisolism (Cushing's syndrome)
- Hypothyroidism

Hypothalamic obesity
- Frohlich's syndrome
- Tumors (and treatment)
- Postinfectious (*i.e.*, encephalitis and tuberculosis)

Iatrogenic causes
- Medications

The diagnosis of either exogenous or secondary obesity can frequently be made by a review of family and personal history as well as by a careful physical examination. Distinguishing between exogenous and secondary obesity can be facilitated by following a diagnostic algorithm (see Fig. 16.1) [2]. A detailed medical history and careful physical examination – including looking for characteristic signs of genetic syndromes or endocrinopathies, accompanied by appropriate laboratory tests, can help diagnose secondary obesity and determine the nature of the underlying medical condition. Evaluation for a genetic syndrome should be considered, especially in an obese child with short stature and developmental delay. However, identification of a genetic syndrome does not alter treatment options, at least in the majority of cases [3].

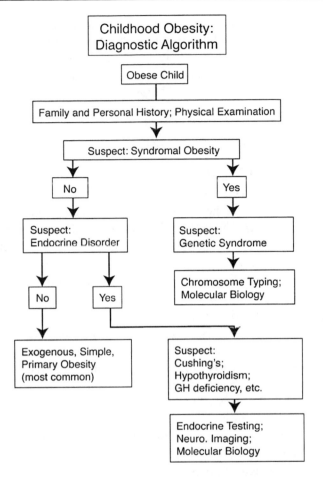

Fig. 16.1. Diagnostic algorithm for the diagnosis of obesity in childhood and adolescence [2]. *GH* growth hormone.

16.2   GENETIC SYNDROMES ASSOCIATED WITH OBESITY

Diverse genetic syndromes are associated with secondary obesity in childhood. Obesity is a central feature in some of these congenital syndromes [4]. These rare diseases may present with characteristic phenotypes that facilitate the diagnostic process [1]. Genetic tests are not available for all syndromes, but, when available, are indicated in the presence of specific findings suggestive of a particular disease, *e.g.*, Prader–Willi syndrome (PWS) [5].

It has been suggested that the central nervous system and the hypothalamic-pituitary axis have a role in the etiology of some genetic syndromes associated with secondary obesity. The pathophysiologic pathways are often not well defined; however, in some cases, the causative mechanisms have been identified and will be described below [4].

16.3   PLEIOTROPIC SYNDROMES

16.3.1   Prader–Willi Syndrome

PWS was first described in 1956 by endocrinologists Prader, Labhart, and Willi [6]. It is one of the most common microdeletion syndromes [7], with a prevalence of 1/15,000–1/30,000 [8] in all ethnic groups, but higher occurrences have been reported in Caucasians [9]. It is the leading known genetic cause of obesity [7].

PWS is caused by a lack of expression of paternally inherited genes imprinted in the chromosome 15 (15q11-q13) region. A deletion of the paternal chromosome 15 (15q11-q13) region accounts for approximately 70% of cases of PWS. Maternal disomy of chromosome 15 is responsible for 25% of cases. The remaining cases are due to defects in the chromosome 15 (15q11-q13) region or to chromosome 15 translocations [9].

Individuals with PWS demonstrate abnormal levels of multiple neuropeptides and hormones involved in eating and neurologic function, such as ghrelin (increased), growth and sex hormones (decreased), and gamma-aminobutyric acid (increased), but the molecular mechanisms underlying these alterations are not understood [9].

Many of the clinical features of PWS are believed to be secondary to hypothalamic insufficiency [7]. Infantile lethargy and hypotonia are among the earliest clinical features observed in individuals with the condition and result in poor feeding and failure to thrive. Hypotonia has a prenatal onset, and mild-to-moderate hypotonia persists throughout life. Other characteristics of PWS, in addition to insatiable appetite (hyperphagia) leading to morbid obesity (if uncontrolled), include developmental and intellectual disability, hypogonadism, characteristic facial appearance and body habitus, and a typical behavioral phenotype that includes temper tantrums and compulsive traits [8]. In addition, individuals with PWS typically exhibit sleep-disordered breathing; sleep apnea as well as excessive daytime sleepiness are observed, especially in older children [7, 9]. Restriction of growth is frequently observed, and approximately 90% of affected individuals have short stature [10].

By the age of 4 years, children with PWS usually become overweight as a consequence of hyperphagia and compulsive eating. While the hyperphagia is hypothalamic in nature, elevated levels of ghrelin have been observed, but the relationship with hyperphagia is unclear [11]. Obesity progresses with age and is likely to be severe, with body mass index (BMI) over 40 kg/m^2. It is typically resistant to dietary, pharmacologic, and behavioral treatments. It is further exacerbated by a low metabolic rate and decreased activity level [12]. Consequently, PWS is also associated with altered body composition: increased body fat mass, decreased lean body mass, and low bone mineral content. About one–third of individuals with the condition are more than twice their ideal body weight [10].

Consensus diagnostic criteria for PWS were developed in 1993 to aid in early recognition and diagnosis [13]. Early diagnosis is critical, because nutritional intervention and growth hormone therapy are frequently prescribed and can improve stature, energy level, and metabolism as well as body composition [9]. It is recommended that all newborns with persistent hypotonia, leading to decreased movement, lethargy with decreased arousal, weak cry and poor reflexes, and poor suck leading to feeding difficulties and ultimately to failure to thrive, be tested for PWS. Testing involves a DNA methylation analysis, followed by fluorescence *in situ* hybridization (FISH) if the DNA methylation analysis is positive, to determine if a deletion is present [7]. Characteristic facial features include narrow temporal distance and nasal bridge, almond-shaped eyes, strabismus, a thin upper lip, and hypopigmentation of hair, eyes, and skin relative to other family members. Problems with thermoregulation and hypogonadism are also evident at birth and throughout life [7].

Treatment of PWS focuses on management of symptoms and providing support to the individual and emphasizes control of food intake and hormone replacement therapies. Treatment also includes special education, behavior management, and ultimately, sheltered employment in adulthood. Multiple studies have demonstrated the benefits of growth hormone therapy in infants, children, and adults [8], including improved linear growth velocity, ultimate height, body composition, muscle function, and level of activity. The use of octreotide, a somatostatin agonist, has been studied in children and adolescents with PWS and has been shown to decrease fasting ghrelin concentrations [14, 15]. Body mass and appetite were not improved, and the investigators concluded that a better understanding of the role of ghrelin in the pathophysiology of appetite in this population was warranted. Furthermore, the effect of the anticonvulsant topiramate has been studied in adults with PWS; no changes were reported however in calories consumed or BMI, and no increase in self-reported appetite was reported [16]. The use of an intragastric balloon for treatment of morbid obesity in PWS patients, as an alternative to failed pharmacotherapy, has also been studied and has demonstrated some success in controlling body weight; careful clinical follow-up and collaboration with parents are critical to avoid severe complications that can result from persistent unrestrained food intake [12].

Complications related to obesity are the major causes of morbidity and mortality in individuals with PWS and include cardiorespiratory insufficiency, obstructive sleep apnea, type 2 diabetes, thrombophlebitis, and chronic leg edema. Up to 25% of obese adults with PWS have type 2 diabetes, with a mean age of onset of 20 years [8]. Obesity-related cardiovascular and respiratory disorders were the most frequent causes of death in both children and adults with PWS. The death rate has been estimated at 3% per year [8, 17].

Weight and dietary management are a major focus in the treatment of PWS, with dietary counseling recommended to be started early in life [7]. Children must also be evaluated and treated for the comorbidities that can be associated with PWS.

16.3.2 Laurence–Moon–Biedl Syndrome

The Laurence–Moon–Biedl syndrome consists of two different syndromes, the Laurence–Moon and the Bardet–Biedl syndromes, but is often considered as one entity. In 1866, J.Z. Laurence and R.C. Moon described four cases of retinitis pigmentosa occurring in the same family, which were accompanied by "general imperfection of development" [18] and were marked by overall impairment, mental disabilities, obesity, and retinal degeneration. Several decades later, Bardet and Biedl added the additional features of polydactyly and hypogenitalism to the list of characteristic phenotypes [19]. The frequency of Bardet–Biedl syndrome is roughly 1:120,000 in the United States and Europe [19], but is much higher in some populations with a high level of consanguinity (e.g., the Middle East or North Africa) or that are geographically isolated [11]. Laurence–Moon syndrome is less common.

Both Laurence–Moon and Bardet–Biedl syndromes are inherited as autosomal recessive traits [20]. Bardet–Biedl syndrome is genetically heterogeneous, and 14 Bardet–Biedl syndrome genes have been described, accounting for approximately 70% of affected families. Bardet–Biedl syndrome is believed to be caused by defects in basal bodies and/or primary cilia. Most of the Bardet–Biedl syndrome defects identified have their genetic code located in the neighborhood of the primary cilia [11].

The Laurence–Moon and Bardet–Biedl syndromes share some common clinical features, including obesity, mental retardation, hypogenitalism, and retinopathy. Polydactyly is rarely found in Laurence–Moon syndrome, but is present in 75% of patients with Bardet–Biedl syndrome. Laurence–Moon syndrome is dominated by progressive neurologic involvement, mainly ataxia and spastic paraplegia, whereas neurologic complications are unusual in Bardet–Biedl syndrome. The most typical clinical manifestations in Bardet–Biedl syndrome are retinal dystrophy; other ocular abnormalities include strabism, cataracts, color blindness, macular edema, and optic atrophy. Night blindness manifests when the child is around 8 years of age, usually progressing to significant blindness by 15 years of age [11]. Additional features of Bardet–Biedl syndrome include renal abnormalities, anosmia, speech disorder/delay, ataxia, increased incidence of hypertension and diabetes mellitus, hearing loss, liver disease, and situs inversus [11].

Diagnosis of Bardet–Biedl syndrome includes identification of at least 4 of the 6 clinical signs: mental retardation (learning disability), obesity, hypogenitalism, polydactyly, tapetoretinal degeneration, or renal abnormalities [19, 21]. The majority of deaths from Bardet–Biedl syndrome are attributed to renal disorders, including cystic tubular disease, lower urinary tract malformations, chronic glomerulonephritis, and defects of tubular concentrating ability [11, 21].

The moderate-to-severe obesity observed in children with Bardet–Biedl syndrome begins to develop at 2–3 years of age and affects mostly the trunk and thighs. The pathogenesis of obesity has been linked to dysfunction of the primary cilium, potentially through defects in vesicular transport to the cilium [11]. There is no evidence of abnormalities in energy expenditure in patients with Bardet–Biedl syndrome compared with normal obese individuals, suggesting no underlying defect in metabolism [11]. Complications arising from obesity include type 2 diabetes, hypertension, and hypercholesterolemia [19].

In a population survey of 109 Bardet–Biedl patients, the majority of whom were under 40 years old, 52% were defined as obese (BMI > 30 kg/m^2) and 16% as morbidly obese (BMI>40 kg/m^2). Furthermore, 6% of the patients had type 2 diabetes (although only a minority of patients had undergone blood glucose testing), and 8% had hypertension [21].

Management of the syndrome involves treatment of the manifestations, including diet, exercise, and behavioral therapy to treat obesity; programs and aids for the visually impaired; special education to address cognitive disability; hormone replacement for hypogonadism; and treatment of renal anomalies or other causes of renal impairment. Renal transplantation has been demonstrated to be a safe and successful procedure in patients with Bardet–Biedl syndrome and end-stage renal failure [22].

16.3.3   Alström Syndrome

Alström syndrome was first described in 1959. The condition is currently listed as a rare disease by the Office of Rare Diseases Research of the National Institutes of Health, with estimates of as few as 500 people affected worldwide [23].

Alström syndrome is an autosomal, recessive, single-gene disorder caused by mutations in *ALMS1*, found on chromosome 2, which is currently of unknown molecular function. The gene encodes a protein composed of 4,169 amino acids, which is ubiquitously expressed [24]. The *ALMS1* protein is known to localize to centrosomes and basal bodies of ciliated cells, essential for proper cilia formation and functioning [25]. While the mechanisms by which the disease alleles of *ALMS1* cause the various pathologies are still unknown, it is currently thought to involve intracellular trafficking [26].

Alström syndrome is a multisystemic disease, which, in addition to eating behavior, affects vision, hearing, the heart, liver, kidneys, bladder, and lungs. Characteristic features of the syndrome include obesity with diabetes mellitus, nystagmus with light sensitivity eventually leading to total blindness, hearing loss, and dilated cardiomyopathy with congestive heart failure—all of which typically can develop and be diagnosed in infancy [24].

The cause of obesity in Alström syndrome is unknown. Rapid weight gain with accelerated childhood growth but reduced final adult height is reported. Although BMI is increased in children compared with age-matched controls, and adults remain obese, BMI usually declines with the onset of other complications [26, 27]. Similarly, severe childhood obesity, waist circumference, and body fat decrease with age, whereas insulin resistance increases [26]. Metabolic disturbances, such as truncal obesity, insulin resistance, hyperinsulinemia (with acanthosis nigricans), hypertriglyceridemia, and hypothyroidism, are all clinical features suggestive of a monogenic cause for metabolic syndrome [26].

A diagnosis of Alström syndrome is difficult, as there is typically a gradual unfolding of the phenotype that can mimic other disorders. Furthermore, the signs and symptoms vary in severity, and not all affected individuals display all of the characteristic features of the disorder. Many of the cardinal features do not become apparent until the teenage years [24]. Children with Alström syndrome frequently complain of chronic respiratory illness and are at risk for developing hepatic dysfunction. As adults, they display a slowly progressive nephropathy and progressive glomerulofibrosis leading to a gradual deterioration of kidney function [24]. Although children with Alström usually have normal intelligence, they typically are delayed in their developmental milestones. Hypogonadism and irregular menses with or without hyperandrogenism are typically present in males and females, respectively.

To date, there are no treatment options to cure Alström syndrome or prevent or reverse its medical complications [24]. A hypocaloric diet and increased physical activity are recommended to aid in weight reduction, and therapeutic options are available for glycemic control. Cardiac, liver, and renal function must be monitored in individuals with Alström syndrome.

Knowledge of the disease's progression from infancy to adulthood can assist in developing an intensive approach to managing systemic manifestations. Anticipating and treating the multiple sensory deficits in young children is crucial, and eventual total loss of vision is expected [24]. Patients should be regularly monitored for cardiac function by electrocardiography, and long-term angiotensin-converting enzyme inhibition is indicated for the patient with cardiomyopathy [24]. Regular monitoring and testing of the potentially affected organs (e.g., thyroid, kidneys) is suggested [24].

16.3.4 Cohen Syndrome

In 1973, Cohen et al. first described a syndrome with the clinical features of mental retardation, obesity, hypotonia, characteristic craniofacial dysmorphism, and abnormalities of the hands and feet [28]. Since its first description, according to the Office of Rare Diseases Research, over 100 cases of Cohen syndrome have been reported worldwide [29]. Cohen syndrome is inherited as an autosomal recessive trait that has considerable variability of expression and has a slightly higher prevalence in the Finnish population [30]. The gene for Cohen syndrome has been mapped to chromosome 8 (8q22-q23). A mutation in the gene COH1 (VPS13B) has been shown in these patients [31]. The gene encodes a protein of 4,022 amino acids, which has a presumed role in vesicle-mediated sorting and intracellular protein transport [31]. The mechanisms of pathogenesis have yet to be determined.

The phenotype in the Finnish population is highly homogeneous and consists of nonprogressive psychomotor retardation, motor clumsiness, childhood hypotonia and hyperextensibility of the joints, myopia, microcephaly, progressive retinochoroidal dystrophy, intermittent isolated neutropenia, and characteristic facial features [32]. Children are sociable and have a cheerful disposition. The typical facial features include high-arched eyelids, a short philtrum, thick hair, and low hairline. These patients also have narrow hands and feet with elongated fingers and toes, ulnar valgus deviation, and mid-childhood onset of truncal obesity [32]. Obesity is not a ubiquitous feature of the syndrome [4]. More than 80% of individuals in the National Cohen Syndrome Database were reported to be underweight during early childhood, but overweight later on in life [33]. Cohen patients who are of non-Finnish descent present with a highly variable phenotype [31].

Due to the high variability of the presenting clinical features, children with Cohen syndrome are frequently misdiagnosed [34]. Patient life-expectancy does not seem to be altered in any way [32]. Currently, no treatments exist to halt the progression of the retinal disease in these patients [34]. However, a multidisciplinary approach to diagnosis and treatment incorporating a pediatrician, ophthalmologist, dentist, orthopedist, psychologist, speech and physical therapist, and endocrinologist helps ensure the best quality of life for the child. Finally, genetic counseling is essential, as siblings have a 25% risk of being affected [32].

16.3.5 Carpenter Syndrome

Carpenter syndrome, first described by George Carpenter in 1909, is a rare autosomal recessive disorder reported in approximately 40 published cases [35]. Also known as acrocephalopolysyndactyly type II (ACPS II), the cardinal features include craniosynostosis, polysyndactyly, obesity, and cardiac defects [36]. Mutations in *RAB23*, mapped to chromosome 6p12.1-q12, are the major causes of Carpenter syndrome. *RAB23* belongs to the RAB family of small guanosine triphosphatases (GTPases) that regulate intracellular trafficking of membrane-associated proteins. *RAB23* acts as a negative regulator of hedgehog signaling [36]. *RAB23* is also believed to act with other intermediaries in the cilium, which supports a link between ciliary function and obesity [37]. Jenkins *et al.* identified 5 different mutations (4 truncating and 1 missense) in the *RAB23* gene in 15 independent families [36].

The clinical picture of Carpenter syndrome can be variable, but most often presents with preaxial polydactyly and syndactyly of the feet, craniosynostosis, and progressive, generalized truncal obesity [37]. Fusion of the midline sutures (metopic and sagittal) is typical in Carpenter syndrome, unlike other syndromes that present with craniosynostosis, where the coronal suture is most commonly affected. Severe cases of the syndrome develop cloverleaf skull [36]. However, Perlyn and Marsh described a variable pattern of craniosynostosis among siblings who were all affected with Carpenter syndrome [38]. Other frequently associated features of the syndrome include mental retardation, congenital heart defects, dental abnormalities, low-set or malformed ears, flat nasal bridge with epicanthal folds, umbilical hernia, and hypogenitalism [39].

Postnatal abdominal obesity is a universal characteristic in patients with Carpenter syndrome. To date, however, the neuroendocrinologic and biochemical pathophysiology of obesity in Carpenter syndrome are unknown. The association of obesity with *RAB23* mutations suggests a possible role of hedgehog signaling in controlling adipocyte metabolism [36]. A few studies have described obesity related to hedgehog signaling, although the molecular mechanisms associated with the development of obesity remain to be elucidated. Based on animal studies, there is evidence that hedgehog signaling inhibits fat formation [40]. To this end, mutations in *RAB23* known to be involved in the hedgehog signaling pathway have the potential to disrupt normal adipogenesis, leading to obesity.

The hedgehog pathway regulates the commitment of cellular precursors into a number of cell fates. Mechanistic studies suggest hedgehog signaling induces antiadipogenic transcription factors [40]. Given the role that hedgehog signaling plays in inhibiting fat formation, this pathway has been considered a potential therapeutic target for obesity [40]. Until molecular therapeutic options are developed, a lifelong diet plan is recommended to maintain a healthy weight. Clinical reports of craniofacial deformations and their subsequent surgical reconstruction have shown that patients with Carpenter syndrome would benefit not only physiologically, allowing for normalized growth of mandibular and maxillary structures as well as other facial bony structures, but also psychologically by correcting facial deformation to improve self-esteem and the associated behavioral problems [41]. It has, however, been shown that early surgical intervention for craniostenosis does not necessarily relate to normal intelligence and that the mental deficiency is secondary to a defect in brain development [42]. Surgery to repair the cardiac defects would undoubtedly help alleviate the potential cardiovascular and/or pulmonary problems these patients typically encounter over their lifespan.

16.3.6 Klinefelter Syndrome

First described in 1942 by Klinefelter *et al.*, Klinefelter syndrome is the most common sex chromosome disorder, affecting approximately 1 in 660 men [43]. As noted by a Danish registry study, it is commonly either underdiagnosed or diagnosed after childhood (postpubertally), as the phenotype of Klinefelter syndrome is quite variable [44]. The syndrome is characterized by the presence of one Y chromosome and two or more X chromosomes in a phenotypic male, leading to the commonest karyotype of 47,XXY [43]. It is currently known that the genetic etiology of Klinefelter's is meiotic nondisjunction, *i.e.*, abnormal separation of chromosomes during meiosis [43]. Since there is no consensus on the correct clinical definition of Klinefelter syndrome, Bojesen and Gravholt recommend that a diagnosis should be based on clinical findings as well as a cytogenetic evaluation [43].

Clinical features of Klinefelter syndrome include small hyalinized testes, hypogonadism, infertility, obesity, increased height, narrow shoulders, gynecomastia, sparse body hair, and reduced intelligence [43, 45]. Many males who have Klinefelter syndrome go through life undiagnosed. This may be due in part to the fact that the physical appearance of a pathologically hypogonadal child is not much different from that of a normal prepubertal boy, thus adding to the difficulty of accurately diagnosing the syndrome without cytogenetic testing [46]. The clinical attributes of Klinefelter change after puberty and can be characterized by small firm testes and varying symptoms of androgen deficiency [46]. Hypogonadism with low testosterone levels and elevated levels of gonadotropin can be associated with metabolic syndrome and type 2 diabetes in men [47].

Conversely, normal testosterone levels increase muscle tissue and decrease abdominal obesity and nonesterified fatty acids, thereby improving insulin sensitivity [48].

The majority of men with Klinefelter syndrome have alterations in body composition that seemingly lead to diabetes mellitus, dyslipidemia, and metabolic syndrome [49]. Both epidemiologic and clinical studies have shown evidence of increased risks of diabetes mellitus and metabolic syndrome in these patients [45, 50]. Truncal obesity in men with Klinefelter's has been shown to be the major determinant of metabolic syndrome and decreased insulin sensitivity, even when controlling for testosterone levels [45]. Furthermore, hypogonadism has also been found to be associated with an adverse cardiovascular profile, including increased C-reactive protein and triglycerides, but decreased high-density lipoprotein (HDL) cholesterol [51].

Early diagnosis and treatment of patients with Klinefelter syndrome can potentially improve quality of life for these patients. Studies investigating the clinical use of testosterone in hypogonadal conditions indicate that early and long-term treatment results in benefits, including, but not limited to, increased lean body mass and decreased body fat [46]. The clinical features of gynecomastia and infertility, however, in these patients are not improved by testosterone replacement therapy, and patients may opt for surgical removal of excess breast tissue and assisted reproductive technologies. Finally, given the connection between low levels of testosterone and a poor metabolic profile, testosterone treatment is a benefit to these patients and hormone therapy should be implemented as soon as androgen levels are low in pubertal and post-pubertal patients [46].

16.3.7   Turner Syndrome

Turner syndrome, affecting approximately one in every 2,500 live female births, is a genetic disorder whereby phenotypic females have one X chromosome missing, with a karyotype of 45,X [52]. The most common clinical features of this syndrome are short stature and premature ovarian failure. Females with Turner syndrome lack spontaneous pubertal development as a result of ovarian sex hormone insufficiency [53]. Characteristic features include neck webbing, infertility, and a high probability of cardiovascular defects [52]. Girls with Turner syndrome typically have normal intelligence, but they may have difficulty with nonverbal, mathematical, social, and psychomotor skills [53]. Given the close association with pubertal development, Turner syndrome can be difficult to recognize before puberty, as the phenotypic features can be quite subtle [53].

Women with Turner syndrome are at an increased risk of ischemic heart disease [52]. Up to 50% of infants with Turner syndrome present with silent cardiac defects, mainly bicuspid aortic valve and other abnormalities such as aortic root dilation, which only become apparent later in life and have the potential to present as catastrophic aortic dissection [52]. Coupled with an increase in cardiovascular heart disease, these girls have an altered body composition, specifically increased fat mass and BMI, while lean body mass is decreased [54]. The combination of these clinical profiles along with short stature commonly manifests as obesity with a Turner-specific metabolic syndrome. The fat mass is typically localized to visceral fat, which predicts a higher risk for developing insulin resistance [54]. Bakalov *et al.* demonstrated reduced insulin secretion, with normal or elevated insulin sensitivity, in women with Turner syndrome. This finding was independent of obesity or hypogonadism, suggesting that beta-cell dysfunction or insufficiency is a primary feature of the Turner-specific metabolic syndrome [55]. Ostberg *et al.* described central adiposity without hyperleptinemia, low fasting glucose, and elevated triglyceride, C-reactive protein, and IL-6 levels as indicators of cardiovascular risk in women with Turner syndrome [56].

Management and treatment of patients with Turner syndrome should include a multidisciplinary approach, including a pediatrician, endocrinologist, cardiologist, and psychologist. Obesity, which contributes to cardiovascular disease risk, and hypertension should be prevented and treated by lifestyle counseling, incorporating a nutritionist or weight-management program [57]. Although girls with Turner syndrome are not typically growth hormone-deficient, many may improve their growth rate and benefit significantly with growth hormone therapy [52]. The long-term risks of growth hormone therapy in Turner syndrome are, however, unknown [52]. Delayed pubertal development, which can negatively impact girls with Turner syndrome psychosocially, can be addressed with early administration of a low-dose estrogen therapy so as not to interfere with growth rate. Continued estrogen use should be emphasized during adulthood to prevent osteoporosis [52]. Finally, due to the serious life-threatening cardiovascular profile seen in many of these females, a comprehensive evaluation by a cardiologist is warranted, commencing at the time of Turner syndrome diagnosis regardless of age [52].

16.4 LEPTIN SIGNALING DISRUPTIONS

16.4.1 *Leptin Deficiency*

Monogenic obesity syndromes result from single-gene defects that affect appetite regulation and lead to severe early-onset obesity. Mutations in the leptin and leptin receptor genes and in the melanocortin-4 receptor (*MC4R*) are prime examples of such defects.

In 1997, a report of two severely obese cousins from a highly consanguineous family of Pakistani origin was published. Both children were found to have a mutation in the leptin gene and had barely detectable levels of serum leptin [58]. The first mutation in the leptin receptor gene was reported in 1998. The mutation results in a leptin receptor that lacks both transmembrane and intracellular domains [59]. The mutant leptin receptor circulates at high concentrations bound to leptin, resulting in elevated serum leptin concentrations [60].

Subjects with leptin and leptin receptor deficiencies exhibit similar clinical phenotypes. Subjects are of normal birth weight, but exhibit rapid weight gain in the first few months of life due to intense hyperphagia, resulting in severe obesity. A preferential deposition of fat mass with excessive amounts of subcutaneous fat over the trunk and limbs is observed [60]. Subjects with leptin deficiency are hyperinsulinemic [61]; some adults have developed type 2 diabetes [60]. No detectable changes in resting metabolic rate have been observed in leptin-deficient subjects [61, 62]. Leptin receptor-deficient subjects in one report by Clement *et al.* showed evidence of mild growth retardation in early childhood with impaired basal and stimulated growth hormone secretion as well as features of hypothalamic hypothyroidism [59]. However, it is not clear whether these features are consistent with leptin receptor deficiency [63].

In addition to obesity and obesity-related complications, leptin and leptin receptor deficiency are also associated with hypothalamic hypothyroidism and hypogonadotropic hypogonadism. While linear growth in childhood and serum insulin-like growth factor-I (IGF-I) levels are normal, final height of adult subjects is reduced due to the absence of a pubertal growth spurt. Impaired linear growth does not appear to be common [64]. Further, children with leptin deficiency have marked abnormalities of T-cell number and function. They have frequent infections, predominantly of the upper respiratory tract [61].

Dramatic and beneficial effects of daily subcutaneous injections of recombinant human leptin leading to reduction in body weight and fat mass in children have been reported, the major effect being on appetite with normalization of hyperphagia [61, 62].

Leptin receptor deficiency should be considered in all patients with hyperphagic obesity of early onset, although the prevalence of leptin receptor mutations is likely to be highest among ethnic groups where consanguinity is common [60].

16.4.2   Melanocortin-4 Receptor Deficiency

Numerous studies have shown that heterozygous mutations in *MC4R* predispose those affected to nonsyndromic obesity [65–67]. Current reports estimate a 1–in–2,000 population prevalence of MC4R deficiency [68]. Melanocortin signaling is known to be one of the pathways involved in the control of body weight by regulating food intake and energy expenditure. The central melanocortin system includes two populations of neurons located in the arcuate nucleus. These neurons are the proopiomelanocortin (POMC)– and cocaine- and amphetamine-regulated transcript prepropeptide (CARTPT)-expressing neurons and the agouti-related peptide (AgRP) and neuropeptide Y (NPY)-expressing neurons. The prohormone, POMC, is posttranslationally cleaved to produce alpha-melanocyte-stimulating hormone (alpha-MSH). This peptide has anorexigenic effects upon activation of the MC4R on the surface of target neurons. Leptin, known to be involved in the control of appetite and metabolism, stimulates POMC expression and eventually results in MC4R stimulation [69]. The hypothalamic neuropeptide AgRP is a potent antagonist of the melanocortin-3 receptor (MC3R) and MC4R. Food intake is increased and energy expenditure is decreased upon activation of the AgRP neurons. In contrast, food intake is decreased and energy expenditure is increased upon activation of the POMC neurons [68].

Mutations in MCR4 are dominantly inherited and are associated with obesity. Individuals carrying homozygous mutations have a more severe phenotype than heterozygous carriers [69]. Children with MC4R deficiency exhibit early-onset hyperphagia, an increase in fat and lean mass, marked increase in bone mineral density, and hyperinsulinemia. There is no evidence of defective energy expenditure, abnormal development of puberty, reduced fertility, and any other major hormonal abnormalities [69]. Most patients are heterozygous carriers and therefore clinically present with a variable phenotype. Dempfle *et al.* showed a greater effect of the MC4R mutation in women than in men [70, 71].

At present, there is no specific therapy for the treatment of MC4R deficiency, although therapeutic research is ongoing [72].

16.5   ENDOCRINE DISORDERS ASSOCIATED WITH OBESITY

16.5.1   Endocrinopathies

Endocrine disorders in rare cases can cause secondary obesity in children (see Table 16.1) [1]. Endocrinopathies resulting both in excess hormonal production, *e.g.*, insulinoma and Cushing's syndrome, and deficient hormone production or activity (growth hormone deficiency, hypothyroidism, pseudohypoparathyroidism [PHP]) can be associated with secondary obesity in childhood. Some endocrinopathies associated with childhood obesity – including growth hormone deficiency, thyroid hormone deficiency, and Cushing's syndrome – are associated with a combination of decreased energy expenditure and decreased growth, resulting in prominent central adiposity in a slowly growing child with short stature [1]. In these diseases, correction of the underlying endocrinopathy can reverse the processes resulting in secondary obesity.

Growth hormone deficiency, other forms of hypopituitarism, hypothyroidism, Cushing's disease or syndrome, or PHP, are associated with increased BMI. However, unlike exogenous obesity, stature and height velocity are decreased, unless there is pubertal acceleration in height velocity. In contrast, stature and height velocity are usually increased with exogenous obesity. Thus, testing for endocrine disorders in a child with obesity is unlikely to be useful unless the child is showing a deceleration in growth velocity and/or has short stature in relation to family background [73].

16.5.2   Insulinoma

Insulinomas are rarely diagnosed in children [1], but are typically identified by symptoms of hypoglycemia resulting from the presence of hyperinsulinism and normal insulin sensitivity. Obesity is a clinical manifestation of insulinoma, primarily due to weight gain resulting from an increased consumption of food to avoid hypoglycemic symptoms. However, the identification of hypoglycemic symptoms and subsequent diagnosis of insulinoma typically occurs before the onset of obesity [20]. Treatment of an insulinoma generally results in weight loss.

16.5.3   Diabetes Mellitus

In contrast to the other endocrine disorders discussed in this chapter, in type 2 diabetes, obesity is a causative factor and not a secondary finding. Being overweight or obese is the most important risk factor for the development of type 2 diabetes in youth [74]. Obesity is strongly associated with insulin resistance and, when coupled with relative insulin deficiency, leads to the development of type 2 diabetes [75]. Type 2 diabetes in youth is now responsible for up to approximately one fifth of new diagnoses of diabetes in pubertal children [1]. As many as 45% of children with newly diagnosed diabetes mellitus have type 2 diabetes rather than type 1 diabetes [3]. The American Diabetes Association (ADA) recommends that all youngsters who are overweight and have at least two other risk factors should be tested for type 2 diabetes beginning at age 10 or at the onset of puberty and every 2 years thereafter [3]. However, some obese children develop type 2 diabetes as well as other comorbidities, such as glucose intolerance, dyslipidemia, and hypertension, even before the onset of puberty [76]. In addition, there is evidence that the complications of diabetes, including atherosclerotic vascular change, often begin before symptoms appear [74].

Standards for the diagnosis of type 2 diabetes are based on values of fasting blood glucose, random blood glucose, and oral glucose tolerance test and are identical for adults and children [74, 77]. Distinguishing between type 1 diabetes and type 2 diabetes as early as possible is important; helpful clinical signs for type 2 diabetes are obesity and signs of insulin resistance (*i.e.*, acanthosis nigricans, hypertension, polycystic ovarian syndrome). Patients with type 2 diabetes frequently have elevated C-peptide levels. The *absence* of autoantibodies to insulin, the islet cell, and/or glutamic acid decarboxylase is also typical in most type 2 diabetes cases [74].

Studies in adults demonstrated the benefits of lifestyle intervention on the prevention of progression from impaired glucose tolerance to T2DM [78, 79]. Weight loss and/or prevention of weight gain is the best way to prevent T2DM among children with risk factors for the disease, primarily through a healthier diet, increased physical activity, and reduced sedentary activity [80]. Although lifestyle changes are always indicated in patients with T2DM, patients presenting with mild hyperglycemia and glycosylated hemoglobin <8.5% or an incidental diagnosis of type 2 diabetes can be treated initially with therapeutic lifestyle changes, in combination with metformin (the only drug FDA-approved for pediatric T2DM). Severe hyperglycemia, an $A_{1C} > 8.5\%$, and/or ketosis should be treated initially with insulin to achieve control [74].

16.5.4 Mauriac Syndrome

Mauriac syndrome was first described in 1930 in a 10-year-old girl with poorly controlled diabetes mellitus, hepatomegaly, protuberant abdomen, dwarfism, moon-shaped face, and fat deposition about the shoulders and abdomen [81]. Often referred to as diabetic dwarfism, Mauriac syndrome is a severe form of growth retardation seen in patients with poorly controlled type 1 diabetes. It is characterized by growth failure, delayed puberty, hepatomegaly, and Cushingoid features.

Mauriac syndrome occurs in both males and females equally, and while there are reports of Mauriac syndrome in toddlers and adults, it is most commonly observed in adolescents. The actual cause is unknown, but is probably a combination of factors, including inadequate glucose in the tissues, decreased IGF-I and growth hormone levels, impaired bioactivity of the hormones, a circulating hormone inhibitor, or resistant or defective hormone receptors. Evidence suggests that periods of supraphysiologic insulin levels are associated with hepatomegaly, because hepatomegaly has not been observed in newly diagnosed patients who have been severely insulin-deficient.

Mauriac syndrome is relatively rare today with the improved knowledge of the importance of glycemic control and the advances made in insulin treatment regimens. Improved glycemic control helps to reverse the growth failure, hepatomegaly, and hyperadrenocorticism, but catch-up growth may not be complete. Aggressive insulin treatment also may cause rapid advancement of retinopathy and nephropathy, so a delicate balance in strict control, but not overcontrol, is necessary [82].

16.5.5 Pseudohypoparathyroidism

PHP, in its broadest sense, is defined as the inability to respond to parathyroid hormone (PTH). The condition was first described in 1942 by Albright *et al.* [83], who observed that several patients with hypocalcemia and hyperphosphatemia (characteristics of hypoparathyroidism) failed to respond to administration of PTH, with correction of the calcium and phosphate metabolic defects. This was then termed "pseudohypoparathyroidism," with later studies describing hyperplasia of the parathyroid glands and PTH elevation in the serum, suggesting inappropriate of PTH resistance [84, 85].

Some patients with PHP were also found to have a convergence of symptoms now referred to as Albright's hereditary osteodystrophy (AHO) [83]. The physical features of AHO include short stature, central obesity, round face, short neck, bradydactyly, subcutaneous ossification, and mental retardation [86, 87]. The prevalence of AHO in European populations is 0.72/100,000 [35].

Five recognized subtypes of PHP have been described since the original report [88, 89]: PHP types 1a, b, and c; type 2; and pseudo-pseudohypoparathyroidism (pseudo-PHP) [90]. Patients with these various PHP syndromes differ in the extent of the effects on physical appearance (*i.e.*, presence of AHO), PTH responses, G-coupled protein responsiveness, and hormone resistance [89, 91–94]. These are summarized briefly in Table 16.2 [88, 89].

Patients with PHP type 1a exhibit AHO, decreased urinary cAMP, and phosphaturic responses to PTH infusion and have decreased Gs activity in the membranes of various cell types (erythrocytes, fibroblasts, and platelets). In addition to PTH resistance, these individuals are also resistant to thyroid-stimulating hormone (TSH), gonadotropins, and growth hormone-releasing hormone (GHRH) [89]. PHP resistance develops within the initial years of life. TSH resistance develops during childhood and adolescence. Thyroid hormone levels are normal or slightly below normal, and serum TSH becomes slightly elevated.

Genetic defects associated with the different forms of PHP involve the alpha-subunit of the stimulatory G protein (Gsα). This signaling protein is essential for the actions of PTH and many other hormones. Patients with PHP type 1a have been shown to have heterozygous-inactivating mutations within Gsα-encoding *GNAS* exons. Normally, when activated by an agonist-occupied G protein-coupled receptor, Gsα stimulates adenyl cyclase, resulting in production of the second messenger cAMP [95–98]. The gene responsible for Gsα expression, *GNAS1*, maps to chromosome 20q13 and

Table 16.2
Pseudohypoparathyroidism subtype characteristics [88, 89]

	PHP type 1a	PHP type 1b	PHP type 1c	PHP type 2	Pseudo-PHP
Physical appearance					
Albright's hereditary osteodystrophy	Yes	No	Yes	No	Yes
Short stature	Yes	No	Yes	No	Yes
Obesity	Yes	No	Yes	No	Yes
Subcutaneous ossification	Yes	No	Yes	No	Yes
Response to PTH					
Urinary cAMP	Defective	Defective	Defective	Normal	Normal
Urinary phosphate	Defective	Defective	Defective	Defective	Normal
Serum calcium	Low, rarely normal	Low	Low	Low	Normal
Hormone resistance	Multiple: PTH, TSH, Gn, GHRH	PTH (TSH has been reported)	Multiple: PTH, TSH, Gn	PTH	No
Genetic					
Gsα activity	Reduced	Normal	Normal	Normal	Reduced
Inheritance	Autosomal dominant	Autosomal dominant/ sporadic	Unknown	Unknown	Autosomal dominant
Molecular defect	Heterozygous *GNAS1* mutations	Specific deletions	Unknown	Unknown	Heterozygous *GNAS1* mutations

PHP pseudohypoparathyroidism; *cAMP* cyclic adenosine monophosphate; *Gsα* alpha-subunit of the stimulatory G protein; *PTH* parathyroid hormone; *TSH* thyroid-stimulating hormone; *Gn* gonadotropin; *GHRH* growth hormone-releasing hormone; *GNAS1* guanine nucleotide binding alpha-subunit 1 is autosomal-dominant. Patients with PHP 1a express a maternally transmitted mutated allele of *GNAS1* that encodes Gsα. There are 50 different loss-of-function *GNAS1* mutations reported [99].

Obesity is a common feature of PHP type 1a. It has been suggested by Germain-Lee *et al.* who reported growth hormone deficiency in 70% of patients whom they evaluated, that growth hormone deficiency, as well as other metabolic factors, may play a role in obesity [92]. Children with PHP 1a attain BMI>95% ile (*i.e.*, ≥30 kg/m²), with standard deviation scores (SDS) typically greater than +3 or +4 [88, 89, 92].

Defective calcium and phosphate processing results in subcutaneous ossification and premature epiphyseal fusion, shortened, blunted phalanges and short stature, where Hand short stature is defined as >2 SDS lower than normal and is typically >3 SDS lower than normal [83]. *GNAS1* is expressed in chondrocytes [92]. Defective renal cAMP and phosphate modulation by PTH affect calcium utilization. It is estimated that 47–75% of children with PHP type 1a suffer from mental retardation [95, 100] due to the defective G-protein signaling.

Corrective hormone therapy has been used in cases of PHP type 1a, but with only modest success. Supplementary growth hormone treatment was successfully used to treat a 7-year-old girl with PHP 1a-related growth hormone deficiency in which her BMI SDS was reduced from 4.4 to 3.7 [99]. Vitamin D and calcium supplements have been used to overcome the defective calcium utilization in PHP type 1a [99, 101, 102]. An interesting approach to treatment of a patient with PHP type 1c was reported [103] in which the cannabinoid receptor-1 inverse-agonist, rimonabant, was used to promote weight reduction. The patient lost 16 kg in 6 months, and BMI was reduced from 40.5 to 33.5kg/m². The treatment ended when the drug was withdrawn from the market.

16.5.6   *Growth Hormone Deficiency*

Growth hormone deficiency in children and adults can be associated with an increase in body fat, especially abdominal fat, and a decrease in lean body mass [20]. Growth hormone deficiency in childhood is characterized by a combination of abnormalities that can be present in varying degrees. These characteristics include auxologic, clinical, genetic, radiologic, metabolic, and hormonal abnormalities. Growth hormone deficiency in children can be caused directly by total or relative absence of growth hormone or by secretion of abnormal growth hormones or indirectly by decreased levels of growth factors that are growth hormone-dependent, such as IGF-I [104].

Different forms of growth hormone deficiency in childhood include idiopathic, organic, familial, or sporadic, or associated with defined genetic defects.

Some cases of growth hormone deficiency have been shown to be secondary to neuroendocrine secretory dysfunction.

In childhood, growth hormone deficiency is characterized by a progressive delay in growth, a delay in skeletal maturation, and a delay in puberty. The growth retardation is disproportional, with the effect on the extremities more notable than on the trunk. The resulting appearance is of a child with a small chin, protruding forehead, and mild truncal adiposity [104]. Growth hormone therapy for children with growth hormone deficiency can both improve growth velocity as well as affect body composition with a reduction in fat and an increase in muscle mass [105].

PHP type 1a is an example of a genetic form of growth hormone deficiency, with 69% of affected patients having growth hormone deficiency compared to the general population, in whom the incidence is 0.029% [92]. This is not present in all PHP type 1a patients, however, and is consistent with the nonuniformity of hormonal deficiencies in PHP type 1a [92]. Growth hormone therapy has been reported to successfully treat a child with growth hormone deficiency due to PHP type 1a [99].

Laron syndrome is a form of dwarfism first reported in 1968 and confirmed by Najjar and coworkers [106, 107]. Affected patients have high levels of growth hormone with end-organ resistance. Patients with Laron syndrome present at birth with lengths that are at least 2 SDS lower than normal. Hands and feet are disproportionally small, and facial characteristics include a saddle nose and defective and irregular teeth. Motor development is slow. Children grow slowly, and height remains below the third percentile. While these children have normal weight, they have a thickened layer of subcutaneous fat in most parts of the body, but mainly in the trunk. This obesity persists past childhood and puberty. Fasting blood glucose is often low, and some exhibit hypoglycemia at birth. Free fasting fatty acids are above normal and rise on growth hormone therapy. Antigrowth hormone antibodies are not present, but the children do *not* respond to growth hormone administration with accelerated growth, indicative of dysfunctional receptor-mediated or other downstream events.

16.5.7   Cushing's Syndrome

Cushing's syndrome is rarely diagnosed in children or adolescents [108]. Cushing's syndrome is caused by excessive circulating glucocorticoid concentrations. Cushing's disease is the most common cause of Cushing's syndrome in children and adolescents and is caused by pituitary adrenocorticotropic hormone (ACTH) secretion from a pituitary microadenoma (or more rarely, a macroadenoma) [109–111] in approximately 80% of cases in this age group [112]. Ectopic ACTH syndrome occurs at a much lower frequency in the pediatric age range than in adults (15%). The majority of pediatric cases with ectopic ACTH syndrome are caused by carcinoid tumors of bronchial or thymic origin [109, 112]. Adrenal cortical tumors (either adenoma or carcinoma), although rare (0.3–0.4% of neoplasms in children), comprise another cause of Cushing's syndrome. Adrenal cortical tumors can be associated with virilization and are seen more commonly in children younger than 4 years of age [109], but have been observed in children ranging from 0.8 to 16 years of age [113]. Adrenal cortical tumors causing chronic hypercortisolism are seen in 20–30% of adults with Cushing's syndrome [114].

Primary Cushing's leads to short stature (−2 SDS in 40% of patients) and obesity that presents as central adiposity involving the trunk, neck, and face. BMI in one study was described as ranging from about +1 to +4 SDS (or greater) [109]. Arms and legs are not hyperadipose, and in the case of the legs, muscle wasting and atrophy can occur. A moon face is a characteristic of hypersteroidism and is often accompanied by other signs of steroid overproduction, that can include inappropriate and premature hirsutism, thinned skin, and bone demineralization. Biochemical diagnosis requires a finding of hypercortisolism, which can be done by testing 24-h urine, late-evening plasma cortisol, or a 48-h dexamethasone suppression test (in which cortisol secretion rises in Cushing's patients, but remains suppressed in normal subjects). Detailed descriptions and complexities of these and other tests are found in reviews by Beauregard *et al.* [115] and Bertagna *et al.* [114]. Positive findings require magnetic resonance imaging (MRI) or other imaging techniques to establish the presence of a tumor.

Transsphenoidal pituitary surgery to remove the pituitary microadenoma is considered to be the first-line treatment for Cushing's disease in the pediatric population [108]. Pituitary radiotherapy is another therapeutic option for children with Cushing's disease. Both therapies carry a risk of hypopituitarism.

Normal body composition is difficult to achieve in children posttherapy for Cushing's disease [108]. In a follow-up study of children and adolescents cured of Cushing's disease, both total body fat and the ratio of visceral to subcutaneous fat were abnormally high in a majority of patients after 7 years [116].

16.5.8 Hypothyroidism

Hashimoto thyroiditis is the most common cause of thyroid disease in children [117]. Hypothyroidism is not a common cause of secondary obesity in children; however, this can be seen. Characteristic findings can include growth delay, above-normal BMI, cold intolerance, fatigue, enlarged thyroid gland, and bradycardia. Goiter is not always obvious, but can become more apparent later in childhood. Diagnostic tests for the evaluation of hypothyroidism secondary to Hashimoto thyroiditis include serum levels of thyroid hormones, TSH, and anti-thyroid peroxidase and anti-thyroglobulin antibodies [118].

In one study of patients with acquired autoimmune thyroiditis [118], 17.5% of subjects had body weight >1 SDS above normal and 7.8% had body weight >2 SDS above normal and only slightly shorter stature that was still within the limits of normal (−0.45 SDS).

In another study of acquired autoimmune hypothyroiditis in a single family, four children had severe obesity (*i.e.*, BMI 35.6–40.8 kg/m^2) [119], three of whom exhibited hypothyroidism. Of the three, two had pituitary enlargements and had insulin resistance that resembled type 2 diabetes. The three children had titers for thyroid peroxidase antibodies ≥20,480 and high serum TSH. In this family, one of the children had primary congenital hypothyroidism, but the other two appeared to have acquired hypothyroidism.

Hashimoto thyroiditis is an autoimmune disorder and is the most prevalent form of autoimmune thyroid disease [120]. It can appear early in childhood and has an incidence reported to be as high as 1–2% during adolescence. It is often associated with other autoimmune diseases, including type 1 diabetes, celiac disease, and rheumatoid arthritis among others [119, 120]. There is also an association with developmental defects that may include Down's syndrome and Turner syndrome. In Hashimoto thyroiditis, autoantibodies to thyroid peroxidase and thyroglobulin are diagnostic, and TSH levels are elevated.

Autoimmune hypothyroidism is inheritable and can be found in immediate as well as extended families [118, 119]. However, it is a product of complex genetics, and a clear human leukocyte antigen system subtype linkage has thus far not been proven to occur in a consistent and predictive manner. There are suggestions, and a body of evidence from isolated populations, to support the idea that environmental factors may come into play [120]. These may include iodine, chemical pollutants, and even viral infection. Causation due to chronic exposure to environmental factors, however, needs to be coupled to susceptibility genes and genetic predisposition, and more extensive epidemiologic studies are needed to firmly establish this concept.

Treatment of hypothyroidism with thyroid hormone increases resting metabolic rate and improves the secretion of growth hormone and IGF-I [1].

16.6   HYPOTHALAMIC OBESITY

Secondary obesity caused by a hypothalamic insult is a devastating complication of cranial injury. Hypothalamic damage is most commonly caused by space-occupying lesions, such as tumors, aneurysms, inflammation, infiltrative diseases, and trauma [121]. The hypothalamus plays a central role in appetite and energy expenditure. Children with hypothalamic damage gain weight either as a result of hypothalamic injury caused by the disease or by its treatment (surgery or radiotherapy). The development of obesity from any of these pathologies or from their subsequent treatment has been termed hypothalamic obesity [122, 123].

16.6.1 The Hypothalamus and Body Weight Regulation

The hypothalamus consists of numerous substructures and nuclei, each with distinct homeostatic functions (Fig. 16.2) [124]. Animal studies in the

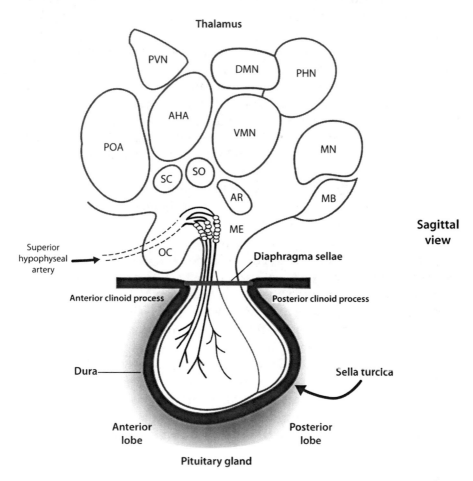

Fig. 16.2. Nuclei of the hypothalamus [124]. *AHA* anterior hypothalamic area; *AR* arcuate nucleus; *DMN* dorsomedial nucleus; *MB* mammillary body; *ME* median eminence; *MN* medial nucleus; *OC* optic chiasm; *PHN* posterior hypothalamic nucleus; *POA* preoptic area; *PVN* paraventricular nucleus; *SCN* suprachiasmatic nucleus; *SO* supraoptic nucleus; *VMN* ventromedial nucleus.

1940s and 1950s implicated medial and lateral hypothalamic nuclei in regulating feeding behavior [125, 126]. The results of those studies gave rise to a dual-center hypothesis of body weight regulation. Namely, the ventromedial hypothalamus (VMH) regulates satiety, while the lateral hypothalamus controls hunger [127].

Physical insult to hypothalamic structures, in particular the VMH, may lead to obesity. Bilateral lesions of the VMH in rats result in hyperphagia and uncontrollable weight gain, *i.e.*, hypothalamic obesity [128, 129]. In humans, VMH damage from tumors, surgery, or radiation promotes uncontrollable weight gain from increased caloric intake and decreased energy expenditure [121, 122]. Causes of hypothalamic injury and subsequent hypothalamic obesity are found in Table 16.3 [121]. Tumors, such as craniopharyngioma, can cause hypothalamic obesity in children. Other causes include radiation, trauma, and infection, *e.g.*, tuberculosis. Frohlich's syndrome (adiposogenital dystrophy) is a rare condition that produces obesity with retarded development of the sex organs in adolescents due to diminished hypothalamic and pituitary function. Children with Frohlich's syndrome often develop normally after puberty [130]. Genetic abnormalities associated with hypothalamic obesity (*e.g.*, PWS) are discussed elsewhere in this chapter.

Table 16.3
Causes of hypothalamic obesity in humans [121]

Structural damage to the hypothalamus
- Craniopharyngioma
- Pituitary macroadenoma with suprasellar extension
- Glioma
- Meningioma
- Teratoma
- Germ cell tumor
- Metastasis
- Aneurysm
- Surgery
- Radiotherapy

Genetic syndromes of obesity with hypothalamic dysfunction
- Prader–Willi syndrome
- Leptin deficiency
- Leptin receptor deficiency
- Proopiomelanocortin mutation
- Melanocortin-4 receptor mutations

16.7 CRANIOPHARYNGIOMA

16.7.1 Epidemiology and Pathology

Craniopharyngioma and/or its treatment is the most frequent cause of acquired hypothalamic damage in children [121]. Craniopharyngiomas are histologically benign tumors that arise in the sellar area of the brain, bordering the optic nerve, pituitary gland, and hypothalamus. Approximately two cases of craniopharyngioma are observed per million persons per year in the United States [131], with approximately 28% of these cases occurring in children under 14 years of age [132]. Overall, craniopharyngiomas account for 80–90% of childhood neoplasms originating in the sellar region of the brain [133]. Virtually all craniopharyngiomas are cystic and contain a thick cholesterol-rich fluid composed of membrane lipids and keratin. Typically, these tumors can grow to 3–4 cm and, because of their location, can physically impact numerous structures, including the optic chiasm, third ventricle, thalamus, hypothalamus, and pituitary.

16.7.2 Clinical Manifestations

Diagnosis of craniopharyngioma is often missed due to presentation of nonspecific symptoms early in the disease. Initially, children typically present with headache and nausea, both due to an increase in intracranial pressure. Patients can also present with oculomotor and visual field defects, the latter from compression of the optic chiasm. As the disease progresses, more serious endocrine symptoms can be observed, so that up to 90% of patients have some form of endocrine pathology at the time of diagnosis [134, 135]. Secretion of growth hormone, luteinizing hormone/follicle stimulating hormone (FSH), ACTH, and TSH are deficient in children with craniopharyngiomas [134, 135]. Growth hormone deficiency is the most common endocrine abnormality in these patients, present in approximately 75% of children with craniopharyngiomas. Consequently, approximately 35–50% of patients have short stature, and 15–25% are obese at diagnosis [136, 137]. Two of the more adverse endocrine effects of craniopharyngioma associated with high mortality, if untreated, are ACTH deficiency (25% of patients) and central diabetes insipidus (9–17% of patients) [136]. However, another study suggested an incidence of central diabetes insipidus of 52% [138].

16.7.3 Treatment Approaches

Treatment of craniopharyngioma follows verification of the tumor by MRI, ophthalmology, and endocrinology. A variety of treatments are available, including surgery, radiation, and pharmacologic intervention.

A catheter can be temporarily implanted to drain the cyst, relieve intracranial pressure, and improve visual defects [139]. In the majority of cases, surgical resection of craniopharyngioma is the favored (and most effective) treatment approach. However, depending on the size and infiltration of the tumor, resection poses a high risk for damage to adjacent structures. Full or partial resection of craniopharyngiomas is associated with 20% morbidity and a 95% prevalence of endocrine dysfunction, especially hypopituitarism [135, 140]. Full resection of the tumor is favorable to partial resection, since partial resection may spare surrounding structures, but is associated with regrowth of the tumor in 71–90% of patients [139]. If a partial resection is done, radiation therapy is usually initiated to limit regrowth of the tumor. After treatment with radiation, patients may develop numerous sequelae, including visual, endocrine, cognitive, psychologic, eating, and sleep disorders [135]. Pharmacologic treatment with antitumor agents, such as bleomycin, through an intracranial catheter has been shown to be successful in some patients in diminishing the size of craniopharyngiomas [141–143]. Complications can occur with this treatment including blindness, endocrine deficits, or death [141, 142, 144].

16.7.4 Treatment Outcomes and Obesity

Hypothalamic obesity has been described in 25–75% of patients after treatment for craniopharyngioma [135]. Damage to the hypothalamus can arise from the tumor itself or from its treatment (surgery and/or radiation). Multiple endocrine abnormalities arise in patients following surgery, including deficiencies in growth hormone (47–100%), corticotropin (57–91%), thyroid hormone (74–97%), and gonadotropin (37–100%) [135]. Postsurgical craniopharyngioma patients are also deficient in melatonin and exhibit severe daytime sleepiness [145].

16.7.4.1 POSTSURGICAL CRANIOPHARYNGIOMA

Treating obesity in postsurgical craniopharyngioma patients has proven difficult. Caloric restriction and exercise are not successful in these patients, and they are often initiated on experimental pharmacologic treatment. Because most patients with hypothalamic obesity also have growth hormone deficiency, early treatment strategies often involved growth hormone replacement. Some morbidly obese patients, however, still maintain normal linear growth (growth without growth hormone deficiency) (Fig. 16.3) [139, 146, 147]. Geffner et al. [148] demonstrated that 3 years of growth hormone treatment in postsurgical children improved growth velocity, but did not improve weight and BMI, compared with children with other causes of organic growth hormone deficiency.

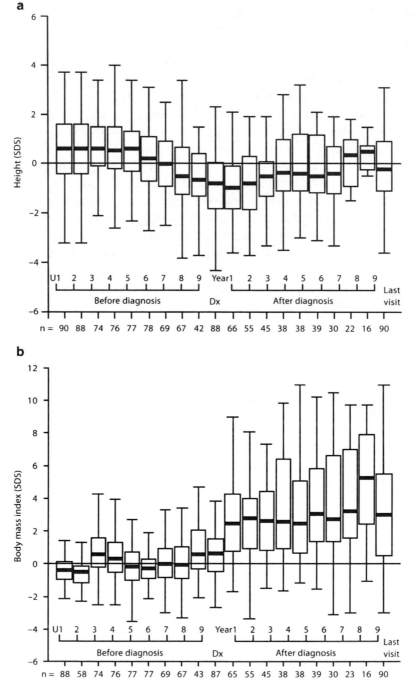

Fig. 16.3. Body height [146] and BMI [147] in craniopharyngioma [139]. Body height/
length (**a**) and BMI (**b**) expressed as standard deviation scores (SDS) at birth (U1), at
routine checkups before diagnosis (U2 – 3rd to 4th day of life; U3 – 3rd to 4th week;

Other approaches have also failed to curb increased weight gain following craniopharyngioma treatment. Such interventions include diet, appetite suppressants, metformin, and behavioral therapy. Recently, however, treatment with the long-acting somatostatin mimetic, octreotide, has been used to stabilize body weight and BMI. In a study by Lustig *et al.* [149], postsurgical craniopharyngioma pediatric patients showed less weight gain (+1.6 vs. +9.1 kg) and a more stable BMI (−0.2 vs. +2.2 kg/m^2) following 6-month treatment with octreotide compared with placebo. Octreotide-treated patients also demonstrated a reduction in insulin hypersecretion associated with hypothalamic obesity and showed an improvement in quality of life.

16.7.4.2 DEXTROAMPHETAMINE

Dextroamphetamine is another experimental therapy that has shown some success in the treatment of craniopharyngioma-induced obesity. Dextroamphetamine, an amphetamine, is a potent appetite suppressant. Treatment of five postsurgical pediatric craniopharyngioma patients with dextroamphetamine stabilized weight gain and increased overall activity [150]. Neither octreotide nor dextroamphetamine is approved for the treatment of obesity in the United States.

16.7.4.3 BARIATRIC SURGERY

Bariatric surgery may also be an option in patients with severe obesity and has been shown to reduce body weight and other comorbidities (*e.g.*, hyperglycemia) in adults and adolescents with nonhypothalamic obesity [151, 152]. A few studies have demonstrated significant weight loss following bariatric surgery in morbidly obese (BMI ≥45 kg/m^2) postsurgical craniopharyngioma patients [153–155]. However, the long-term safety of bariatric surgery in this patient population is unknown. One patient in these studies developed chronic pain and fatigue, while another developed intestinal stenosis [154]. Bariatric surgery may also lead to nutritional deficiencies [156]. It is important to note that patients with hypothalamic obesity will require hormone replacement following bariatric surgery due to permanent hypothalamic damage.

Fig. 16.3 (continued) U4 – 3rd to 4th month; U5 – 6th to 7th month; U6 – 10th to 12th month; U7 – 21st to 24th month; U8 – 3.5–4 years; U9 – 5th year), at the time of diagnosis (Dx), at annual intervals after the diagnosis of craniopharyngioma, and at the time of the last visit (*n*=90).

16.8   IATROGENIC CAUSES OF OBESITY

16.8.1   Medications

Weight gain is a common side effect of many drugs (Table 16.4) [157]. It is well known that high-dose, chronic glucocorticoid treatment is associated with a distinctive pattern of centripetal weight gain, with visceral fat accumulation predisposing to cardiovascular risk. This pattern of weight gain may closely resemble the clinical feature of Cushing's syndrome, as both exogenous and spontaneous Cushing's syndrome are caused by prolonged exposure to high levels of cortisol [158]. Other drugs used in children and adolescents associated with weight gain include cyproheptadine, valproate, and progestins [1]. Mounting evidence suggests that treatment with some of the newer antipsychotic drugs can cause rapid increase in body weight, but there is considerable variability among the drugs in their effect on weight gain, lipid profile, and the risk of diabetes mellitus [159]. Table 16.5 [157] lists potential mechanisms involved in drug-induced obesity.

As a result of the unwanted weight gain, comorbidities associated with increasing weight and obesity, including T2DM and hyperlipidemia, may begin to develop, and medication compliance and the success of treatment may suffer, all of which can lead to dire consequences for the patient.

Table 16.4
Drugs causing obesity [157]

Drug class	Drug or subclass
Antipsychotics	All subgroups
Antidepressants	Tricyclic antidepressants
	Lithium
	Monoamine oxidase inhibitors
Anticonvulsants	Valproate, carbamazepine
Antimigraine and antihistaminergic drugs	Cyproheptadine, flunarizine, pizotifen
Antidiabetic agents	Sulfonylurea agents, all insulin preparations, glitazones
Glucocorticoids	Pharmacologic doses
Beta blockers	Nonspecific (e.g., propranolol)
Sex hormones	Estrogen (high dose), megestrol acetate, tamoxifen
Other	Some antineoplastic agents

Table 16.5
Putative mechanisms involved in drug-induced obesity [157]

Decreased serotoninergic and dopaminergic activity
Impaired mitochondrial beta-oxidation of fatty acids and other changes
    in substrate oxidation
Reduced sympathetic nervous system activity
Decreased energy expenditure
Sedation
Anticholinergic side effects causing dry mouth and increased intake
    of caloric beverages
Altered activity of hypothalamic leptin and neuropeptide Y

REFERENCES

1. Speiser PW, Rudolf MC, Anhalt H *et al.* (2005) Consensus statement: childhood obesity. J Clin Endocrinol Metab 90:1871–1887
2. Kiess W, Galler A, Reich A *et al.* (2001) Clinical aspects of obesity in childhood and adolescence. Obes Rev 2:29–36
3. Barlow SE (2007) Expert committee recommendations regarding the prevention, assessment, and treatment of child and adolescent overweight and obesity: summary report. Pediatrics 120(Suppl 4):S164–S192
4. Stefan M, Nicholls RD (2004) What have rare genetic syndromes taught us about the pathophysiology of the common forms of obesity? Curr Diab Rep 4:143–150
5. Krebs NF, Himes JH, Jacobson D, Nicklas TA, Guilday P, Styne D (2007) Assessment of child and adolescent overweight and obesity. Pediatrics 120(Suppl 4):S193–S228
6. Prader A, Labhart A, Willi H (1956) Ein syndrom von adipositas, kelinwuchs, kryptorchismus und oligophrenie nach myatonieartigem zustand im neugeborenenalter. Schweiz Med Wochenschr 86:1260–1261
7. Chen C, Visootsak J, Dills S, Graham JM Jr (2007) Prader–Willi syndrome: an update and review for the primary pediatrician. Clin Pediatr (Phila) 46:580–591
8. Cassidy SB, Driscoll DJ (2009) Prader–Willi syndrome. Eur J Hum Genet 17:3–13
9. Bittel DC, Butler MG (2009) Prader–Willi syndrome. In: Squire LR (ed) Encyclopedia of neuroscience. Academic Press, London, pp 873–883
10. Burman P, Ritzen EM, Lindgren AC (2001) Endocrine dysfunction in Prader–Willi syndrome: a review with special reference to GH. Endocr Rev 22:787–799
11. Kousta E, Hadjiathanasiou CG, Tolis G, Papathanasiou A (2009) Pleiotropic genetic syndromes with developmental abnormalities associated with obesity. J Pediatr Endocrinol Metab 22:581–592
12. De Peppo F, Di Giorgio G, Germani M *et al.* (2008) BioEnterics intragastric balloon for treatment of morbid obesity in Prader–Willi syndrome: specific risks and benefits. Obes Surg 18:1443–1449
13. Holm VA, Cassidy SB, Butler MG *et al.* (1993) Prader–Willi syndrome: consensus diagnostic criteria. Pediatrics 91:398–402
14. Haqq AM, Stadler DD, Rosenfeld RG *et al.* (2003) Circulating ghrelin levels are suppressed by meals and octreotide therapy in children with Prader–Willi syndrome. J Clin Endocrinol Metab 88:3573–3576

15. De Waele K, Ishkanian SL, Bogarin R et al. (2008) Long-acting octreotide treatment causes a sustained decrease in ghrelin concentrations but does not affect weight, behaviour and appetite in subjects with Prader–Willi syndrome. Eur J Endocrinol 159:381–388

16. Shapira NA, Lessig MC, Lewis MH, Goodman WK, Driscoll DJ (2004) Effects of topiramate in adults with Prader–Willi syndrome. Am J Ment Retard 109:301–309

17. Whittington JE, Holland AJ, Webb T, Butler J, Clarke D, Boer H (2001) Population prevalence and estimated birth incidence and mortality rate for people with Prader–Willi syndrome in one UK health region. J Med Genet 38:792–798

18. Laurence JZ, Moon RC (1866) Four cases of retinitis pigmentosa occurring in the same family accompanied by general imperfections of development. Ophthalmol Rev 2:32–41

19. Klysik M (2008) Ciliary syndromes and treatment. Pathol Res Pract 204:77–88

20. Kokkoris P, Pi-Sunyer FX (2003) Obesity and endocrine disease. Endocrinol Metab Clin North Am 32:895–914

21. Beales PL, Elcioglu N, Woolf AS, Parker D, Flinter FA (1999) New criteria for improved diagnosis of Bardet–Biedl syndrome: results of a population survey. J Med Genet 36:437–446

22. Waters AM, Beales PL (2010) Bardet–Biedl syndrome. Available at: http://www.ncbi.nlm.nih.gov/bookshelf/br.fcgi?book=gene&partid=1363. Accessed 24 March 2010

23. National Library of Medicine, Genetics Home Reference (2010) Alstrom syndrome. Available at: http://ghr.nlm.nih.gov/condition=alstromsyndrome. Accessed 24 March 2010

24. Marshall JD, Beck S, Maffei P, Naggert JK (2007) Alstrom syndrome. Eur J Hum Genet 15:1193–1202

25. Li G, Vega R, Nelms K et al. (2007) A role for Alstrom syndrome protein, Alms1, in kidney ciliogenesis and cellular quiescence. PLoS Genet 3:e8

26. Minton JA, Owen KR, Ricketts CJ et al. (2006) Syndromic obesity and diabetes: changes in body composition with age and mutation analysis of ALMS1 in 12 United Kingdom kindreds with Alstrom syndrome. J Clin Endocrinol Metab 91:3110–3116

27. Marshall JD, Bronson RT, Collin GB et al. (2005) New Alstrom syndrome phenotypes based on the evaluation of 182 cases. Arch Intern Med 165:675–683

28. Cohen MM Jr, Hall BD, Smith DW, Graham CB, Lampert KJ (1973) A new syndrome with hypotonia, obesity, mental deficiency, and facial, oral, ocular, and limb anomalies. J Pediatr 83:280–284

29. NIH Office of Rare Diseases Research, Genetic and Rare Diseases Information Center (2010) Cohen syndrome. Available at: http://rarediseases.info.nih.gov/GARD/Condition/6126/Cohen_syndrome.aspx. Accessed 24 March 2010

30. Kivitie-Kallio S, Eronen M, Lipsanen-Nyman M, Marttinen E, Norio R (1999) Cohen syndrome: evaluation of its cardiac, endocrine and radiological features. Clin Genet 56:41–50

31. Kolehmainen J, Black GC, Saarinen A et al. (2003) Cohen syndrome is caused by mutations in a novel gene, COH1, encoding a transmembrane protein with a presumed role in vesicle-mediated sorting and intracellular protein transport. Am J Hum Genet 72:1359–1369

32. Ballesta CG, Lajarin LP, Lillo OC (2010) Cohen syndrome. Available at: http://www.orpha.net/data/patho/GB/uk-cohen.pdf. Accessed 24 March 2010

33. Falk MJ, Wang H, Traboulsi EI (2010) Cohen syndrome. In: GeneReviews at GeneTests: medical genetics information resource (database online). Available at: http://www.ncbi.nlm.nih.gov/bookshelf/br.fcgi?book=gene&part=cohen. Accessed 24 March 2010

34. Taban M, Memoracion-Peralta DS, Wang H, Al-Gazali LI, Traboulsi EI (2007) Cohen syndrome: report of nine cases and review of the literature, with emphasis on ophthalmic features. J AAPOS 11:431–437

35. Ayme S, Olry A. Prevalence of rare diseases: bibliographic data listed in alphabetical order of diseases. Orphanet Report Series, Rare Diseases Collection. November 2009, Number 1. Available at: http://www.orpha.net/orphacom/cahiers/docs/GB/Prevalence_ of_rare_diseases_by_alphabetical_list.pdf. Accessed 24 March 2010

36. Jenkins D, Seelow D, Jehee FS *et al.* (2007) RAB23 mutations in Carpenter syndrome imply an unexpected role for hedgehog signaling in cranial-suture development and obesity. Am J Hum Genet 80:1162–1170

37. Goldstone AP, Beales PL (2008) Genetic obesity syndromes. Front Horm Res 36:37–60

38. Perlyn CA, Marsh JL (2008) Craniofacial dysmorphology of Carpenter syndrome: lessons from three affected siblings. Plast Reconstr Surg 121:971–981

39. Ramos JM, Davis GJ, Hunsaker JC III, Balko MG (2009) Sudden death in a child with Carpenter Syndrome. Case report and literature review. Forensic Sci Med Pathol 5:313–317

40. Suh JM, Gao X, McKay J, McKay R, Salo Z, Graff JM (2006) Hedgehog signaling plays a conserved role in inhibiting fat formation. Cell Metab 3:25–34

41. Hidestrand P, Vasconez H, Cottrill C (2009) Carpenter syndrome. J Craniofac Surg 20:254–256

42. Robinson LK, James HE, Mubarak SJ, Allen EJ, Jones KL (1985) Carpenter syndrome: natural history and clinical spectrum. Am J Med Genet 20:461–469

43. Bojesen A, Gravholt CH (2007) Klinefelter syndrome in clinical practice. Nat Clin Pract Urol 4:192–204

44. Bojesen A, Juul S, Gravholt CH (2003) Prenatal and postnatal prevalence of Klinefelter syndrome: a national registry study. J Clin Endocrinol Metab 88:622–626

45. Bojesen A, Kristensen K, Birkebaek NH *et al.* (2006) The metabolic syndrome is frequent in Klinefelter's syndrome and is associated with abdominal obesity and hypogonadism. Diabetes Care 29:1591–1598

46. Lanfranco F, Kamischke A, Zitzmann M, Nieschlag E (2004) Klinefelter's syndrome. Lancet 364:273–283

47. Laaksonen DE, Niskanen L, Punnonen K *et al.* (2004) Testosterone and sex hormone-binding globulin predict the metabolic syndrome and diabetes in middle-aged men. Diabetes Care 27:1036–1041

48. Marin P, Holmang S, Jonsson L *et al.* (1992) The effects of testosterone treatment on body composition and metabolism in middle-aged obese men. Int J Obes Relat Metab Disord 16:991–997

49. Bojesen A, Host C, Gravholt CH (2010) Klinefelter's syndrome, type 2 diabetes and the metabolic syndrome – the impact of body composition. Mol Hum Reprod 16:396–401

50. Swerdlow AJ, Higgins CD, Schoemaker MJ, Wright AF, Jacobs PA (2005) Mortality in patients with Klinefelter syndrome in Britain: a cohort study. J Clin Endocrinol Metab 90:6516–6522

51. Laaksonen DE, Niskanen L, Punnonen K *et al.* (2003) Sex hormones, inflammation and the metabolic syndrome: a population-based study. Eur J Endocrinol 149:601–608

52. Bondy CA (2009) Turner syndrome 2008. Horm Res 71(Suppl 1):52–56

53. Morgan T (2007) Turner syndrome: diagnosis and management. Am Fam Physician 76:405–410

54. Gravholt CH, Hjerrild BE, Mosekilde L *et al.* (2006) Body composition is distinctly altered in Turner syndrome: relations to glucose metabolism, circulating adipokines, and endothelial adhesion molecules. Eur J Endocrinol 155:583–592

55. Bakalov VK, Cooley MM, Quon MJ *et al.* (2004) Impaired insulin secretion in the Turner metabolic syndrome. J Clin Endocrinol Metab 89:3516–3520

56. Ostberg JE, Attar MJ, Mohamed-Ali V, Conway GS (2005) Adipokine dysregulation in turner syndrome: comparison of circulating interleukin-6 and leptin concentrations with measures of adiposity and C-reactive protein. J Clin Endocrinol Metab 90:2948–2953

57. Rubin KR (2008) Turner syndrome: transition from pediatrics to adulthood. Endocr Pract 14:775–781

58. Montague CT, Farooqi IS, Whitehead JP et al. (1997) Congenital leptin deficiency is associated with severe early-onset obesity in humans. Nature 387:903–908

59. Clement K, Vaisse C, Lahlou N et al. (1998) A mutation in the human leptin receptor gene causes obesity and pituitary dysfunction. Nature 392:398–401

60. Farooqi IS (2008) Monogenic human obesity. Front Horm Res 36:1–11

61. Farooqi IS, Matarese G, Lord GM et al. (2002) Beneficial effects of leptin on obesity, T cell hyporesponsiveness, and neuroendocrine/metabolic dysfunction of human congenital leptin deficiency. J Clin Invest 110:1093–1103

62. Farooqi IS, Jebb SA, Langmack G et al. (1999) Effects of recombinant leptin therapy in a child with congenital leptin deficiency. N Engl J Med 341:879–884

63. Farooqi IS, O'Rahilly S (2005) Monogenic obesity in humans. Annu Rev Med 56:443–458

64. Farooqi IS, Wangensteen T, Collins S et al. (2007) Clinical and molecular genetic spectrum of congenital deficiency of the leptin receptor. N Engl J Med 356:237–247

65. Mergen M, Mergen H, Ozata M, Oner R, Oner C (2001) A novel melanocortin 4 receptor (MC4R) gene mutation associated with morbid obesity. J Clin Endocrinol Metab 86:3448–3451

66. Lubrano-Berthelier C, Dubern B, Lacorte JM et al. (2006) Melanocortin 4 receptor mutations in a large cohort of severely obese adults: prevalence, functional classification, genotype-phenotype relationship, and lack of association with binge eating. J Clin Endocrinol Metab 91:1811–1818

67. Branson R, Potoczna N, Kral JG, Lentes KU, Hoehe MR, Horber FF (2003) Binge eating as a major phenotype of melanocortin 4 receptor gene mutations. N Engl J Med 348:1096–1103

68. Farooqi IS (2005) Genetic and hereditary aspects of childhood obesity. Best Pract Res Clin Endocrinol Metab 19:359–374

69. Santini F, Maffei M, Pelosini C, Salvetti G, Scartabelli G, Pinchera A (2009) Melanocortin-4 receptor mutations in obesity. Adv Clin Chem 48:95–109

70. Stutzmann F, Tan K, Vatin V et al. (2008) Prevalence of melanocortin-4 receptor deficiency in Europeans and their age-dependent penetrance in multigenerational pedigrees. Diabetes 57:2511–2518

71. Dempfle A, Hinney A, Heinzel-Gutenbrunner M et al. (2004) Large quantitative effect of melanocortin-4 receptor gene mutations on body mass index. J Med Genet 41:795–800

72. Rivera G, Bocanegra-Garcia V, Galiano S et al. (2008) Melanin-concentrating hormone receptor 1 antagonists: a new perspective for the pharmacologic treatment of obesity. Curr Med Chem 15:1025–1043

73. August GP, Caprio S, Fennoy I et al. (2008) Prevention and treatment of pediatric obesity: an endocrine society clinical practice guideline based on expert opinion. J Clin Endocrinol Metab 93:4576–4599

74. Hannon TS, Rao G, Arslanian SA (2005) Childhood obesity and type 2 diabetes mellitus. Pediatrics 116:473–480

75. Jones KL (2008) Role of obesity in complicating and confusing the diagnosis and treatment of diabetes in children. Pediatrics 121:361–368

76. Weiss R, Dziura J, Burgert TS et al. (2004) Obesity and the metabolic syndrome in children and adolescents. N Engl J Med 350:2362–2374
77. Expert Committee on the Diagnosis and Classification of Diabetes Mellitus (2003) Report of the expert committee on the diagnosis and classification of diabetes mellitus. Diabetes Care 26(Suppl 1):S5–S20
78. Tuomilehto J, Lindstrom J, Eriksson JG et al. (2001) Prevention of type 2 diabetes mellitus by changes in lifestyle among subjects with impaired glucose tolerance. N Engl J Med 344:1343–1350
79. Knowler WC, Barrett-Connor E, Fowler SE et al. (2002) Reduction in the incidence of type 2 diabetes with lifestyle intervention or metformin. N Engl J Med 346:393–403
80. Barlow SE, Dietz WH (1998) Obesity evaluation and treatment: expert committee recommendations. The Maternal and Child Health Bureau, Health Resources and Services Administration and the Department of Health and Human Services. Pediatrics 102:E29
81. Mauriac P (1930) Gros ventre, hepatomegalie. Troubles de al croissance chez les enfants diabetiques traits depuis plusieurs annees par l'insuline. Gaz Hebd Sci Med Bordeaux 51:402–404
82. Kim MS, Quintos JB (2008) Mauriac syndrome: growth failure and type 1 diabetes mellitus. Pediatr Endocrinol Rev 5(Suppl 4):989–993
83. Albright F, Burnett CH, Smith PH, Parson W (1942) Pseudohypoparathyroidism: an example of Seabright-Bantam syndrome. Endocrinology 30:922–932
84. Tashjian AH Jr, Frantz AG, Lee JB (1966) Pseudohypoparathyroidism: assays of parathyroid hormone and thyrocalcitonin. Proc Natl Acad Sci U S A 56:1138–1142
85. Mann JB, Alterman S, Hills AG (1962) Albright's hereditary osteodystrophy comprising pseudohypoparathyroidism and pseudo-pseudohypoparathyroidism. With a report of two cases representing the complete syndrome occurring in successive generations. Ann Intern Med 56:315–342
86. Eyre WG, Reed WB (1971) Albright's hereditary osteodystrophy with cutaneous bone formation. Arch Dermatol 104:634–642
87. Farfel Z, Brothers VM, Brickman AS, Conte F, Neer R, Bourne HR (1981) Pseudohypoparathyroidism: inheritance of deficient receptor-cyclase coupling activity. Proc Natl Acad Sci USA 78:3098–3102
88. Levine MA (2000) Clinical spectrum and pathogenesis of pseudohypoparathyroidism. Rev Endocr Metab Disord 1:265–274
89. Mantovani G, Spada A (2006) Mutations in the Gs alpha gene causing hormone resistance. Best Pract Res Clin Endocrinol Metab 20:501–513
90. Albright F, Forbes AP, Henneman PH (1952) Pseudo-pseudohypoparathyroidism. Trans Assoc Am Physicians 65:337–350
91. Wemeau JL, Balavoine AS, Ladsous M, Velayoudom-Cephise FL, Vlaeminck-Guillem V (2006) Multihormonal resistance to parathyroid hormone, thyroid stimulating hormone, and other hormonal and neurosensory stimuli in patients with pseudohypoparathyroidism. J Pediatr Endocrinol Metab 19(Suppl 2):653–661
92. Germain-Lee EL (2006) Short stature, obesity, and growth hormone deficiency in pseudohypoparathyroidism type 1a. Pediatr Endocrinol Rev 3(Suppl 2):318–327
93. Weinstein LS, Yu S, Warner DR, Liu J (2001) Endocrine manifestations of stimulatory G protein alpha-subunit mutations and the role of genomic imprinting. Endocr Rev 22:675–705
94. Levine MA, Downs RW Jr, Moses AM et al. (1983) Resistance to multiple hormones in patients with pseudohypoparathyroidism. Association with deficient activity of guanine nucleotide regulatory protein. Am J Med 74:545–556

95. Mantovani G, de Sanctis L, Barbieri AM *et al.* (2010) Pseudohypoparathyroidism and GNAS epigenetic defects: clinical evaluation of Albright hereditary osteodystrophy and molecular analysis in 40 patients. J Clin Endocrinol Metab 95:651–658

96. Bastepe M (2008) The GNAS locus and pseudohypoparathyroidism. Adv Exp Med Biol 626:27–40

97. Hayward BE, Barlier A, Korbonits M *et al.* (2001) Imprinting of the G(s)alpha gene GNAS1 in the pathogenesis of acromegaly. J Clin Invest 107:R31–R36

98. Mantovani G, Ballare E, Giammona E, Beck-Peccoz P, Spada A (2002) The Gs-alpha gene: predominant maternal origin of transcription in human thyroid gland and gonads. J Clin Endocrinol Metab 87:4736–4740

99. Nwosu BU, Lee MM (2009) Pseudohypoparathyroidism type 1a and insulin resistance in a child. Nat Rev Endocrinol 5:345–350

100. Farfel Z, Friedman E (1986) Mental deficiency in pseudohypoparathyroidism type I is associated with Ns-protein deficiency. Ann Intern Med 105:197–199

101. Drezner MK, Neelon FA, Haussler M, McPherson HT, Lebovitz HE (1976) 1, 25-Dihydroxycholecalciferol deficiency: the probable cause of hypocalcemia and metabolic bone disease in pseudohypoparathyroidism. J Clin Endocrinol Metab 42: 621–628

102. Metz SA, Baylink DJ, Hughes MR, Haussler MR, Robertson RP (1977) Selective deficiency of 1, 25-dihydroxycholecalciferol. A cause of isolated skeletal resistance to parathyroid hormone. N Engl J Med 297:1084–1090

103. Al-Salameh A, Despert F, Kottler ML, Linglart A, Carel JC, Lecomte P (2010) Resistance to epinephrine and hypersensitivity (hyperresponsiveness) to CB1 antagonists in a patient with pseudohypoparathyroidism type Ic. Eur J Endocrinol 162:819–824

104. Sizonenko PC, Clayton PE, Cohen P, Hintz RL, Tanaka T, Laron Z (2001) Diagnosis and management of growth hormone deficiency in childhood and adolescence. Part 1: diagnosis of growth hormone deficiency. Growth Horm IGF Res 11:137–165

105. Carrel AL, Allen DB (2000) Effects of growth hormone on body composition and bone metabolism. Endocrine 12:163–172

106. Laron Z, Pertzelan A, Karp M (1968) Pituitary dwarfism with high serum levels of growth hormone. Isr J Med Sci 4:883–894

107. Najjar SS, Khachadurian AK, Ilbawi MN, Blizzard RM (1971) Dwarfism with elevated levels of plasma growth hormone. N Engl J Med 284:809–812

108. Savage MO, Storr HL, Chan LF, Grossman AB (2007) Diagnosis and treatment of pediatric Cushing's disease. Pituitary 10:365–371

109. Storr HL, Chan LF, Grossman AB, Savage MO (2007) Paediatric Cushing's syndrome: epidemiology, investigation and therapeutic advances. Trends Endocrinol Metab 18: 167–174

110. Fahlbusch R, Honegger J, Buchfelder M (1994) Neurosurgical management of Cushing's disease in children. In: Savage MO, Bourguignon J-P, Grossman AB (eds) Frontiers in paediatric neuroendocrinology. Blackwell Scientific Publications, Oxford, pp 68–72

111. Storr HL, Afshar F, Matson M *et al.* (2005) Factors influencing cure by transsphenoidal selective adenomectomy in paediatric Cushing's disease. Eur J Endocrinol 152:825–833

112. Chan LF, Storr HL, Grossman AB, Savage MO (2007) Pediatric Cushing's syndrome: clinical features, diagnosis, and treatment. Arq Bras Endocrinol Metab 51:1261–1271

113. Mayer SK, Oligny LL, Deal C, Yazbeck S, Gagne N, Blanchard H (1997) Childhood adrenocortical tumors: case series and reevaluation of prognosis – a 24-year experience. J Pediatr Surg 32:911–915

114. Bertagna X, Guignat L, Groussin L, Bertherat J (2009) Cushing's disease. Best Pract Res Clin Endocrinol Metab 23:607–623

115. Beauregard C, Dickstein G, LaCroix A (2002) Classic and recent etiologies of Cushing's syndrome: diagnosis and therapy. Treat Endocrinol 1:79–94

116. Leong GM, Abad V, Charmandari E et al. (2007) Effects of child- and adolescent-onset endogenous Cushing syndrome on bone mass, body composition, and growth: a 7-year prospective study into young adulthood. J Bone Miner Res 22:110–118

117. Lorini R, Gastaldi R, Traggiai C, Perucchin PP (2003) Hashimoto's thyroiditis. Pediatr Endocrinol Rev 1(Suppl 2):205–211

118. de Vries L, Bulvik S, Phillip M (2009) Chronic autoimmune thyroiditis in children and adolescents: at presentation and during long-term follow-up. Arch Dis Child 94:33–37

119. Reutrakul S, Hathout EH, Janner D et al. (2004) Familial juvenile autoimmune hypothyroidism, pituitary enlargement, obesity, and insulin resistance. Thyroid 14:311–319

120. Duntas LH (2008) Environmental factors and autoimmune thyroiditis. Nat Clin Pract Endocrinol Metab 4:454–460

121. Pinkney J, Wilding J, Williams G, MacFarlane I (2002) Hypothalamic obesity in humans: what do we know and what can be done? Obes Rev 3:27–34

122. Bray GA, Gallagher TF Jr (1975) Manifestations of hypothalamic obesity in man: a comprehensive investigation of eight patients and a review of the literature. Medicine (Baltimore) 54:301–330

123. Bray GA (1984) Syndromes of hypothalamic obesity in man. Pediatr Ann 13:525–536

124. Nussey SS, Whitehead SA (2010) Chapter 7: the pituitary gland. In: Endocrinology: an integrated approach. Available at: http://www.ncbi.nlm.nih.gov/bookshelf/br.fcgi?book=endocrin&part=A1257&renertype=box&id=A1272. Accessed 23 March 2010

125. Hetherington AW, Ranson S (1940) Hypothalamic lesions and adiposity in the rat. Anat Rec 78:149–172

126. Anand BK, Brobeck JR (1951) Localization of a "feeding center" in the hypothalamus of the rat. Proc Soc Exp Biol Med 77:323–324

127. Elmquist JK, Elias CF, Saper CB (1999) From lesions to leptin: hypothalamic control of food intake and body weight. Neuron 22:221–232

128. Berthoud HR, Jeanrenaud B (1979) Acute hyperinsulinemia and its reversal by vagotomy after lesions of the ventromedial hypothalamus in anesthetized rats. Endocrinology 105:146–151

129. Rohner-Jeanrenaud F, Jeanrenaud B (1980) Consequences of ventromedial hypothalamic lesions upon insulin and glucagon secretion by subsequently isolated perfused pancreases in the rat. J Clin Invest 65:902–910

130. Werner SC (1941) A study of untreated Frohlich's Syndrome without brain tumor: adiposogenital dystrophy. J Clin Endocrinol Metab 1:134–137

131. U.S. Cancer Statistics Working Group (2010) United States cancer statistics: 2004 incidence and mortality. Available at: http://www.cdc.gov/cancer/npcr/npcrpdfs/US_Cancer_Statistics_2004_Incidence_and_Mortality.pdf. Accessed 23 March 2010

132. Bunin GR, Surawicz TS, Witman PA, Preston-Martin S, Davis F, Bruner JM (1998) The descriptive epidemiology of craniopharyngioma. J Neurosurg 89:547–551

133. Lafferty AR, Chrousos GP (1999) Pituitary tumors in children and adolescents. J Clin Endocrinol Metab 84:4317–4323

134. Sklar CA (1994) Craniopharyngioma: endocrine abnormalities at presentation. Pediatr Neurosurg 21(Suppl 1):18–20

135. May JA, Krieger MD, Bowen I, Geffner ME (2006) Craniopharyngioma in childhood. Adv Pediatr 53:183–209

136. Sorva R (1988) Children with craniopharyngioma. Early growth failure and rapid postoperative weight gain. Acta Paediatr Scand 77:587–592
137. Muller HL, Emser A, Faldum A et al. (2004) Longitudinal study on growth and body mass index before and after diagnosis of childhood craniopharyngioma. J Clin Endocrinol Metab 89:3298–3305
138. de Vries L, Lazar L, Phillip M (2003) Craniopharyngioma: presentation and endocrine sequelae in 36 children. J Pediatr Endocrinol Metab 16:703–710
139. Muller HL (2008) Childhood craniopharyngioma. Recent advances in diagnosis, treatment and follow-up. Horm Res 69:193–202
140. Yasargil MG, Curcic M, Kis M, Siegenthaler G, Teddy PJ, Roth P (1990) Total removal of craniopharyngiomas. Approaches and long-term results in 144 patients. J Neurosurg 73:3–11
141. Hader WJ, Steinbok P, Hukin J, Fryer C (2000) Intratumoral therapy with bleomycin for cystic craniopharyngiomas in children. Pediatr Neurosurg 33:211–218
142. Mottolese C, Stan H, Hermier M et al. (2001) Intracystic chemotherapy with bleomycin in the treatment of craniopharyngiomas. Childs Nerv Syst 17:724–730
143. Voges J, Sturm V, Lehrke R, Treuer H, Gauss C, Berthold F (1997) Cystic craniopharyngioma: long-term results after intracavitary irradiation with stereotactically applied colloidal beta-emitting radioactive sources. Neurosurgery 40:263–269
144. Savas A, Erdem A, Tun K, Kanpolat Y (2000) Fatal toxic effect of bleomycin on brain tissue after intracystic chemotherapy for a craniopharyngioma: case report. Neurosurgery 46:213–216
145. Muller HL, Handwerker G, Wollny B, Faldum A, Sorensen N (2002) Melatonin secretion and increased daytime sleepiness in childhood craniopharyngioma patients. J Clin Endocrinol Metab 87:3993–3996
146. Prader A, Largo RH, Molinari L, Issler C (1989) Physical growth of Swiss children from birth to 20 years of age. First Zurich longitudinal study of growth and development. Helv Paediatr Acta Suppl 52:1–125
147. Rolland-Cachera MF, Cole TJ, Sempe M, Tichet J, Rossignol C, Charraud A (1991) Body mass index variations: centiles from birth to 87 years. Eur J Clin Nutr 45:13–21
148. Geffner M, Lundberg M, Koltowska-Haggstrom M et al. (2004) Changes in height, weight, and body mass index in children with craniopharyngioma after three years of growth hormone therapy: analysis of KIGS (Pfizer International Growth Database). J Clin Endocrinol Metab 89:5435–5440
149. Lustig RH, Hinds PS, Ringwald-Smith K et al. (2003) Octreotide therapy of pediatric hypothalamic obesity: a double-blind, placebo-controlled trial. J Clin Endocrinol Metab 88:2586–2592
150. Mason PW, Krawiecki N, Meacham LR (2002) The use of dextroamphetamine to treat obesity and hyperphagia in children treated for craniopharyngioma. Arch Pediatr Adolesc Med 156:887–892
151. Collins J, Mattar S, Qureshi F et al. (2007) Initial outcomes of laparoscopic Roux-en-Y gastric bypass in morbidly obese adolescents. Surg Obes Relat Dis 3:147–152
152. Nadler EP, Youn HA, Ginsburg HB, Ren CJ, Fielding GA (2007) Short-term results in 53 US obese pediatric patients treated with laparoscopic adjustable gastric banding. J Pediatr Surg 42:137–141
153. Inge TH, Pfluger P, Zeller M et al. (2007) Gastric bypass surgery for treatment of hypothalamic obesity after craniopharyngioma therapy. Nat Clin Pract Endocrinol Metab 3:606–609

154. Rottembourg D, O'Gorman CS, Urbach S *et al.* (2009) Outcome after bariatric surgery in two adolescents with hypothalamic obesity following treatment of craniopharyngioma. J Pediatr Endocrinol Metab 22:867–872
155. Schultes B, Ernst B, Schmid F, Thurnheer M (2009) Distal gastric bypass surgery for the treatment of hypothalamic obesity after childhood craniopharyngioma. Eur J Endocrinol 161:201–206
156. Davies DJ, Baxter JM, Baxter JN (2007) Nutritional deficiencies after bariatric surgery. Obes Surg 17:1150–1158
157. Breum L, Fernstrom MH (2001) Drug-induced obesity. In: Bjorntorp P (ed) International textbook of obesity. Wiley, Chichester, pp 269–281
158. Hopkins RL, Leinung MC (2005) Exogenous Cushing's syndrome and glucocorticoid withdrawal. Endocrinol Metab Clin North Am 34:371–384, ix
159. American Diabetes Association (2004) Consensus development conference on antipsychotic drugs and obesity and diabetes. Diabetes Care 27:596–601

Index

From: *Nutrition and Health: Management of Pediatric Obesity and Diabetes*,
Edited by: R.J. Ferry, Jr., DOI 10.1007/978-1-60327-256-8
© Springer Science+Business Media, LLC 2011

CPSIA information can be obtained at www.ICGtesting.com

226975LV00005B/27/P